REAL-WORLD NURSING SURVIVAL GUIDE:
CRITICAL CARE & EMERGENCY NURSING

REAL WORLD NURSING SURVIVAL GUIDE SERIES

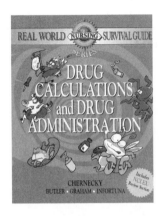

REAL WORLD NURSING SURVIVAL GUIDE SERIES

DRUG CALCULATIONS and DRUG ADMINISTRATION

Includes NCLEX Review Section

CHERNECKY
BUTLER • GRAHAM • INFORTUNA

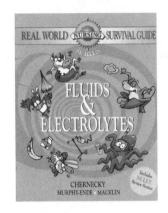

REAL WORLD NURSING SURVIVAL GUIDE SERIES

FLUIDS & ELECTROLYTES

Includes NCLEX Review Section

CHERNECKY
MURPHY-ENDE • MACKLIN

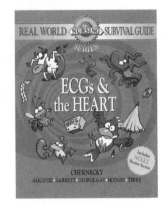

REAL WORLD NURSING SURVIVAL GUIDE SERIES

ECGs & the HEART

Includes NCLEX Review Section

CHERNECKY
ALICHNIE • GARRETT • GEORGE-GAY • HODGES • TERRY

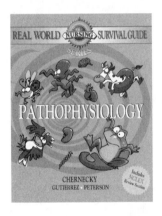

REAL WORLD NURSING SURVIVAL GUIDE SERIES

PATHOPHYSIOLOGY

Includes NCLEX Review Section

CHERNECKY
GUTIERREZ • PETERSON

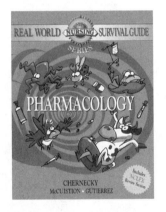

REAL WORLD NURSING SURVIVAL GUIDE SERIES

PHARMACOLOGY

Includes NCLEX Review Section

CHERNECKY
McCUISTION • GUTIERREZ

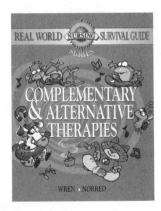

REAL WORLD NURSING SURVIVAL GUIDE SERIES

COMPLEMENTARY & ALTERNATIVE THERAPIES

WREN • NORRED

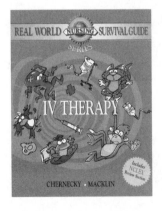

REAL WORLD NURSING SURVIVAL GUIDE SERIES

IV THERAPY

Includes NCLEX Review Section

CHERNECKY • MACKLIN

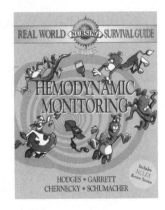

REAL WORLD NURSING SURVIVAL GUIDE SERIES

HEMODYNAMIC MONITORING

Includes NCLEX Review Section

HODGES • GARRETT
CHERNECKY • SCHUMACHER

REAL-WORLD NURSING SURVIVAL GUIDE:

CRITICAL CARE
&
EMERGENCY
NURSING

LORI SCHUMACHER, PhD, RN, CCRN
Assistant Professor
Medical College of Georgia, School of Nursing
Augusta, Georgia

CYNTHIA CHERNECKY, PhD, RN, CNS, AOCN
Professor
Medical College of Georgia, School of Nursing
Augusta, Georgia

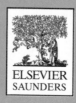

ELSEVIER
SAUNDERS

ELSEVIER
SAUNDERS

11830 Westline Industrial Drive
St. Louis, Missouri 63146

REAL-WORLD NURSING SURVIVAL GUIDE:
CRITICAL CARE & EMERGENCY NURSING

NOTICE

Nursing is an ever-changing field. Standard safety precautions must be followed, but as new research and clinical experience broaden our knowledge, changes in treatment and drug therapy may become necessary or appropriate. Readers are advised to check the most current product information provided by the manufacturer of each drug to be administered to verify the recommended dose, the method and duration of administration, and contraindications. It is the responsibility of the licensed prescriber, relying on experience and knowledge of the patient, to determine dosages and the best treatment for each individual patient. Neither the publisher nor the author assumes any liability for any injury and/or damage to persons or property arising from this publication.

ISBN-13: 978-0-7216-0374-2

ISBN-10: 0-7216-0374-2

Acquisitions Editor: Sandra Clark Brown
Senior Developmental Editor: Cindi Anderson
Publishing Services Manager: Melissa Lastarria
Design Manager: Amy Buxton

Printed in the United States of America

Last digit is the print number: 9 8 7 6 5 4 3

About the Authors

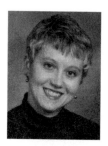 **Lori Schumacher** earned her degrees at Duquesne University (PhD), the University of Minnesota (MS), and Creighton University (BSN). She has over 15 years of experience in critical care and neuroscience nursing and maintains CCRN certification. She is active in her church and an accomplished flutist. Lori enjoys giving flute lessons and spending time with her family, friends, and four cats.

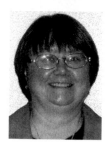 **Dr. Cynthia Chernecky** earned her degrees at the Case Western Reserve University (PhD), the University of Pittsburgh (MN), and the University of Connecticut (BSN). She also earned an NCI fellowship at Yale University and a postdoctorate visiting scholarship at UCLA. Her clinical area of expertise is critical care oncology with publications including *Laboratory Tests and Diagnostic Procedures* (fourth edition) and *Advanced and Critical Care Oncology Nursing: Managing Primary Complications*. She is a national speaker, researcher, and published scholar in cancer nursing. She is also active in the Orthodox Church and enjoys life with family, friends, colleagues, and two West Highland white terriers.

Contributors

John Aiken, RN, BSN
Nurse Anesthesia Student
School of Nursing, Nurse Anesthesia Program
Louisiana State University Health Sciences
    Center
New Orleans, Louisiana

Robert Dee Bledsoe, MSN, RN, CDE, CWOCN
Department of Learning Resources
St. Joseph Hospital
Augusta, Georgia

Julie M. Brown, MSN, CRNA, BSN, RN
Department of Nursing Anesthesia
Medical College of Georgia
Augusta, Georgia

James A. Cleveland, BSN, MSN, RN
Major, Army Nurse, Director-Phase 1,
    Licensed Practical Nurse Course
    (91WM6)
Department of Nursing Science
Academy of Health Sciences
Ft. Sam Houston, Texas

Kimberly D. Davis, MN, CRNA
Nurse Anesthesia Program
Medical College of Georgia
Augusta, Georgia

Juanita L. Derouen, BSN, RN
Nurse Anesthesia Student
School of Nursing, Nurse Anesthesia Program
Louisiana State University Health Sciences
    Center
New Orleans, Louisiana

Lillian Fogarty, BSN, RN, MN, CRNA
School of Nursing, Nurse Anesthesia Program
Louisiana State University Health Sciences
    Center
New Orleans, Louisiana

Brenda L. Garman, RN, BSN, MEd
Education Specialist
Department of Learning Resources
St. Joseph Hospital
Augusta, Georgia

Kitty M. Garrett, RN, MSN, CCRN
Critical Care Clinical Nurse Specialist
Department of Learning Resources
St. Joseph Hospital
Augusta, Georgia

Renee B. Guidry, MN, MSN, CRNA, CCRN,
    APRN
Certified Registered Nurse Anesthetist
Department of Anesthesia
Parish Anesthesia and Associates
East Jefferson General Hospital
Metairie, Louisiana

Kathleen M. Hall, MN, MSN, ATCN, CPAN,
    CRNA
Certified Registered Nurse Anesthetist
School of Nursing, Nurse Anesthesia Program
Louisiana State University Health Sciences
    Center
New Orleans, Louisiana

Walter H. Harwood, III, RN
Nurse Manager
Emergency Department
St. Joseph Hospital
Augusta, Georgia

Rebecca K. Hodges, MSN, RN, CCRN
Critical Care Clinical Nurse Specialist
Department of Learning Resources
St. Joseph Hospital
Augusta, Georgia

Robin Foell Johns, MSN, RN
Assistant Professor
School of Nursing—Athens Campus
Medical College of Georgia
Athens, Georgia

Thomas B. Johnson, CRNA
Surgical Anesthesia Associates
Jackson, Mississippi

Rosalind Gail Jones, MSN, APRN
Instructor
Department of Undergraduate Studies
Medical College of Georgia
Augusta, Georgia

Matthew W. Kervin, MN, CRNA
Associate Director
Mercer University School of Medicine
    Program in Nurse Anesthesia
Medical Center of Central Georgia
Macon, Georgia

Jane E. Kwilecki, MSN, ARNP, CCRN
Trauma Program Coordinator
Department of Trauma Services
Halifax Medical Center
Daytona Beach, Florida

Christine Langer, CRNA
Assistant Program Director
School of Nursing, Nurse Anesthesia Program
School of Nursing
Louisiana State University Health Sciences
    Center
New Orleans, Louisiana

Nancy J. Newton, RN, BSN
Nurse Anesthesia Student
School of Nursing, Nurse Anesthesia Program
Louisiana State University Health Science
    Center
New Orleans, Louisiana

Lyza Reddick, MSN, CRNA
Nurse Anesthesia Program
Medical College of Georgia
Augusta, Georgia

Carl A. Ross, PhD, RN, CRNP
Associate Professor and Director
Center for International Nursing
Duquesne University School of Nursing
Pittsburgh, Pennsylvania

Jeanne R. Russell, RN, BSN, SNP
Student Nurse Practitioner
Louisiana State University School of
    Nursing
New Orleans, Louisiana

Brenda K. Shelton, RN, MS, CCRN, AOCN
Clinical Nurse Specialist
The Sidney Kimmel Comprehensive Cancer
    Center at Johns Hopkins
The Johns Hopkins Hospital
Baltimore, Maryland

Lynn C. Simko, PhD, RN, CCRN
Associate Professor
School of Nursing
Duquesne University
Pittsburgh, Pennsylvania

Nancy Stark, RN, MSN
Instructor
Department of Undergraduate Studies
Medical College of Georgia
Augusta, Georgia

Kathryn Thornton Tinkelenberg, MS, RN
Assistant Professor
Department of Nursing
Lenoir-Rhyne College
Hickory, North Carolina

Kathleen R. Wren, CRNA, PhD
Associate Professor of Nursing
School of Nursing
Louisiana State University Health Sciences
    Center
New Orleans, Louisiana

Timothy L. Wren, RN, MS
Assistant Professor
Department of Adult Nursing
Louisiana State University Health Sciences
    Center
New Orleans, Louisiana

Diane Salentiny Wrobleski, PhD, RN,
    APRN, BC, CEN
Staff Nurse
Department of Nursing
Olmstead Medical Center
Rochester, Minnesota

Faculty and Practitioner Reviewers

Theresa L. Culpepper, PhD, CRNA
Director of Clinical Anesthesia Services
Department of Nurse Anesthesia
Ida V. Moffett School of Nursing
Samford University
Birmingham, Alabama

Carmencita C. Mercado-Poe, EdD, RN, APN, CS, OCN, CHPN
Clinical Nurse Manager, Oncology/Medical-Surgical Nursing
Bon Secours De Paul Medicine Center
Norfolk, Virginia

Louise Diehl-Oplinger, RN, MSN, CCRN, APRN, BC, CLNC
Advanced Practice Nurse
PopKave-Mascarenhas Cardiology
Phillipsburg, New Jersey

Preface

The Real-World Nursing Survival Guide series was created with your input. Nursing students told us about topics they found difficult to master, such as critical care and emergency and hemodynamics. Based on information from focus groups at the National Student Nurses Association meeting, this series was developed on your recommendations. You said to keep the text to a minimum; to use an engaging, fun approach; to provide enough space to write on the pages; to include a variety of activities to appeal to the different learning styles of students; to make the content visually appealing; and to provide NCLEX review questions so you could check your understanding of key topics and review as necessary. This series is a result of your ideas!

Understanding the concepts and principles of critical care and emergency nursing provides a solid foundation for the nurse who works with critically ill patients to guide drug therapy, who monitors hemodynamic parameters, and who is expected to make sound clinical decisions. It is essential for any nurse working in critical care and emergency nursing to be aware of the assessment and technical skills and nursing knowledge associated with the nursing management for these types of patients.

Critical Care & Emergency Nursing in the *Real World Nursing Survival Guide Series* was developed to explain difficult concepts in an easy-to-understand manner and to assist nursing students in the mastery of these concepts. A basic understanding of pathophysiology, anatomy, and physiology is assumed because the content in this text builds on previous nursing knowledge and provides the fundamental introduction to critical care and emergency nursing. *Critical Care & Emergency Nursing* can also serve as a valuable guide and resource for the novice and the experienced nurse who want to review concepts and principles of critical care and emergency nursing.

We include many features in the margins to help you focus on the vital information you will need to succeed in the classroom and in the clinical setting. **TAKE HOME POINTS** are made up of both study tips for classroom tests and "pearls of wisdom" to assist you in caring for patients. Both are drawn from our many years of combined academic and clinical experience. Content marked with a **Caution icon** is vital and usually involves nursing actions that may have life-threatening consequences or may significantly affect patient outcomes. The **Lifespan icon** and the **Culture icon** highlight variations in treatment that may be necessary for specific age or ethnic groups. A **Calculator icon** will draw your eye to important formulas. A **Web Links icon** will direct you to sites on the Internet that will give more detailed information on a given topic. Each of these icons is designed to help you focus on real-world patient care, the nursing process, and positive patient outcomes.

We also use consistent headings that emphasize specific nursing actions. **What It IS** provides a definition of a topic. **What You NEED TO KNOW** provides the explanation of the topic. **What You DO** explains what you do as a practicing nurse. **Do You UNDERSTAND?** provides questions and exercises that are both entertaining and useful to reinforce the topic's concepts. This four-step approach provides you with information and helps you learn how to apply it to the clinical setting.

Our inspirations and goals for *Critical Care & Emergency Nursing* were to make difficult topics easier. We have used real-world clinical experiences and expertise to bring you a text that will help you understand critical care and emergency nursing to facilitate better patient care. The art and science of nursing is based on understanding, which is the key to critical thinking and clinical decision making. Our hope is for you to share your new insights and understanding with others and apply this information to affect nursing care positively.

Lori Schumacher, PhD, RN, CCRN
Cynthia C. Chernecky, PhD, RN, CNS, AOCN

Acknowledgments

I would like to extend grateful appreciation to my family, colleagues, and students who have provided me with continuous support and encouragement through this endeavor. To my students, who, without them and their desire to learn critical care nursing, none of this would have been possible. I also want to express special thanks to the doctoral faculty at Duquesne University, especially Dr. Joannie Lockhart and Dr. Gladys Husted, for their inspiration and encouragement through my doctoral studies and the publishing of this book. I especially wish to extend my deepest gratitude to my family. To my sister, Julie, and my father and mother, Stan and Sandy, who have continually inspired me in all my nursing endeavors. I wish to dedicate this book to them. Thank you to all the critical care and emergency nurses at Buffalo General Hospital, Medical College of Georgia Health Inc., and WCA Hospital for your diligence and care that you provided to my father during his numerous visits to your nursing units—without you, great things would not be possible! I appreciate and will never forget all the encouragement that Dad gave me through the writing and editing process of this book, although he was ill and not feeling his best. Through his illness, he always strived and was determined to make life better and to live to the best of his abilities.

Dad, it is your determination, strength, love, wisdom, and encouragement that I will always cherish and will attempt to foster in my nursing endeavors and those of my students.

Lori Schumacher

Vision and unselfishness are qualities of the true professional. These qualities are indeed part of Lori's life and have made it a pleasure to work with her on such a worthwhile project. We have many nursing colleagues to thank for supporting us and, of course, nursing students for challenging us. We could not have completed this book from idea to print without a professional environment that encouraged and supported us in our educational efforts, both in our jobs and from the many experts at Elsevier.

Special thanks for the support and continuous encouragement to my mother, Olga, the nuns of Saints Mary and Martha Orthodox Monastery, and Cindi Anderson at Elsevier. Professional thanks to Drs. Linda Sarna, Ann Kolanowski, Jean Brown, Geri Padilla, Mary Cooley, Leda Danao, Rich Haas, Fred Lupien, and Lucy Marion (Dean) for their support and encouragement.

And, finally, to my dogs, Joshua and Buffy, who gave up long walks so I could write and edit.

Cynthia (Cinda) Chernecky

Contents

Review of Hemodynamics

What IS Hemodynamics?

Hemodynamics is the study of forces involved in the flow of blood through the cardiovascular and circulatory systems. The components of hemodynamics include blood pressure (BP), central venous pressure (CVP), and right and left heart pressures.

The physiologic principles of hemodynamics include factors that affect myocardial function, regulate BP, and determine cardiac performance and cardiac output (CO). Understanding the basic concepts of pressure, flow, and resistance provides an insight into the understanding of hemodynamic values. Assessing ventricular function through the evaluation of hemodynamic variables enables the nurse to identify cardiovascular problems and to determine appropriate interventions. This chapter provides a basis for the interpretation of hemodynamic values and clinical application.

What IS the Circulatory System?

The body has a complex network of veins and arteries within a continuous circuit that makes up the *circulatory system*. The heart pumps a constant volume of blood through this system to maintain balance between oxygen delivery and demand.

What You NEED TO KNOW

Several mechanisms regulate the flow of blood through the system. When the body's metabolic demands increase, the blood vessels constrict in an attempt to force blood back to the heart. When the metabolic demand decreases, the veins dilate. This dilation causes pooling of blood in the periphery and reduces venous return to the heart. Other mechanisms that control flow are the result of the ability of the heart to increase or decrease heart rate (HR) and strength of contraction.

How Does the Heart Work?

The function of the heart is to pump blood through the body. The heart is composed of two upper chambers called the *atria* and two lower chambers called the *ventricles*. The atria serve as reservoirs for incoming blood, and the ventricles are the main pumping chambers of the heart. The atria are separated from the ventricles by **atrioventricular valves** (AV valves). The tricuspid valve separates the right atrium from the right ventricle, and the mitral valve separates the left atrium from the left ventricle. Two other valves, the **pulmonic** semilunar and the **aortic** semilunar, help control the flow of blood from the ventricles to the lungs and systemic circulation. The pulmonic semilunar valve controls the flow of blood from the right ventricle to the lungs, and the aortic semilunar valve controls the flow of blood from the left ventricle to the aorta.

The electrical conduction system is specialized tissue that allows electrical impulses to travel very efficiently from the atria to the ventricles. **Depolarization** is the electrical activation of the muscle cells of the heart and stimulates cellular contraction. Once the cells are depolarized, they return to their original state of electrolyte balance, which is called **repolarization.**

Cardiac Cycle

The right atrium receives venous blood from the systemic circulation while the left atrium receives reoxygenated blood from the lungs. While both atria are filling with blood, the sinoatrial (SA) node in the electrical conduction system fires and starts the process of depolarization. As the atria fill with blood, the pressure within the atria increases, forcing the AV valves to open. The majority of ventricular filling (diastole) passively occurs when the AV valves open. After atrial depolarization, the atria contract, forcing the remaining atrial blood into the ventricles. This contraction is referred to as the **atrial kick** and is responsible for as much as a 30% contribution to CO.

After atrial contraction, the atria begin to relax and atrial pressure decreases. The electrical impulses from the atria now travel through the remainder of the conduction system and cause ventricular depolarization, which is the beginning of ventricular contraction. Ventricular pressure now exceeds atrial pressure, and the AV valves close and the semilunar valves open. Desaturated blood is ejected from the right ventricle into the lungs, where it drops off carbon dioxide and

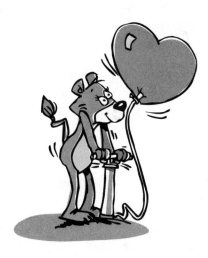

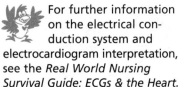

For further information on the electrical conduction system and electrocardiogram interpretation, see the *Real World Nursing Survival Guide: ECGs & the Heart.*

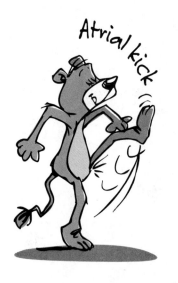

Atrial kick

picks up oxygen. Oxygenated blood from the left ventricle is ejected into the systemic circulation via the aorta. The ejection of blood from the ventricles is referred to as **systole.**

   Stroke volume (SV) is the volume of blood that is ejected during systole. Left ventricular end–*systolic* volume (LVESV) is the amount of blood that remains in the left ventricle at the end of systole. Left ventricular end–*diastolic* volume (LVEDV) is the amount of blood that is in the ventricle just before ejection occurs. The left ventricle never ejects the entire volume it receives during diastole. The portion of the volume it does eject is referred to as **ejection fraction** (EF), which is approximately 70% of the total volume at the end of diastole.

Do You UNDERSTAND?

DIRECTIONS: **Fill in the blanks to complete the following statements.**

1. The cardiac conduction system provides electrical activation to cause the

   heart to _____.

2. During systole, the _____ valves are

   open and the _____ are closed.

3. During diastole, the _____ valves are open and the

   _____ _____ are closed.

4. Atrial contraction is referred to as atrial _____ and

   is responsible for as much as _____% contribution to CO.

5. The left ventricle never ejects the entire volume it receives during systole.

   The portion of blood the left ventricle ejects during systole is referred to as

   _____ _____.

6. The volume of blood that is in the ventricle just before ejection occurs is

   called _____ _____ _____–

   _____ _____.

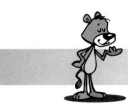

What IS Blood Pressure?

If flow or resistance is altered, then pressure is affected. This principle of physics can be applied to BP. Narrowed vessels increase resistance and increase pressure. Conversely, dilated vessels decrease resistance and decrease pressure.

BP is defined as the tension exerted by blood on the arterial walls. Monitoring BP is based on the following equation:

$$Pressure = Flow \times Resistance$$

BP = CO × SVR
Normal values:
Systolic: 100 to 139 mm Hg
Diastolic: 60 to 90 mm Hg

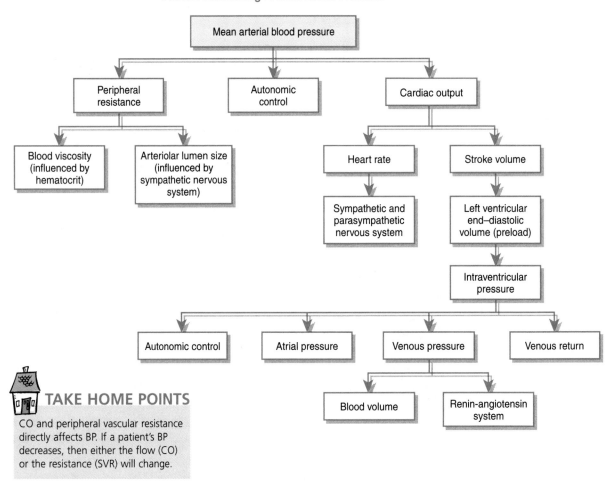

Factors Influencing Arterial Blood Pressure

TAKE HOME POINTS

CO and peripheral vascular resistance directly affects BP. If a patient's BP decreases, then either the flow (CO) or the resistance (SVR) will change.

SVR is a reflection of peripheral vascular resistance and is the opposition to blood flow from the blood vessels. It is affected by the tone of the blood vessels, blood viscosity, and resistance from the inner lining of the blood vessels. SVR is also the resistance against which the left ventricle pumps; it usually has an inverse relationship with CO.

TAKE HOME POINTS

If the SVR decreases, then the CO increases. SVR increases to maintain BP when the CO decreases.

$$SVR = \frac{Mean\ Arterial\ Pressure\ (MAP) - CVP \times 80}{CO}$$

The diameter of the blood vessel is one of the major factors that influence SVR. SVR decreases when the blood vessels relax, and it increases with the narrowing of the blood vessels. Vasoactive drugs are often used in the critical care setting to change the size of the arterioles to decrease or increase BP.

Normal value:
800 to 1200 dynes/sec/cm^{-5}

What You NEED TO KNOW

TAKE HOME POINTS

- Common medications and habits can often change SVR. For example, smoking and stress can cause vasoconstriction.
- Vasodilators enlarge **(dilate)** the size of the arterioles in an attempt to decrease BP. Vasoconstrictors shrink **(constrict)** the size of the arterioles in an attempt to increase BP.

Elevations of Systemic Vascular Resistance

The two primary reasons for elevations in SVR are vascular disturbances, such as vasoconstriction caused by hypertension, or excessive catecholamine release and compensatory responses to maintain BP in decreased CO. In addition, elevations of SVR increase the workload of the heart and myocardial oxygen consumption.

Decreases in Systemic Vascular Resistance

Several potential causes for decreased SVR exist, including sepsis and neurologically mediated vasomotor tone loss. When SVR decreases, CO increases in an attempt to maintain BP.

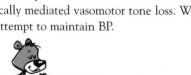

What IS Cardiac Output?

CO is the amount of blood ejected from the heart in 1 minute. CO has two components: SV and HR. A major goal in assessing CO is ensuring adequate oxygenation.

CO = SV × HR
Normal values: 4 to 8 L/min

What IS Stroke Volume?

SV is the amount of blood ejected from the heart with each beat. The three factors that influence SV are preload, afterload, and contractility.

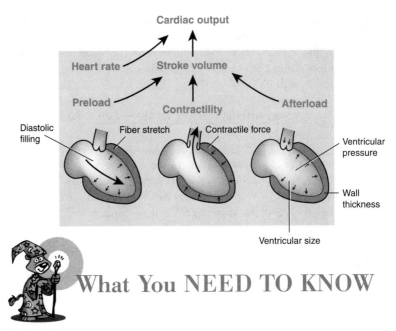

What You NEED TO KNOW

Preload

Preload is the filling volume of the ventricle at the end of diastole. It reflects the amount of cardiac muscle stretch at end diastole just before contraction. Preload is dependent on the volume of blood returning to the heart. Venous tone and the actual amount of blood in the venous system influence this volume. Preload is measured by obtaining a pressure measurement with a pulmonary artery (PA) catheter. This pressure is referred to as a *pulmonary artery occlusion pressure/pulmonary artery wedge pressure* (PAOP/PAWP).

TAKE HOME POINTS

- Preload is directly related to the force of myocardial contraction.
- An enlarged heart will increase preload and is measured by an elevated PAWP.

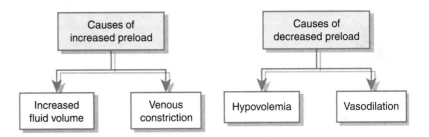

TAKE HOME POINTS

Vasoconstriction results from an increase in systemic arterial tone, which increases BP and causes an increase in afterload.

Afterload

Afterload is the amount of resistance against which the left ventricle pumps. It is primarily influenced by the blood vessels, but blood viscosity, flow patterns, and valves can also have an effect. The greater the resistance, the more the myocardium has to work to overcome the resistance. Afterload is determined by BP and arterial tone.

Left ventricular afterload is measured by the assessment of the SVR. Pulmonary vascular resistance (PVR) measures the resistance against which the right ventricle works.

Contractility

Contractility is defined as the strength of myocardial fiber shortening during systole. It allows the heart to work independently, regardless of changes in preload, afterload, or fiber length. Because contractility is a determinant of SV, it affects ventricular function. Preload is one factor that directly influences contractility because of the physiologic principle referred to as the **Frank-Starling law,** which states, "The greater the stretch, the greater the force of the next contraction."

Increases in preload (end-diastolic volume) maximally increase SV. However, in cases of compromised cardiac or pulmonary function, volume and pressure relationships are not directly linear. Ventricular stroke work index (VSWI) is a useful measurement of myocardial contractility.

Heart Rate

The number of heartbeats per minute is important in maintaining CO and is included in the CO formula. When contractility is depressed or if CO is decreased, then the HR will increase to maintain sufficient blood flow for metabolic demand.

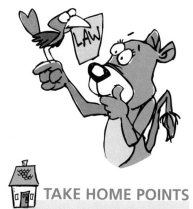

TAKE HOME POINTS

As resistance to left ventricular ejection (afterload) increases, left ventricular work increases and SV may decrease.

- **Left VSWI = MAP − PCWP × SV Index (SVI) × 0.0136**
  Normal value:
  40 to 70 gm/m²/beat
- **SVI = CO ÷ Body Surface Area (BSA)**
  Normal value: 33 to 47 ml/beat/m²

Manipulation of Cardiac Output

STROKE VOLUME					HEART RATE	
PRELOAD		AFTERLOAD (SYSTEMIC VASCULAR RESISTANCE)		CONTRACTILITY		
Increased	Decreased	Increased	Decreased	Decreased Contractility	Increased	Decreased
Diuretics Venodilators	Fluids Vasoconstrictors	Arterial vasodilators	Vasoconstrictors	Positive inotropes	Beta blockers and calcium channel blockers to decrease heart rate	Sympathometics Cardiac pacing

Physiologic Principles that Affect Cardiac Performance

Factors that influence cardiac performance include the Frank-Starling law of the heart, the ability to influence contractility of the muscle fibers of the heart (inotropism), any changes in HR or regularity of rhythm (force-frequency ratio), and miscellaneous influences such as the sympathetic or parasympathetic nervous system responses.

Frank-Starling law of the heart. Augmenting ventricular filling during diastole before the onset of a contraction will increase the force of contraction during systole.

Normal HR: 60 to 100 beats/min
Bradycardia: <60 beats/min (lengthens diastolic filling time)
Tachycardia: >100 beats/minute (shortens diastolic filling time)

Inotropism. Inotropism is the ability to influence contractility of muscle fibers. A positive inotrope enhances contractility. A negative inotrope depresses contractility.

Force-frequency ratio. Any changes in HR or rhythm can change diastolic filling time of the ventricles, therefore altering fiber stretch and the force of the next contraction. This ratio influences SV and CO. In addition, the majority of coronary artery filling occurs during diastole. When HRs increase, myocardial oxygen demand increases; however, when diastolic filling time is shortened, coronary artery filling decreases. This ratio results in an imbalance between the supply and demand of myocardial oxygen.

Miscellaneous influences. Factors such as hypoxia, hyperkalemia, hypercarbia, hyponatremia, and myocardial scar tissue also can decrease myocardial contractility. Sympathetic stimulation increases myocardial contractility, and parasympathetic stimulation (via the vagus nerve) depresses the SA node, atrial myocardium, and AV junctional tissue.

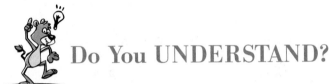

Do You UNDERSTAND?

DIRECTIONS: **Fill in the blanks to complete the following statements.**

1. CO = _____ _____ × _____ _____.

2. Preload, afterload, and contractility are determinants of

   _____ _____.

3. Preload is defined as _____

   _____.

4. Afterload is defined as _____

   _____.

5. PAWP measures _____.

6. SVR measures _____.

DIRECTIONS: **Match the descriptions in Column A with the terms in Column B.**

Column A

_____ 7. Decreases myocardial contractility
_____ 8. Increases myocardial contractility
_____ 9. Inotropism
_____ 10. "The greater the stretch, the greater the next force of contraction"

Column B

a. Sympathetic stimulation
b. Influencing contraction
c. Frank-Starling law
d. Hyperkalemia, hypoxia, hypercarbia, hyponatremia

What IS Hemodynamic Monitoring?

Hemodynamics or pressures of the cardiovascular and circulatory system can be measured by invasive methods such as direct arterial BP monitoring, CVP monitoring, and indirect measurements of left ventricular pressures via a flow-directed, balloon-tipped catheter (e.g., PA catheters, Swan-Ganz catheters).

The goals of hemodynamic monitoring include ensuring adequate perfusion, detecting inadequate perfusion, titrating therapy to specific end point, qualifying the severity of illness, and differentiating system dysfunction (e.g., differentiating between cardiogenic and noncardiogenic pulmonary edema).

Direct Arterial Blood Pressure Monitoring

Direct intraarterial monitoring allows for accurate, continuous monitoring of arterial BPs. It also provides a system for continuous sampling of blood for arterial blood gases without repeated arterial punctures. Clinical considerations include the potential complications of thrombosis, embolism, blood loss, and infection. Invasive intraarterial monitoring is considered to be more accurate and reliable than noninvasive types of BP monitoring.

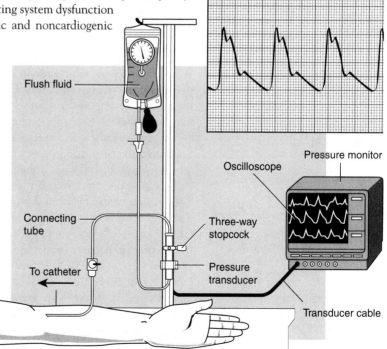

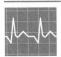

Monitoring: Normal CVP or RAP values are 0 to 6 mm Hg.

TAKE HOME POINTS

Low RAP or CVP measurements can reflect hypovolemia or extreme vasodilation. High RAP measurements can reflect hypervolemia, or severe vasoconstriction, or conditions that reduce the ability of the right ventricle to contract (i.e., pulmonary hypertension and right ventricular failure).

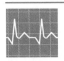

Monitoring: Normal PA catheter values:
• **Right ventricular pressures:**
Systolic 15 to 25 mm Hg
Diastolic 0 to 6 mm Hg
• **PA pressures:**
Systolic 15 to 25 mm Hg
Diastolic 8 to 15 mm Hg
• **PA occlusion pressure:**
6 to 12 mm Hg

TAKE HOME POINTS

It is important to remember that changes in PCWP are not always equal to volume changes because the PCWP is not the only parameter involved in muscle stretch. Patients who have compliant left ventricles can have large volume changes without large changes in pressure; conversely patients with noncompliant ventricles may have extreme volume changes without PCWP increases.

Right Atrial Pressure Monitoring

Measuring pressures from the right atrium can be referred to as right atrial pressures (RAP) or CVPs. Measuring pressure from the superior or inferior vena cava (CVP) or from the right atrium (RAP) is a direct method. The pressures between these two areas are essentially equal. Because the tricuspid valve (i.e., AV valve between the right atria and right ventricle) is open during diastole, a RAP measurement can reliably reflect right ventricular end–diastolic pressure (RVEDP). Any condition that changes venous tone, blood volume, or contractility of the right ventricle can cause an abnormality in RAP values. (See the inside back cover for waveform and catheter placement.)

Left Atrial Pressure Monitoring

Direct left atrial pressure (LAP) monitoring is not routinely used except in cardiac surgical procedures, cardiac catheterization laboratories, and after open-heart procedures. Most often, a catheter is inserted during cardiac surgery with the distal end tunneled through an incision in the chest wall. LAP monitoring provides the ability to observe the pressures in the left atrium; however, air embolism and system debris are major complications that can obstruct a coronary or cerebral artery. To prevent the possibility of complications, connections must be tight and caps should be on stopcocks to avoid air entering or administering medications and fluids through this line.

Pulmonary Artery Monitoring

The PA catheter is a multilumen, balloon-tipped catheter that is inserted through the venous system into the right side of the heart and into the PA. The catheter may be inserted at the bedside from an antecubital vein, external jugular vein, subclavian artery, or any other peripheral vein into the PA through a percutaneous introducer. Fluoroscopy is not required because the pressure tracing can identify the positioning on the monitor. The catheter is inserted with the balloon deflated; however, when the catheter enters the right atrium, the balloon is inflated, allowing it to float with the flow of blood into the PA. When the balloon is deflated, the catheter directly measures PA pressures. With balloon inflation, the catheter floats into a pulmonary arteriole and wedges itself in a smaller lumen. The opening of the catheter beyond the inflated balloon reflects pressures distal to the PA (i.e., passive runoff of pulmonary venous blood in the left atrium). This PCWP, also referred to as the PAOP, indirectly measures left ventricular function because the mean PCWP or PAOP and left atrial pressures closely approximate LVEDP in patients with normal mitral valve function. (See back inside cover for waveform and catheter placement.)

The other lumen of the catheter allows for monitoring of right atrial pressures (CVP). An additional port, referred to as the *thermistor*, allows for the measurement of CO. PA catheters may also have additional lumens, which allow for intravenous administration of solutions or insertion of pacemaker electrodes for the purpose of transvenous pacing. Other catheters also have the ability to monitor CO or mixed venous oxygen saturation continuously. The PA catheter is used to monitor high-risk, critically ill patients with goals that include the detection of adequate perfusion and the diagnosis and evaluation of the effects of therapy. This at-risk patient group also includes those with a variety of cardiopulmonary problems, including acute myocardial infarction, severe angina, cardiomyopathy, right and left ventricular failure, and pulmonary diseases. In addition, PA monitoring is a valuable tool for observing fluid balance in the critically ill patient at risk for other cardiopulmonary problems.

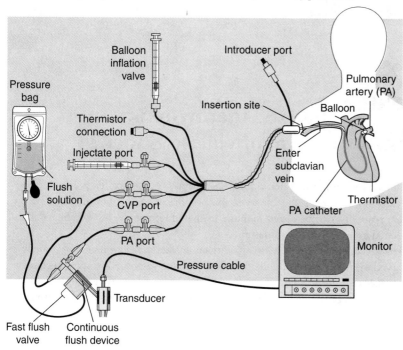

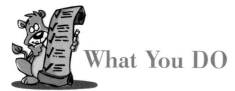

What You DO

To monitor hemodynamics, the equipment must include a transducer, amplifier, display monitor, catheter system, and tubing filled with fluid. This system provides the ability to monitor a pressure waveform that is displayed as a digital readout on the oscilloscope.

Nursing interventions for hemodynamic monitoring include (1) providing patient education about the procedure, (2) ensuring that the appropriate procedure consent forms are signed, (3) setting up the equipment, (4) preparing the line, (5) assisting the physician with catheter insertion, (6) monitoring the pressures, and (7) making clinical decisions per institutional policy. The nurse should also be alert to potential complications.

For further information on hemodynamic monitoring and values, see the *Real World Nursing Survival Guide: Hemodynamic Monitoring.*

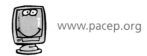

www.pacep.org

Shock Trauma

What IS Anaphylaxis and Anaphylactic Shock?

Anaphylaxis is a life-threatening hypersensitivity or pseudoallergic reaction to an exogenous agent, often observed in the critical care environment. These severe reactions can be either immune mediated (anaphylactic) or chemically mediated (anaphylactoid) in nature.

Anaphylaxis is the result of an antigen-antibody reaction and is usually observed in individuals with allergies. The immune response is directed against substances that are not inherently harmful to the body and that enter through either the skin or the respiratory tract. Substances such as foods, food additives, environmental agents (e.g., pollens, molds, animal dander), diagnostic agents, medications, blood or blood products, or venoms (e.g., bee stings, snakebites) can trigger an immune-mediated reaction.

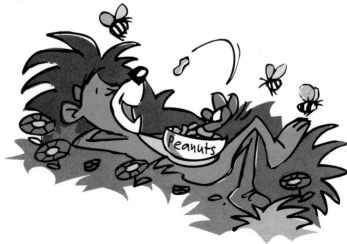

Typically, the initial exposure to the allergy-inducing agent (allergen) results in the formation of an antibody called *immunoglobulin E* (IgE) specific for that allergen. This first exposure to the antigen is known as the *primary immune response*. No clinical evidence of the exposure is usually observed at this time. The antibodies accumulate and attach themselves to the membrane of mast cells, which contain large amounts of histamine, and to the basophils in the plasma. The mast cells and basophils are both dispersed throughout the body where they wait for the next allergen exposure. Subsequent exposures to the allergen produce a *secondary immune response*. The antigen and the IgE antibody interact to trigger the rupture of the mast cells, which is called *degranulation*. The mast cells then release chemical mediators such as histamine, eosinophilic chemotactic factor of anaphylaxis (ECF-A), leukotrienes (formerly known as slow-reacting substance of anaphylaxis [SRS-A]), platelet-activating factors (PAF), kinins, and prostaglandins. Histamine is believed to be the most important cause of the symptoms associated with allergic reactions. The substances released cause vasodilation, increased capillary permeability, and smooth muscle contraction. This reaction is followed by evidence of symptomatic clinical changes, which precipitates **anaphylactic shock.**

Anaphylactoid reactions reflect the release of histamine from mast cells and basophils in response to the administration of a drug (chemical mediator). The histamine released is independent of an antigen-antibody interaction, but the signs and symptoms are exactly the same. In contrast to anaphylactic reactions that need prior exposure, anaphylactoid reactions may occur without prior exposure to a drug. Although anaphylactoid reactions can be as life threatening as anaphylactic reactions, they tend to be self-limiting (5 to 10 minutes) because of the short half-life of histamine in the plasma (see Color Plate 1 of the insert for mediator response and clinical manifestations).

TAKE HOME POINTS

- Anaphylactic reactions need prior exposure; anaphylactoid reactions may occur without prior exposure.
- Anaphylactic reactions have the possibility of increasing with each exposure.

What You NEED TO KNOW

Anaphylactic and anaphylactoid reactions, which are clinically indistinguishable, may become rapidly fatal if appropriate therapy is not promptly initiated.

Symptoms of anaphylaxis usually occur within seconds to minutes of injection of the causative agent, although symptoms may be delayed up to 1 hour after exposure. Histamine triggers physiologic changes by promoting vasodilation and increasing capillary-venous permeability, clinically evidenced by redness, warmth, and swelling.

The first dermatologic symptoms to typically appear include pruritus, generalized erythema, urticaria (usually on the chest, and then on the face), and angioedema. Angioedema is a result of fluid leaking into the interstitial space, which causes a swelling of the face, oral cavity, and lower pharynx. The patient may become restless, anxious, and apprehensive with the complaint of a sense of impending doom—the most ominous sign that should never be taken lightly by a critical care nurse. Gastrointestinal (GI) and genitourinary signs may also

Anaphylactic and anaphylactoid reactions are associated with acute medical emergencies that ultimately involve compromised cardiovascular and respiratory systems.

develop because of smooth muscle constriction and may include vomiting, diarrhea, cramping, abdominal pain, urinary incontinence, or vaginal bleeding.

Pulmonary manifestations may also include laryngeal edema, bronchoconstriction, bronchorrhea, or pulmonary edema. Clinical signs and symptoms of laryngeal edema include inspiratory stridor, hoarseness, dysphonia, or difficulty swallowing. The patient may complain of the feeling of a lump in his or her throat, which is caused by soft-tissue swelling. Bronchoconstriction can cause chest tightness, dyspnea, and wheezing, which can be quite frightening for the patient.

With cardiovascular involvement, the patient may complain of dizziness or changes in his or her level of consciousness (LOC). The patient may feel faint, weak, or complain of palpitations. Typically, the electrocardiogram (ECG) shows tachycardia, supraventricular arrhythmias, myocardial ischemia, and possibly infarction. Tachycardia and syncope may lead to the development of hypotension and severe cardiovascular compromise.

The net effect of this downward spiral is significant hypotension and a decreased systemic vascular resistance (SVR) because of the leaky capillaries and postcapillary venules. Anaphylactic shock occurs as a result of an extreme decrease in venous return from the vasodilation and lowered intravascular volume. Assessment of the patient in anaphylactic shock shows hemodynamic compromise of cardiac function, including decreased SVR, decreased stroke volume, decreased afterload, decreased end-diastolic volume, and decreased mixed venous oxygenation saturation. These hemodynamic responses lead to an overall decrease in cardiac output (CO) with ineffective tissue perfusion. Once the patient has reached the level of shock, any number of organ systems can be affected. During the time of decreased CO with a drop in blood volume, the body protects itself by diverting oxygenated blood to organs of highest priority. These organs include the heart, brain, and kidneys. Although the major organs are receiving most of the blood volume at this time, ineffective tissue perfusion is still taking place, which leads to cell death and lactic acidosis. Depending on the extent of hypoperfusion, the body's organs may or may not recover with appropriate therapy. Rapid recognition and treatment is the mainstay of preventing the morbidity and mortality that can occur.

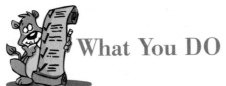

What You DO

Medical Management and Treatment

The key to successful treatment of anaphylactic and anaphylactoid reactions is an astute clinician that recognizes the problem early and takes immediate life-saving actions. Both anaphylactic and anaphylactoid reactions require rapid identification with an immediate and purposeful reaction from the critical care nurse. Because an anaphylactic or anaphylactoid reaction can be life threatening, it is important to recognize that steps taken to treat this reaction may need to be done simultaneously to ensure patient safety. Primary treatment for an

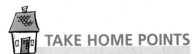

For further information on ECG interpretation, see the *Real World Nursing Survival Guide: ECGs & the Heart.*

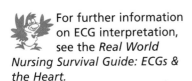

TAKE HOME POINTS

Anaphylactic shock occurs as a result of an extreme decrease in venous return from the vasodilation and lowered intravascular volume, which results in severe cardiovascular and respiratory compromise.

anaphylactic reaction should first include immediately discontinuing the causative agent, even when the product is only under suspicion and not a definitive cause of the reaction. This discontinuation prevents any further recruitment of mast cells and the release of their mediators. The second step, which is the hallmark of treatment for anaphylaxis, is the administration of epinephrine (Adrenaline). If the adult patient does not have an existing intravenous (IV) device in place, epinephrine (Adrenaline) should be subcutaneously administered as soon as possible at a dose of 0.3 to 0.5 ml of a 1:1000 solution. This dose may be repeated every 5 to 10 minutes as needed. If the patient does have an IV in place, then the required dose should be 3 ml of a 1:10,000 solution in an adult. Epinephrine (Adrenaline) promotes vasoconstriction, inhibits bronchoconstriction, and inhibits the release of mediators from stimulated mast cells or basophils by stimulating the production of cyclic adenosine monophosphate (cAMP). Epinephrine can also be administered via the endotracheal tube in smaller doses, 3 to 5 ml of a 1:10,000 solution for an adult.

FIRST-LINE AND INITIAL TREATMENT
FOR ANAPHYLACTIC AND ANAPHYLACTOID REACTIONS

- Find the cause and discontinue it.
- Administer epinephrine (Adrenaline).
- Provide oxygen.
- Administer antihistamines or beta-2 agonists.
- Administer corticosteroids.

The third step involves the very well-regarded ABCs of patient care: *airway, breathing,* and *circulation.* The nurse must support the patient's airway while administering supplemental oxygen up to 100%. The most appropriate oxygen-delivery device available should be used, whether it is via a nasal canula or facemask. Changes in pulmonary capillary leakage with mismatching ventilation and perfusion can take place for several days after an allergic reaction; therefore the nurse should consider endotracheal intubation with mechanical ventilation until the patient's situation stabilizes. Oral tracheal intubation can be unsuccessful—even in the most experienced hands—in the patient with severe laryngeal edema. If the patient cannot be orally intubated, immediate action should be taken to provide oxygen to the patient. An experienced professional can perform emergency measures (e.g., cricothyrotomy, surgical tracheotomy) to establish an airway. If cardiac arrest or a total loss of blood pressure (BP) or pulse occurs, resuscitative doses of epinephrine are administered at a dose of 0.01 mg/kg along with rapid volume expansion and cardiopulmonary resuscitation (CPR). If the patient's condition is such that airway, respiratory, or cardiovascular compromise is present, the patient should be admitted to an intensive care unit (ICU) for treatment and monitoring. Vital signs including BP, heart rate and rhythm, oxygen saturation, and neurologic status must be frequently assessed. Often the patient needs a pulmonary artery catheter to monitor cardiac function, an arterial line for continuous monitoring of BP, and frequent blood sampling to evaluate arterial blood gases.

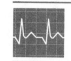

Monitoring the patient's ABCs is crucial.

Secondary treatment for anaphylaxis takes place once the patient's condition improves and measures to prevent further compromise can be initiated. Secondary therapy may include administering antihistamines or beta-2 agonists. If the patient experiences bronchospasms, albuterol inhalation treatments should be initiated to keep the airways open. Diphenhydramine (Benadryl) is used to inhibit the histamine response, and corticosteroids may also be used to prevent a delayed allergic reaction and to stabilize the capillary membranes. Fluid replacement and positive inotropic agents may need to be ongoing if hypotension persists as a result of increased capillary permeability. The vasoactive agents may help reverse the effects of the myocardial depression and vasodilation from the chemical mediators.

The management of a patient with an anaphylactic reaction should always include an investigation to find the causative agent. To prevent future reactions, the nurse should take every measure to avoid further exposure. Because the allergic reaction may return, the patient should be observed in the ICU even after he or she has recovered from an anaphylactic reaction.

Nursing Management and Prevention

Because it is not possible to predict which patient may experience an anaphylactic reaction, the critical care nurse should become suspicious of any change in behavior or patient presentation when administering medications, blood products, or diagnostic products. The critical care nurse should take a thorough admission assessment of all patients, including any history of allergies to foods, environmental agents, or medications. It is possible that patients may not have an anaphylactic reaction to the antigen with the second exposure but will to a third. Many times the repeating exposures are less severe than the initial event; however, once again, this outcome is not predictable. Unfortunately, most severe allergic reactions leading to anaphylactic shock unexpectedly occur.

Prevention is the ideal way for the nurse to manage severe anaphylactic and anaphylactoid reactions. Nurses in the critical care areas are responsible for identifying patients with allergies along with the type of reaction the patient experiences with exposure. Factors that improve a patient's survival during an anaphylactic episode include (1) decreasing the length of time between exposure and onset of symptoms, (2) determining route and dose of the agent, (3) identifying length of time between onset of symptoms and initiation of therapy, and (4) determining overall sensitivity of the patient.

Depending on the patient's symptoms, the critical care nurse should prioritize interventions to manage the patient's care successfully. Nursing interventions should first include recognizing the problem and instituting measures to prevent further compromise such as anaphylactic shock. With knowledge that the hallmark of management for anaphylaxis is the administration of epinephrine (Adrenaline), the nurse should be prepared to deliver the correct dose through the appropriate route. Priority should be taken to maintain the patient's ABCs. The nurse should position the patient to optimize breathing and determine whether the patient needs any assistance. Oxygen should be administered to improve saturation and tissue oxygenation. The astute critical care nurse also knows that an anaphylactic reaction ultimately produces leaky capillaries and that the patient will require fluid volume replacement. Therefore it is wise to

TAKE HOME POINTS

Life-threatening situations may occur up to 8 hours without symptoms.

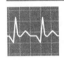

Continued vigilance on the part of the critical care nurse provides the patient with the needed attention should any signs of an allergic reaction return. These signs may include only mild dermatologic changes or more severe respiratory or cardiovascular compromise.

TAKE HOME POINTS

A thorough admission history can be obviously helpful, but the astute nurse must also keep in mind that exposure without symptoms does not eliminate the possibility of an anaphylactic reaction.

establish two large-bore peripheral IV lines in the patient. Overall, the critical care nurse should provide the patient comforting measures including emotional support during the crisis until subsequent treatment is determined. Finally, thorough documentation and a patient alert bracelet for allergies are essential.

 Do You UNDERSTAND?

DIRECTIONS: Complete the following crossword puzzle.

Across

3. Anaphylactic reactions are immune-mediated responses by IgE bound to mast cell membranes and _____.

6. Anaphylactic reactions need prior exposure, _____ reactions may occur without prior exposure.

8. Anaphylactic reactions are _____-mediated responses.

9. _____ is the hallmark of management for anaphylaxis.

10. Classic signs of a histamine-triggered reaction include _____, warmth, and swelling.

Down

1. The first step in treating a possible anaphylactic reaction is to _____ the causative agent.

2. _____ triggers physiologic changes in the body by promoting vasodilation and increasing capillary-venous permeability.

4. _____ is a life-threatening hypersensitivity or pseudoallergic reaction to an exogenous agent.

5. When treating anaphylaxis, the nurse should maintain the patient's airway while administering _____.

7. Common causes of an anaphylactic reaction include foods, environmental agents, medications, _____ or blood products, or venoms.

Answers: *Across:* 3. basophils; 6. anaphylactoid; 8. immune; 9. epinephrine; 10. redness. *Down:* 1. discontinue; 2. histamine; 4. anaphylaxis; 5. oxygen; 7. blood.

What IS Cardiogenic Shock?

Maintaining tissue oxygenation is crucial, otherwise cells begin to die.

Cardiogenic shock is a special kind of shock during which the heart does not adequately pump enough blood to the body's tissues. When the heart does not contract adequately, blood flow to tissues decreases and oxygen delivery falls. When oxygen delivery falls below critical levels, tissues fail to function and eventually break down (cellular destruction) and die. When enough tissues die, the entire body dies.

Pathophysiology

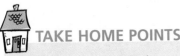

TAKE HOME POINTS

Acute myocardial infarction is the main cause for cardiogenic shock.

Cardiogenic shock is due to decreased functioning of the heart, which leads to decreased forward flow of oxygenated blood to the tissues. The most common cause of cardiogenic shock is a heart attack (myocardial infarction) that can damage 40% or more of the ventricle.

Ventricular function is very important to cardiac function because this chamber of the heart performs most of the work in moving the blood forward in the body. When the ventricle is damaged, it does not empty completely, which causes a decreased stroke volume. Stroke volume is the amount of blood pumped out of the heart during each contraction or heart beat. The CO, or the amount of blood pumped out of the heart every minute, also decreases. As stroke volume and CO decrease, blood builds up in the heart. When blood builds up in the heart, the left ventricular end–diastolic volume (LVEDV) increases. An increased LVEDV increases the amount of oxygen the heart needs (oxygen demand) to do its work. This increased demand occurs because the heart, among other things, has to now try and pump out a larger volume of blood.

TAKE HOME POINTS

Hypoxia in cardiac tissues leads to a further decrease in cardiac functioning and continues to compromise cardiovascular function.

An increased LVEDV also decreases the amount of blood that flows through the coronary arteries. This happens because the blood in the ventricle increases the pressure in the heart muscle. As pressure increases in the heart muscle, the coronary artery decreases in size, which results in decreased blood flow in the coronary arteries. This decreased blood flow decreases the amount of oxygen that is delivered to the heart muscle. Once again, decreased oxygen delivery to the heart can lead to cardiac hypoxia.

As the stroke volume and CO decrease, blood also backs up into the pulmonary system. When blood backs up into pulmonary system, fluid leaks out of the pulmonary capillaries into the lung tissue and alveoli, which causes pulmonary edema. Pulmonary edema hinders the movement of oxygen from the alveoli to the blood in the pulmonary capillaries. Decreased movement of oxygen from the alveoli to the blood reduces the oxygen contained in arterial blood (oxygen content). Decreased oxygen content in arterial blood can lead to tissue hypoxia.

As the cardiovascular system becomes more damaged, a vicious cycle develops, which may lead to patient deterioration and death if left untreated.

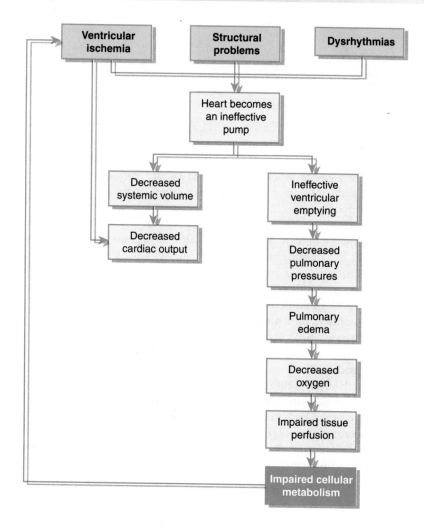

At-Risk Populations

Patients at risk for developing cardiogenic shock often have one of the following pathologic conditions:

- Acute myocardial infarction
- Atrial thrombus
- Cardiac contusion
- Cardiac tamponade
- Cardiac tumor
- Cardiomyopathic conditions
- Cardiopulmonary arrest
- Dysrhythmias
- Myocarditis
- Open heart surgery
- Pneumothorax
- Pulmonary embolus
- Valvular dysfunction
- Ventricular aneurysm

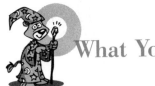

What You NEED TO KNOW

Clinical Manifestations

Many clinical manifestations can appear in the patient with cardiogenic shock; these manifestations depend on the severity of the shock, other underlying conditions in the patient, and cause of the pump failure. Some clinical manifestations are a result of the pump's failure, whereas others are the result of the body's response to the shock.

Cardiovascular signs of cardiogenic shock include a low BP of less than 90 mm Hg systolic initially. Tachycardia develops in response to the low BP and decreased CO. As the heart continues to fail, the pulse becomes "weak and thready." Catecholamines are released in response to the low BP. The catecholamines cause the BP to rise as a result of an increase in the heart rate and peripheral vascular constriction. Severe vasoconstriction causes the pulses to feel weak and thready. Capillary refill is sluggish, and peripheral tissues begin to show signs of hypoxia as a result of decreased blood flow and oxygen delivery. The heart cannot continue to respond to the catecholamines because of a lack of oxygen, which is needed for heart contraction. Oxygen is also needed to maintain vessel constriction. If oxygen delivery is not restored, the heart becomes more hypoxic, experiences more damage, and becomes even less able to pump blood. The CO continually falls and leads to a continual increase of tissue hypoxia.

As the heart becomes more hypoxic, ischemic changes may be observed on an ECG. These changes are often seen as ST segment changes or premature ventricular contractions (PVCs). The patient may also complain of chest pain or tightness.

 For further information on ECG interpretation, see the *Real World Nursing Survival Guide: ECGs & the Heart.*

www.sprojects.
mmip.mcgill.ca/
cardiophysio/default.
htm

ST segment depression

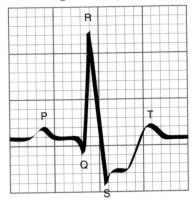

T wave inversion

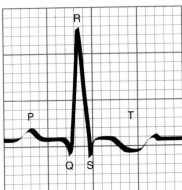

ST segment elevation

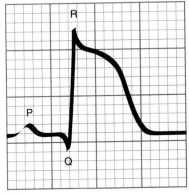

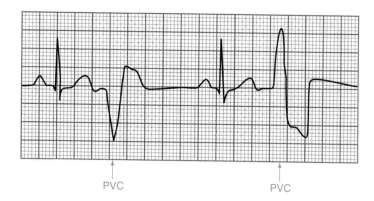

PVC   PVC

As CO decreases, blood backs up into the heart and lungs. Fluid leaks out from the pulmonary capillaries into the lungs. Fluid in the lungs causes crackles and diffuse rales when the patient breathes. Oxygen does not cross as easily from the alveoli into the blood because of the fluid in the alveoli and capillary membrane. As a result, arterial blood is less oxygenated and oxygen saturation falls. Oxygen saturation may be measured by direct arterial blood sampling or estimated through pulse oximetry measurements. In instances of severe hypoxia, the patient may have dark-colored nail beds and mucous membranes.

The central nervous system (CNS) is dependent on blood flow and oxygen for proper functioning. Decreased blood flow and hypoxia can lead to anxiety, confusion, lethargy, and coma. The first sign that a patient may be experiencing decreased blood flow and hypoxia is often a change in mental status.

Cardiogenic shock also affects the GI system. Patients are often nauseated and experience decreased bowel sounds because of a lowered BP. As the shock becomes severe, blood flow can fall so low as to cause bowel ischemia and infarction (death).

The renal system is also very sensitive to decreases in blood flow and oxygen supply. The kidneys require a constant supply of oxygen from the blood to do their job. The kidneys have the ability to regulate a constant blood flow in spite of a range of BPs. This ability is termed *autoregulation*. Autoregulation allows the kidneys to have a constant blood flow, though the mean arterial BP may range from 50 to 150 mm Hg. If the mean arterial BP falls below 50 mm Hg, blood flow to the kidneys also falls and the kidneys become hypoxic. During times of hypoxia, the kidneys are less able to regulate the body's fluids and electrolytes, as well as excrete waste products and metabolize medications. Decreased blood flow in the kidneys causes urine output to fall, and peripheral edema may become apparent. The kidneys can be damaged by the decrease in blood flow and lack of oxygen. Vasoconstriction in the kidneys from catecholamines often worsens kidney damage. Severe or prolonged decreases in blood flow and oxygenation can lead to renal insufficiency and failure.

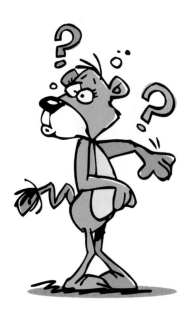

 TAKE HOME POINTS

The prognosis is poor for patients who develop cardiogenic shock. The risk of dying is between 70% and 80%.

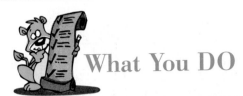

What You DO

To prevent cardiogenic shock, all treatments must be aimed at restoring blood flow and oxygenation. Treatments must be quickly administered and early to limit tissue and organ damage. Emergent cardiac revascularization through thrombolytic therapy, angioplasty, or bypass surgery is often needed to decrease mortality in patients experiencing myocardial ischemia. To prepare the patient for thrombolytic therapy, the nurse should review the patient history to determine patient age, onset of symptoms, medications, allergies, presence of hypertension, and recent history of surgery, trauma, bleeding, or stroke. Preparing for angioplasty or bypass surgery requires the standard preoperative assessment and work-up unless emergency circumstances preclude an in-depth surgical preoperative work-up.

Patients at risk for or experiencing cardiogenic shock may require circulatory support from mechanical devices such as an intraaorta balloon pump (IABP), a left ventricular assist device (LVAD), or pharmacologic interventions. Additionally, oxygen therapy and respiratory support may assist in increasing oxygen supply to a failing heart.

Intraaorta Balloon Pump and Left Ventricular Assist Device

The IABP works by inflating during diastole and deflating during systole. Systolic deflation helps move blood out of the heart by reducing the afterload or the resistance against which the heart has to pump. When the balloon deflates, a space is created that has less resistance, enabling the heart to send blood. By decreasing afterload, the workload of the heart is decreased and the amount of oxygen needed to do the work is decreased (see Color Plate 2 for IABP placement and balloon effects).

When the balloon inflates during diastole, blood is "pushed" into the coronary arteries on either side of the aorta. This action increases the blood flow through the coronary arteries to the heart muscle. By increasing blood flow to the heart muscle, oxygen delivery is also increased. Increasing oxygen delivery to the heart muscle increases the oxygen supply to the heart and helps reduce cardiac hypoxia. Thus by decreasing afterload and increasing coronary artery perfusion, the IABP decreases cardiac workload, decreases myocardial oxygen demand (MVO_2), and increases myocardial oxygen supply, which allows the heart to function more efficiently.

An LVAD increases CO by helping the left ventricle pump blood to the periphery. By helping the heart work, the LVAD allows the heart to rest and not work so hard while the body tries to repair the damage. An LVAD is often used as a last resort in patients with severe cardiogenic shock.

LVADs and IABP are inserted surgically. The use of these devices requires that the patient be anticoagulated to prevent blood clot formation that could cause an embolus around the device. Nursing care involves monitoring the coagulation status of the patient so that clotting is adequately reduced. The patient, surgical site, and equipment connections should also be monitored for bleeding and exsanguination. Both the IABP and LVAD are not permanent solutions but are used to help the heart recover from the shock phase.

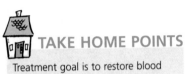

TAKE HOME POINTS

Treatment goal is to restore blood flow and oxygenation to the tissues.

The patient's coagulation status must be closely monitored to prevent the LVAD or IABP catheters from becoming clotted.

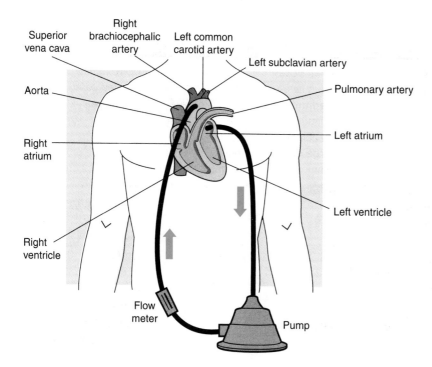

Superior
vena cava

Right
brachiocephalic
artery

Left common
carotid artery

Left subclavian artery

Pulmonary artery

Aorta

Left atrium

Right
atrium

Left ventricle

Right
ventricle

Flow
meter

Pump

Pharmacologic Intervention

The cause of cardiogenic shock may be left heart failure (most common), right heart failure, or cardiac tamponade. A number of available pharmacologic agents for treatment are available, and the best combination is determined by the cause of the pump's failure and the patient's response. Some of the more common agents include the following:

- **Dopamine (Intropin):** Increases renal perfusion at lower doses and causes an increase in CO, heart rate, and systemic arterial pressure at higher doses, which increases the pumping action of the heart (positive inotropic).
- **Dobutamine (Dobutrex):** Increases the pumping action of the heart (positive inotropic) and CO and decreases ventricular filling pressure.
- **Norepinephrine (Levophed):** A profound peripheral vasoconstrictor that is used in patients with extremely low systolic pressure (<70 mm Hg) to prevent total circulatory collapse.
- **Milrinone (Primacor):** Promotes arterial vasodilation and reduces preload and afterload while increasing the pumping action of the heart (positive inotropic).
- **Sodium nitroprusside (Nipride):** Decreases arterial resistance and is often used to decrease SVR, afterload, and systolic BP.
- **Nitroglycerin (Nitrol, Tridil):** Decreases venous resistance and increases coronary artery dilation to assist with decreasing anginal pain.
- **Diuretics:** Decrease body water, pulmonary edema, and systemic fluid overload.

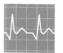 The patient needs to be monitored carefully for effect while medications are being adjusted and titrated. Attention must be paid to the effects on the patient's heart rate, BP, and hemodynamic readings to optimize cardiac function.

Medication, Doses, and Sites of Action

MEDICATION	ACTION	RECEPTOR	DOSE RANGE
Dopamine (Intropin)	Increases blood pressure, cardiac output, urine output	**Small doses:** <2 µg/kg/min—stimulates dopaminergic sites **Medium doses:** 3-10 µg/kg/min—stimulates dopamine and β-adrenergic sites **Large doses:** >10 µg/kg/min—stimulates α-adrenergic sites	0.5-10 µg/kg/min, titrated based on hemodynamic response
Dobutamine (Dobutrex)	Positive inotrope with minimal heart rate increase	β-1 agonist	Starting with 0.5-1.0 µg/kg/min, titrated to 40 µg/kg/min
Epinephrine (Adrenaline)	Positive inotrope, positive chronotrope, bronchodilator, vasoconstrictor	β-1, β-2, and α-adrenergic agonist	Resuscitation: 0.5-1 mg every 3-5 min Maintenance: 1-4 µg/min
Milrinone (Primacor)	Positive inotrope	Vascular smooth muscle dilator	Loading dose: 50 µg/kg over 10 min Infusion: 0.375-0.750 µg/kg/min
Nitroglycerin (Nitrol, Tridil)	Decreases blood pressure, decreases angina	Dilates coronary arteries, dilates peripheral veins	IV: Start 5 µg/min, titrated upward, based on hemodynamic response
Sodium nitroprusside (Nipride)	Lowers blood pressure, decreases cardiac preload and afterload	Peripheral arteriole and venous smooth muscle dilator	0.3-10.0 µg/kg/min

Oxygen Therapy

The goal of oxygen therapy is to improve arterial blood oxygenation to help increase oxygen supply to the tissues. A measurement of oxygen tension in the arterial blood (PaO_2) of >80 mm Hg on blood gas analysis and an oxygen saturation of >90% are both therapeutic goals. Patients experiencing myocardial ischemia or at risk for cardiogenic shock should receive supplemental oxygen. The patient's condition may require use of mechanical ventilation with the addition of positive-end expiratory pressure to help meet the goals of adequate oxygenation.

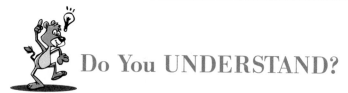

Do You UNDERSTAND?

DIRECTIONS: Complete the following crossword puzzle.

Across
2. Embolus
4. Type of shock
8. He has had three _____ bats
9. What the heart does
10. James Bond
11. Contracting ability
13. Has four chambers
15. Not enough oxygen in the tissues causes this

Down
1. Candy _____
3. Diplomacy
5. Chest pain
6. Increases pumping action of the heart
7. Decreases afterload (*abbreviation*)
10. Cardiogenic _____
12. Dynamite (*abbreviation*)
14. Hazard

Answers: Across: 2. clot; 4. cardiogenic; 8. at; 9. pump; 10. spy; 11. inotropic; 13. heart; 15. ischemia.
Down: 1. bars; 3. tact; 5. angina; 6. dopamine; 7. IABP; 10. shock; 12. TNT; 14. risk.

What IS Hypovolemic Shock?

Hypovolemic shock, the most common form of shock, is caused from an inadequate circulating blood volume in the intravascular bed. As with all forms of shock, circulating oxygenated blood flow to the body organs decreases. This lack of oxygenated blood leads to inadequate tissue perfusion, which causes cellular hypoxia, subsequent organ failure, and death.

What You NEED TO KNOW

The causes of hypovolemic shock can be divided into two categories: *absolute hypovolemia* and *relative hypovolemia*. Absolute hypovolemia occurs as a result of external losses of fluid; relative hypovolemia occurs as a result of the internal shifting of fluid between the body's two compartments, which is known as *third spacing*. Third spacing is when the fluid of the intravascular space relocates to the extravascular space, causing edema.

Causes of Hypovolemic Shock

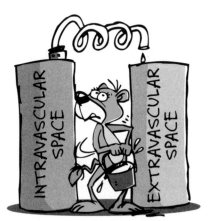

ABSOLUTE AND DIRECT LOSSES	RELATIVE AND INDIRECT LOSSES
GI status (diarrhea, vomiting, GI suction, ostomies, fistulas)	Hemoperitoneum or hemorrhagic pancreatitis
Hemorrhage (trauma, surgery, GI bleeding, DIC, thrombocytopenia, hemophilia)	Hemothorax
	Increase capillary membrane permeability (sepsis, anaphylaxis, thermal injuries, spinal shock)
Plasma losses (thermal injuries, exudative lesions, decreased oral fluid intake)	Laceration of great vessels
	Long bone fractures, pelvic fractures
Renal losses (massive diuresis, hyperglycemic osmotic diuresis, diabetes insipidus, Addison's disease)	Loss of intravascular integrity as a result of internal hemorrhage
	Rupture of spleen or liver
	Sequestration of fluid as a result of decrease colloidal osmotic pressure (cirrhosis, intestinal obstruction, ileus, peritonitis, severe sodium depletion, hypopituitarism)

GI, Gastrointestinal; *DIC,* disseminated intravascular coagulation.

Pathophysiology of Hypovolemic Shock

As the circulating blood volume decreases, the venous return to the right side of the heart also decreases. This action leads to a decrease in cardiac filling pressure and volume, which is known as the *preload* or the *end–diastolic volume*. A decrease in preload results in a decrease in stroke volume and CO. The decrease in CO leads to hypotension and a subsequent decrease in oxygenated blood flow to the organs and inadequate tissue perfusion. The baroreceptors in the aortic notch and carotid sinuses sense a decrease in circulating blood volume, which stimulates the sympathetic branch of the autonomic nervous system. The fibers of the sympathetic nervous system (SNS), as well as the medullary portion of the adrenal glands, release two neurotransmitter substances—epinephrine and norepinephrine.

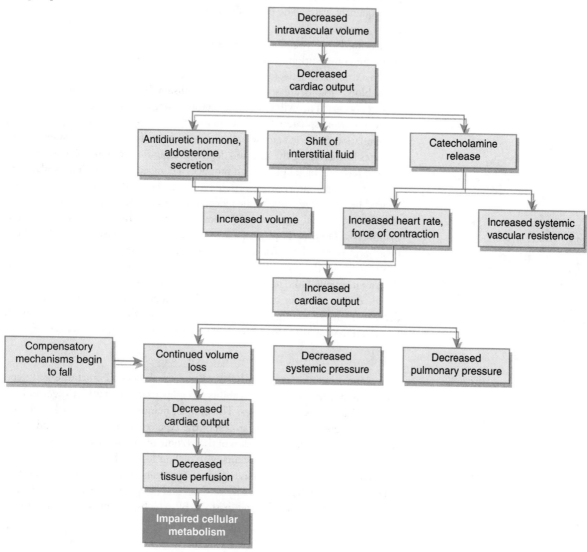

Epinephrine and norepinephrine cause an increase in heart rate and strengthen the contractile force of the heart in an attempt to increase the CO. These neurotransmitter substances also cause systemic vasoconstriction to maintain arterial BP. The vasoconstriction shunts much needed blood flow away from nonvital organs such as the skin, GI tract, kidneys, and musculoskeletal system. This vasoconstriction is part of the body compensatory mechanism, which maintains oxygenated blood flow and tissue perfusion to the vital organs, specifically to the brain and heart.

The kidneys contribute to this vasoconstriction by releasing a substance called *renin*, which stimulates the lungs to produce a powerful vasoconstrictor substance called *angiotensin II*. Angiotensin II stimulates the adrenal cortex to produce *aldosterone*, which acts on the renal tubules by reabsorbing sodium and, consequently, water. The posterior pituitary releases a vasoconstrictor substance called *antidiuretic hormone* (ADH) (vasopressin) in response to the decreased circulating blood volume. This action causes renal reabsorption of water and therefore conservation of fluid, as well as an increase in intravascular volume that is exhibited as a decrease in urinary output.

As blood flow decreases and tissue perfusion becomes inadequate, cellular hypoxia occurs. The cells resort to anaerobic metabolism in an effort to produce adenosine triphosphate (ATP) for energy. This type of metabolism produces an accumulation of lactic acid, which causes acidosis. The respiratory system compensates by increasing the rate and depth of respirations to blow off carbon dioxide and raise the blood pH, which produces a compensatory respiratory alkalosis.

In the compensatory stage of hypovolemic shock, the SNS outflow is evidenced by tachycardia, tachypnea, decreased urinary output, apprehension, and restlessness, as well as cutaneous vasoconstriction, which produces pallor and diaphoresis. These pathophysiologic responses protect perfusion to the brain and heart and restore homeostasis. However, the compensatory mechanisms are short lived. As the patient's compensatory mechanisms fail and the condition deteriorates, metabolic acidosis and hypoxia are produced, which leads to cell death, organ ischemia and failure, and eventually death. The hypoxia and decrease perfusion to organs such as the brain cause the patient to be confused, restless, uncooperative, maybe even combative, and perhaps comatose.

Clinical Manifestations of Hypovolemic Shock

The clinical manifestations of hypovolemic shock depend on the severity and rate of volume loss, the patient's ability to compensate, the patient's age, and the presence of preexisting illnesses. The clinical manifestations of shock will continue to progress in stages, regardless of the type of shock. The signs and symptoms of each stage are a reflection of the volume of loss and the body's response.

The compensatory stage occurs with a fluid loss of 15% to 30% or 750 to 1500 ml. The goal of this stage is to restore oxygenation and perfusion to the cells. The patient may exhibit normal BP readings and narrowed pulse pressure (the difference between the systolic and diastolic BP, which is normally 40 mm Hg). In addition, the patient may also develop tachycardia, tachypnea (creating a respiratory alkalosis), hypoxia, decreased urinary output, thirst, pale and cool skin, delayed capillary refill (less than 2 seconds), and changes in the LOC (e.g., confusion, restless, anxiousness).

If the underlying problem is not corrected, the patient then enters the progressive stage of shock. This stage begins with a fluid loss of 30% to 40% or 1500 to 2000 ml. In this stage the compensatory mechanisms fail and tissue perfusion becomes ineffective for the body organs to function. The heart rate continues to increase. Cardiac dysrhythmias develop because of myocardial ischemia. The CO and cardiac index, the right atrial pressure, and pulmonary artery wedge pressure decrease. The SVR increases as a result of the continued vasoconstriction of the arterial system. The prolonged vasoconstriction decreases capillary blood flow to the tissues, which contributes to the cellular hypoxia, anaerobic metabolism, and acidosis. The prolonged capillary vasoconstriction causes the vessels to become clogged, which impedes blood flow. Eventually, the capillary hydrostatic pressure increases, leading to third spacing of fluid and the presentation of edema. The fluid shift is further aggravated as capillary permeability is increased and the colloidal osmotic pressure is decreased from loss of proteins. As fluid shifts out of the intravascular space into the extravascular space, hypovolemia increases. The patient becomes hypotensive with a narrowed pulse pressure.

As the respiratory system fails, the patient can develop pulmonary edema and the arterial blood gases can deteriorate to reflect a respiratory and metabolic acidosis with continued hypoxemia. The oliguria progressively worsens and becomes unresponsive to treatment. As the kidneys lose function, the blood urea nitrogen (BUN) and creatinine levels increase. The patient's LOC continues to deteriorate as cerebral perfusion decreases. The patient becomes increasingly lethargic, confused, and eventually comatose. During this stage, organs become dysfunctional and all body systems are affected. As one organ system fails, the others eventually become dysfunctional, leading to multiorgan dysfunction syndrome (MODS). (Refer to the discussion on MODS later in Chapter 12.)

Once the body systems are no longer responsive to treatment and multiple-organ failure ensues, the patient is in the refractory or irreversible stage of shock. This final stage of shock occurs with a fluid volume loss of greater than 40% or more than 2000 ml. In this stage the compensatory mechanisms have been completely exhausted and organ failure has occurred. Death is imminent in this stage. Once brain damage occurs, sympathetic tone is lost. The severe tachycardia becomes bradycardia with continued hypotension until cardiopulmonary arrest. The patient becomes unresponsive. The acidosis, fluid shifts, edema, oliguria to anuria also become severe. A variety of clinical manifestations may occur in response to the failure of other body systems. All systems do not have to fail for death to ensue. The patient has a 90% to 100% mortality rate when only three body systems fail.

> **During the compensatory stage, it is very easy to overlook the occurring manifestations as hypovolemic shock.**

> **Hypotension is a late sign. Patients can lose 30% or more of their intravascular volume before signs and symptoms appear.**

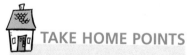

TAKE HOME POINTS

The outcome of the irreversible stage of shock is death.

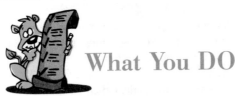

What You DO

Treatment of the patient in hypovolemic shock is focused on identifying and treating the underlying cause. The care of these patients involves maintaining oxygenation and perfusion by keeping the mean arterial pressure (MAP) equal to or greater than 60 mm Hg. These patients are treated according to their BP, urine output, hemodynamic parameters, laboratory results, and clinical status. The patient in hypovolemic shock may require massive fluid resuscitation and diligent monitoring of the patient's intake and output to stay ahead of the patient's fluid needs. The goal of fluid resuscitation is to restore intravascular volume, maintain oxygen-carrying capacity, and restore venous return and CO necessary for adequate tissue perfusion.

Equation for calculating MAP:

$$MAP = \frac{\text{Systolic BP} + 2(\text{Diastolic BP})}{3}$$

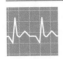

The patient's BP, heart rate, urine output, and laboratory and hemodynamic readings must be monitored to evaluate the effectiveness of treatments and to adjust as necessary.

FIRST-LINE AND INITIAL TREATMENT FOR HYPOVOLEMIC SHOCK

Goal: Restore homeostasis and intravascular volume.
Intervention: Infuse IV fluids or blood products or both.

The patient requires at least two large-bore (14- or 16-gauge) IV catheters, preferably in the antecubital veins for rapid administration of fluid. These fluids may need pressure-bagged or rapid-infusion devices. The patient may also need a central line for administering fluids and vasoactive drugs, as well as for monitoring the central venous pressure (CVP).

Because renal blood flow is sensitive to the CO, an increase or decrease in CO affects the urinary output. It is imperative to monitor the urinary output of the patient with hypovolemic shock; it is a valuable indicator of the patient's fluid status. Adequate fluid replacement should yield a urinary output of at least 0.5 ml/kg/hr.

Crystalloids, colloids, and blood and blood products are used to treat hypovolemic shock. Crystalloids, the first-line choice of treatment, are inexpensive and move rapidly and freely within the intravascular and extravascular spaces. The recommended initial treatment is 1 to 2 L bolus rapidly infused for adults. When given in sufficient amounts according to the patient's underlying condition and needs, crystalloids can be just as effective as colloids in restoring intravascular volume. Crystalloids may be given in large volumes, but evaluation is needed because greater than 4 to 5 L can cause internal and external edema. The crystalloid of choice is Ringer's lactate. Normal saline can be used as a second choice, but it can potentially cause hyperchloremic acidosis, which is made worse in the presence of renal impairment.

The patient's urinary output should be at least 0.5 ml/kg/hr when determining the adequacy of the replacement of fluid volume.

Colloids, a more expensive choice than crystalloids, contain proteins that increase the intravascular osmotic pressure and pull fluid out of the extravascular space into the intravascular space to expand the plasma volume. Colloids stay in the intravascular space longer than crystalloids; they have a half-life between 3 to 6 hours. General indications for colloid administration include patients with severe intravascular fluid deficits and severe hypoalbuminemia or conditions associated with large protein losses. Colloids are sometimes used with crystalloids when volume replacement has exceeded 3 to 4 L of crystalloids.

Unlike crystalloids, colloids are given in small volumes. Albumin and Plasmanate are colloid solutions that are administered when volume loss is due to a loss of plasma proteins and volume rather than a loss of blood volume. Other synthetic colloids that act as volume expanders include dextran and hetastarch. Dextran is contraindicated in patients with hemorrhagic shock because it decreases platelet adhesiveness and therefore increases bleeding. Additional complications with dextran include allergic reactions and renal damage. Hetastarch has no effect on the renal function and is not as likely to cause an allergic reaction; however, it does alter bleeding times. No more than 1 L of either dextran or hetastarch should be administered in a 24-hour period because both produce coagulopathic results.

If bleeding causes hypovolemic shock, then the patient can be initially treated with crystalloids. A three-to-one rule is used when replacing blood loss with crystalloids. For every 1 ml of blood loss, 3 ml of crystalloid should be given. Once the blood loss has reached 1500 ml, blood transfusion with packed red blood cells should be administered along with other blood products such as fresh-frozen plasma (FFP) and platelets as needed to restore clotting factors. Clinicians must understand that a loss in total blood volume—not the loss of red blood cells—causes the patient to develop hypovolemic shock (impaired tissue oxygenation and perfusion). A transfusion with packed red blood cells should be initiated when the danger of anemia places the patient at risk for organ ischemia. Transfusions are recommended when the hemoglobin is 7 to 8 g/dl (hematocrit of 21% to 24%); even then the clinician must take into account the rate of blood loss, the presence of cardiovascular or pulmonary disease, and the patient's age. A higher limit of 10 g/dl may be needed if the patient is older or has a co-morbid illness such as cardiac disease. If blood loss is expected to continue at a rapid rate, then higher limits for a transfusion may be indicated or surgical intervention may be needed. Normal saline is the fluid of choice for administering blood.

If volume replacement does not adequately support CO and MAP to ensure and maintain tissue perfusion, then pharmacologic therapy may be used. Vasopressors such as dopamine (Intropin) and norepinephrine (Levophed) can be used to support the BP and increase cardiac contractility. It must be noted that volume loading is the major intervention in the treatment of hypovolemic shock and that drug therapy should be used as a last choice. It is imperative that intravascular volume be replaced with fluids to ensure the effectiveness of the vasopressors. The vasoconstriction from the pharmacologic effect can worsen cellular hypoxia and anaerobic metabolism by decreasing capillary blood flow to the tissues if the vascular bed has not been volume loaded and CO sustained with fluids.

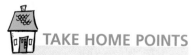

TAKE HOME POINTS

The intravascular half-life of crystalloids is 20 to 30 minutes.

- **Dextran may cause an allergic reaction or renal damage (or both) in some patients.**
- **Dextran and hetastarch infusions alter bleeding times and may produce coagulopathic results.**

TAKE HOME POINTS

To ensure the effectiveness of vasopressors in the treatment of hypovolemia (i.e., causing vasoconstriction and increasing BP), the patient must have adequate intravascular volume and not be severely vasoconstricted as a compensatory mechanism.

Managing the patient's respiratory status is also part of the treatment for hypovolemic shock. All patients should receive 100% oxygen via a nonrebreather mask. Ideally, the patient's oxygen saturation should be 95%, which yields 85% to 100% PaO_2. Arterial blood gases should be frequently monitored for oxygen saturation and acidosis. The patient's respiratory status is affected by the volume loss, and the patient may require mechanical ventilation. If the patient is hemodynamically unstable with a large volume deficit, then early initiation of mechanical ventilation is necessary to influence the best outcome. Mechanical ventilation is the most effective way to improve the patient's oxygenation and acid-base status.

These patients require frequent monitoring of vital signs. Once the patient becomes hypotensive, BP levels should be monitored continuously with an arterial line. Temperature is another important vital sign to monitor. Patients receiving large volumes of fluid or cold blood from the blood bank are at risk for hypothermia. Body temperature should be monitored at least every hour in those with hypovolemic shock—every 30 minutes if needed. *Hypothermia* is defined as a body temperature less than 36° C (96° F). When the patient is hypothermic, physiologic changes occur in all body systems. Hypothermia is a cardiac depressant and can predispose the patient to cardiac dysrhythmias. Hypothermia can alter the clotting mechanisms and place the patient at risk for coagulopathic consequences. The best treatment for hypothermia is prevention. All fluids should be warmed. The use of external warming devices such as overhead heat lamps, warming blankets, or thermal caps should be used in patient care. The clinician must also keep in mind that shivering increases metabolic demands for oxygen up to 400%. This additional demand for oxygen is crucial in the patient who is already suffering from tissue hypoxia.

Positioning is another important aspect of patient care. If the patient with mild hypovolemia is stable, the best position is supine with the head of the bed elevated 30 to 60 degrees to maintain pulmonary ventilation. Turning the patient every 2 hours has also been shown to improve oxygenation and pulmonary function. However, when the patient is unstable and hypotensive, the best position is supine and flat. The Trendelenburg position should not be used in the management of the patient in hypovolemic shock. The Trendelenburg position causes an increase in mediastinal pressure from the increase in blood volume and the shifting of abdominal contents against the diaphragm. These actions stimulate the baroreceptors, which leads to a decrease in CO, peripheral vascular resistance, heart rate, and BP. The Trendelenburg position also causes a decrease in the functional residual capacity and pulmonary compliance, which increases the patient's hypoxia. Furthermore, the Trendelenburg position increases cerebral venous congestion and intracranial pressure, resulting in decreased cerebral perfusion pressure and worsening cerebral hypoxia.

The patient in hypovolemic shock requires the vigilance of a critical care nurse with frequent monitoring of vital signs, oxygen saturation, fluid intake, and urine output. These patients need cardiac monitoring, CVP monitoring, and a pulmonary artery catheter for measuring hemodynamic parameters. Monitoring laboratory series (e.g., chemistry profile; hematocrit, hemoglobin and platelet counts; coagulation studies; arterial blood gases) is necessary.

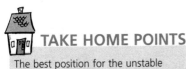

TAKE HOME POINTS

The best position for the unstable patient in hypovolemic shock is supine or flat.

Do NOT attempt to place the patient with hypovolemic shock in the Trendelenburg (head down) position because it stimulates the baroreceptor response and aggravates hypoxia and cerebral venous congestion.

The hypovolemic patient is a critically ill individual; even patients with mild hypovolemia can rapidly deteriorate. The hypovolemic patient requires vigilant nursing care. The nurse must remember that hypovolemia affects all organs. The treatment of hypovolemia is volume load and oxygenation.

Do You UNDERSTAND?

DIRECTIONS: **Identify the following statements as** *true* **(T) or** *false* **(F).**

_____ 1. Inadequate tissue perfusion, which causes cellular hypoxia, subsequent organ failure, and death from decreased circulating oxygenated blood flow, is the underlying pathophysiologic cause of all forms of shock.

_____ 2. Intestinal obstruction can cause sequestration of fluid as a result of a decrease in colloidal osmotic pressure leading to hypovolemic shock.

_____ 3. The Trendelenburg position is the best position for a patient in hypovolemic shock.

_____ 4. Hypotension is a late sign of shock.

DIRECTIONS: **Fill in the blanks to complete each of the following statements.**

5. Renal blood flow is sensitive to CO. The _____

_____ is the most sensitive indicator of a patient's fluid status

that a nurse must monitor when caring for the patient with hypovolemia.

6. The fluid of choice for the initial treatment of hypovolemic shock is

_____ _____.

7. The initial goal in the resuscitation of a patient in hypovolemic shock is

accomplished with fluid volume loading to preserve oxygen perfusion to

the tissues by sustaining the _____ _____

and the _____ greater than _____ mm Hg.

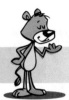

What IS Neurogenic Shock?

Neurogenic shock is also known as *spinal shock*. Neurogenic shock is a rare shock state that is a result of a loss of peripheral vasomotor tone, which leads to a decrease in tissue perfusion. The cause of neurogenic shock is anything that disrupts the SNS impulse transmission and may be attributed to a spinal cord injury, spinal anesthesia, autonomic blocking medications, pain, emotional stress, or CNS dysfunction. The onset of neurogenic shock can follow anywhere from minutes to months—all depending on the underlying cause.

What You NEED TO KNOW

In neurogenic shock, the SNS is disrupted, which results in a cascade of events.

Normally, the body attempts to compensate from the massive vasodilation by becoming tachycardic in an attempt to increase the amount of blood flow and oxygen being delivered to the tissues. However, in neurogenic shock, the SNS becomes disrupted; consequently, the parasympathetic influence takes over and bradycardia results. Although the heart is pumping, the CO as a result of bradycardia is not sufficient, and thus the patient shows signs of decreased tissue perfusion:

- Bradycardia
- Decreased CO
- Decreased pulmonary artery pressure (PAP), pulmonary capillary wedge pressure (PCWP)
- Decreased SVR (as a result of vasodilation)
- Hypotension
- Hypothermia

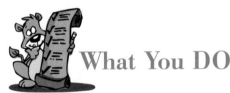

What You DO

The management goal for the patient in neurogenic shock is to improve tissue perfusion. One of the first interventions is to find the cause and remove it, if possible. While investigating the cause or attempting to correct the cause of the neurogenic shock state, promoting tissue perfusion and correcting any cardiovascular instability that the patient might be exhibiting are important. To promote tissue perfusion and manage cardiovascular instability, infusing IV fluids for volume replacement

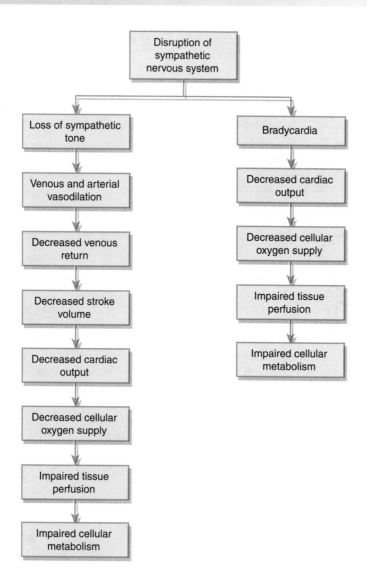

and initiating vasopressors to control BP levels might be necessary. In addition, if the patient is exhibiting symptomatic bradycardia, then it is necessary to administer atropine sulfate or apply a transcutaneous pacemaker that will increase the patient's heart rate and hopefully improve tissue perfusion.

If the patient is hypothermic, then the goal is to maintain normothermia through various warming measures without causing large fluctuations that could cause more vasodilation and worsen the circulatory instability. An appropriate intervention includes covering the patient with warm blankets. The patient should also be monitored for hypoxia because altered tissue perfusion leads to decreased tissue oxygenation. Therefore the patient should be placed on a continuous pulse oximeter, and astute respiratory assessment is needed to alert the

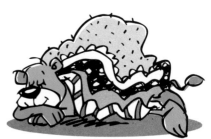

To avoid possible fluid overload, use caution when fluid resuscitating in an attempt to replace intravascular volume. Remember that the underlying dilemma is a distributive and vasomotor tone problem.

nurse to a problem or impending problem with hypoxia. If the patient is hypoxic or exhibiting difficulties in maintaining an airway, then the patient most likely needs to be intubated and placed on a ventilator.

FIRST-LINE AND INITIAL TREATMENT FOR NEUROGENIC SHOCK

- Maintain the patient's ABCs.
- Place the patient on a continuous pulse oximeter.
- Intubate and secure an airway, if necessary.
- Infuse IV fluids for volume replacement.
- Administer vasopressors.
- Administer atropine sulfate, if necessary.
- Provide rewarming measures.

Do You UNDERSTAND?

DIRECTIONS: **Identify the following statements as** *true* **(T) or** *false* **(F).**

_____ 1. Neurogenic shock is an intravascular volume problem.

_____ 2. A patient with a T2 spinal cord injury is at risk for neurogenic shock.

_____ 3. Tachycardia results from the massive vasodilation and the response of the parasympathetic nervous system.

_____ 4. A patient in neurogenic shock who is hemodynamically unstable most likely needs to be treated with IV fluid boluses, vasopressors, and atropine sulfate.

What IS Septic Shock?

Septic shock is a shock state that occurs when sepsis is present in a patient. Sepsis occurs when a microbial infection is present in the blood and signs and symptoms of severe infection such as fever, tachycardia, and tachypnea are present. The presence of sepsis is complicated when an overwhelming microbial infection occurs, which releases endotoxins into the bloodstream, and the patient's status degenerates into septic shock. Gram-negative microorganisms most often cause septic shock, but it can also occur with infections stemming from gram-positive microorganisms, fungi, or yeasts.

In the past, it was theorized that the endotoxins released from these microorganisms were the cause of the septic shock state. It is now believed that excessive activation of the host's defense mechanisms cause the clinical syndrome of sepsis rather than the microorganisms themselves. Signs and symptoms of early sepsis can be subtle; therefore careful monitoring is essential. For this reason, identifying the patients who are at the greatest risk is important.

What You NEED TO KNOW

Septic shock is a distributive shock and characterized by tachycardia, hyperthermia or hypothermia, and hypotension caused by decreased SVR. The blood volume is adequate but misplaced. Vasodilation occurs, capillary permeability increases, and fluid is lost in the interstitial space. A decline in SVR is one of the first indications of shock. In addition, the patient develops compromised CO and index as a result of decreased vascular tone. Ascertaining this state without invasive hemodynamic monitoring may be difficult because the body compensates by increasing the heart rate. In this early or preshock state, CO increases and the arterial pressures lower but are not necessarily in the "shock" range, which is typically a systolic pressure of less than 90 mm Hg or a decrease in 40 points from a previously hypertensive systolic pressure. Because of this compensation and vasodilation, the patient will have pink, warm skin with rapid capillary refill and a bounding pulse.

Compensatory mechanisms include baroreceptor reflex, which causes increased heart rate, and an increase in vasomotor tone. The SNS is stimulated, which results in the release of epinephrine and norepinephrine that causes systemic vasoconstriction. This release causes blood to be shunted to the vital organs. Because of a decrease in blood flow to the kidneys, a decrease in glomerular filtration rate occurs, which activates the renin-angiotensin (I and II) and aldosterone system and results in sodium and water retention. The retention of sodium and water is the body's attempt to compensate for the decrease in blood flow by increasing the venous return to the heart and possibly increasing the patient's BP Progression of the shock state causes the compensatory mechanisms to be no longer effective and causes the patient to become hemodynamically compromised.

Continued decrease in blood flow to the vital organs ultimately results in tissue ischemia and acidosis from anaerobic metabolism. Anaerobic metabolism leads to depletion of cellular ATP and the failure of the sodium-potassium pump, which results in further hemodynamic compromise and an inability to maintain BP.

Respiratory failure is another complication and occurs in 30% to 80% of patients in septic shock. Tachypnea is observed in patients with and without fever and may be a result of endotoxins released by the invading microorganisms or by defense mechanisms mediated by the body in an attempt to maintain tissue oxygenation. With the progression of sepsis comes increased fluid in the lungs from the higher alveolar capillary permeability; the result is an even higher respiratory rate and hypoxia. Fatigue of breathing may ensue as the body attempts

 TAKE HOME POINTS

Patients at the greatest risk for septic shock include the following:
- Very young children
- Older adults
- Immunocompromised individuals
- Chronically ill patients
- Patients with malignancies

 Invasive monitoring lines, indwelling catheters, or venous access devices may predispose a patient to acquiring a nosocomial sepsis.

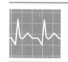 SVR decreases and CO increases.

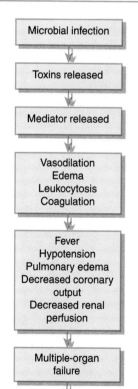

Microbial infection

↓

Toxins released

↓

Mediator released

↓

Vasodilation
Edema
Leukocytosis
Coagulation

↓

Fever
Hypotension
Pulmonary edema
Decreased coronary output
Decreased renal perfusion

↓

Multiple-organ failure

↓

Death

One of the first signs of inadequate tissue perfusion is a decreased level of consciousness that may be exhibited as confusion.

TAKE HOME POINTS

- Respiratory failure in septic shock is associated with a higher mortality rate than in patients without respiratory failure.
- A common cause of TSS is the use of tampons.
- Prolonged hypotension causes tissue hypoperfusion and results in ischemia and end-organ damage.

to maintain oxygenation. This fatigue leads to more shallow, less effective respirations that cause hypocarbia (decreased carbon dioxide), which triggers the CNS to further increase the respiratory rate, eventually causing exhaustion. The patient may progress into acute respiratory distress syndrome (ARDS).

The effect of septic shock on the kidneys can be profound. Renal involvement during sepsis can vary from a minor proteinuria to acute tubular necrosis (ATN) in septic shock. It is unknown whether the ATN is due to the decreased blood supply to the kidneys as a result of the hypotension or by the endotoxins released by the offending microorganism. Regardless of the cause, ATN can lead to renal failure. (For more information about ATN, refer to the discussion in Chapter 8.)

The patient in septic shock can exhibit skin lesions that are most often located on the lower extremities. These lesions can be associated with the development of disseminated intravascular coagulation (DIC), which is another complication of septic shock; the lesions can be associated with the causative bacteria. Toxic shock syndrome (TSS) can produce a profound septic shock and has a very distinctive cutaneous component. *Staphylococcus aureus* or a severe streptococcal infection causes TSS. The rash can be localized or generalized and appears in the form of a macular erythema that blanches with pressure.

Serum glucose increases with septic shock as a result of gluconeogenesis and insulin resistance. Hyperglycemia may be the first indicator of sepsis in the patient with diabetes. Control of the hyperglycemia may be difficult until the infection is under control. Hypoglycemia is relatively uncommon in sepsis, but it does occasionally occur in patients with other underlying problems.

Septic encephalopathy occurs in 70% of patients in septic shock. The patient may be agitated, confused, lethargic, disoriented, or even unarousable, but seizures are rare. Infection of the CNS may be considered; however, most patients in septic shock do not have infections of the CNS. Recovery from septic encephalopathy hinges on the control of the underlying septic shock.

MODS may develop in patients with septic shock and involves two or more organ systems. The release of endotoxins causes a massive inflammatory response, which leads to microvascular injury to various organs. To complicate matters further, hypotension leads to tissue hypoperfusion and end-organ damage. Early intervention and the identification and treatment of the underlying infection are imperative in halting this destructive event (see Chapter 12 for more information).

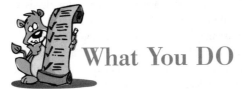

What You DO

Maintaining a patent airway is the first and foremost intervention with the critically ill patient. An assistive device, such as an oral or a nasal airway, may be needed. In the event of respiratory failure, the nurse should be prepared to assist with intubation, which is usually performed by the attending physician, nurse anesthetist, or other qualified professional. Initial intervention is oxygen delivery at 5 to 6 L via nasal cannula. To assess the adequacy of oxygenation, pulse oximeter readings, arterial blood gases, and mixed venous gases should be monitored. Higher concentrations of oxygen may become necessary, depending on arterial oxygen saturation (SaO_2) and arterial blood gas values. Mechanical ventilation may become necessary as a result of respiratory muscle fatigue. Frequent assessment of breath sounds for rate, character, and quality indicate adequacy of the patient's ventilation.

FIRST-LINE AND INITIAL TREATMENT FOR SEPTIC SHOCK

- Maintain a patent airway.
- Administer oxygen.
- Monitor hemodynamics.
- Provide IV access.
- Support BP with fluids and medications.
- Obtain cultures.
- Administer appropriate antibiotic therapy.

Optimal cardiac contractility and output is necessary to provide blood, which is rich in oxygen and nutrients, to the tissues and may be accomplished by administering prescribed IV fluids and pharmacologic agents. Careful monitoring of the patient's BP, pulses, and cardiovascular and hemodynamic status is essential. If the patient becomes hemodynamically unstable, the critical care nurse should anticipate the use of inotropic agents and vasoactive drugs. If hemodynamic monitoring is available, the patient's filling pressures (CVP) should be monitored to assess adequacy of fluid replacement and pulmonary wedge pressures. Fluid replacement is an important step in the treatment of the patient in septic shock. In sepsis, massive vasodilation and increased capillary permeability occurs, which results in fluid moving into the interstitial space. Because the patient requires IV fluids and possible pharmacologic agents, a good IV access site is essential; further, the patient often needs central venous access.

Frequent vital sign monitoring helps the nurse assess the patient's response to therapy. Monitoring BP by means of an arterial line should be anticipated. MAP should be closely monitored because of the variable pressures in the patient in septic shock. A MAP of <60 mm Hg negatively affects perfusion of the brain and kidneys and should be immediately addressed. The nurse should promptly notify the physician if a trend of a decreasing MAP develops. PAPs and CVPs enable the nurse to assess the effectiveness of the patient's treatment and to help prevent fluid overload by monitoring the patient's intravascular fluid status. Urinary output is also another important response to monitor and indicates adequacy of renal perfusion.

Some debate continues over the management and treatment of fever for the patient in septic shock. Few studies exist relating the control of temperature to the mortality or morbidity rate. Fever is usually treated because of the increased demands that the hypermetabolic state of septic shock places on the body. Some studies show that decreasing fever also decreases oxygen demand for organs and

TAKE HOME POINTS
- A nasogastric tube might be needed in an intubated patient to prevent aspiration of gastric contents and to decompress the stomach.
- The blood volume is adequate in the patient in septic shock, but it is misplaced.

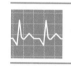 SVR will be decreased.

TAKE HOME POINTS
During hypotensive states, an arterial line measurement of BP is more precise than a manual or automatic cuff pressure.

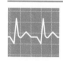 Observe the patient for changes in LOC because it may indicate hypoxia or decreased cerebral perfusion.

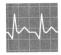

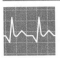 To assess nutritional adequacy, serum electrolytes, blood glucose, serum albumin, weight, and fluid volume status are closely monitored. Trace elements, vitamins, and glucose are added as prescribed.

 The desired urinary output is 0.5 ml/kg/hr.

 Indwelling urinary catheters place patients at risk for developing a nosocomial urinary tract infection.

TAKE HOME POINTS

Since prompt identification of the infecting organisms is essential, blood cultures can sometimes be simultaneously drawn while initiating IV access.

tissues and promotes patient comfort; others suggest that fever itself may provide some protection from the microbial pathogens. Fever, however, is always treated in the immunosuppressed patient.

FIRST-LINE AND INITIAL TREATMENT FOR FEVER

- Administer an antipyretic agent such as acetaminophen.

Another major aim in the treatment of septic shock is to improve the patient's nutritional status. The use of enteral nutrition is indicated unless contraindicated by the presence of acute pancreatitis, which requires parental nutrition. The patient needs increased nutrition because of the hypermetabolic state superimposed by the infection or disease state.

Maintaining renal perfusion is a priority and is monitored by urine output. A urine output >30 ml/hr or >0.5 ml/kg/hr indicates adequate renal perfusion. Indwelling urinary catheters are usually used to monitor hourly outputs. Catheter care is essential because the catheter can be a direct entry point for microorganisms. Therefore catheters must be closely monitored for change in the color and consistency or odor of urine, which may indicate myoglobinuria, hemoglobinuria, or possible urinary tract infection.

Proper isolation of the infective organisms is usually identified by blood, urine, sputum, or other cultures. For this reason, obtaining these cultures before initiating prescribed antibiotic therapy is important. The patient's outcome hinges on rapid identification and proper treatment of the infecting organism.

Do You UNDERSTAND?

DIRECTIONS: **Using the words listed below, fill in the blanks to complete the sentences on the following page. Words are used only once, and some words are not used at all.**

>30 ml/hr	less precise
>60 mm Hg	mechanical ventilation
<60 mm Hg	more precise
distributive shock	proper antibiotic treatment
hypovolemic shock	rapid identification
invasive monitoring lines	urinary catheterization

1. _____ _____

   _____ may predispose a patient to acquiring a nosocomial sepsis.

2. Septic shock is a _____ _____.

3. A MAP of _____ leads to decreased renal and cerebral perfusion.

4. _____ _____ may

   become necessary for respiratory muscle fatigue.

5. Arterial line BP monitoring is _____ _____

   than cuff pressures during hypotensive states.

6. The outcome of the patient in septic shock often depends on

   _____ and _____

   _____ _____ of

   the infectious organism.

CHAPTER

3 Trauma and Emergency Care

What IS Rapid Sequence Intubation?

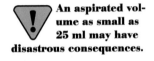

An aspirated volume as small as 25 ml may have disastrous consequences.

Rapid sequence intubation (RSI) is a specialized form of placing an endotracheal tube (ETT) in a patient to provide ventilation via a secure airway. Patients in respiratory distress or those unable to maintain a patent airway often require the placement of an ETT to allow some form of assisted or controlled ventilation. When the potential for gastric content regurgitation exists, an RSI is used to reduce the risk of aspiration. An RSI is designed to ensure that no gastric contents are aspirated into the tracheal tree, which could result in pneumonia or acute respiratory distress syndrome (ARDS).

At-Risk Populations

Although prescribed most frequently for emergency and trauma patient populations, RSI is also used in any case in which there is a potential for aspiration or when the patient is assumed to have a "full stomach" (e.g., obstetrics [OB] and labor and delivery).

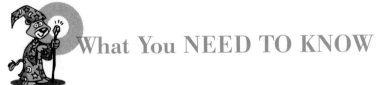

What You NEED TO KNOW

Clinical Technique

RSI differs from normal intubations in several key ways. Similar to all intubations, the patient should first be preoxygenated to fill the functional residual capacity (FRC) with 100% oxygen. However, unlike standard intubation procedure, RSI calls for the use of the Sellick maneuver (cricoid pressure) while the

42

patient is induced with anesthetic medications. Further, once induced the patient with RSI is **not** ventilated before administering neuromuscular-blocking agents or before attempting direct laryngoscopy. A period of apnea is intentionally instituted to prevent forcing air into the stomach via positive-pressure ventilation, which would increase intragastric pressure and potentiate regurgitation and aspiration. During a normal intubation, at least one attempt is made at controlled positive-pressure mask ventilation (test breath) between the administration of the anesthetic induction agent and the neuromuscular-blocking agent. This ventilation provides the health care provider with the knowledge that the patient can be mask ventilated in the event that intubation attempts are not successful. RSI does not allow for this ventilatory check, which increases the risk for hypoxia in the apneic patient. Thus the major risk involved in performing an RSI is the inability to ventilate the patient should intubation fail.

 Hypoxia, hypercarbia, and airway trauma are also potential hazards with any RSI attempt.

Assembly of all required equipment is essential before attempting any intubation. Suction must always be available to remove secretions, blood, and regurgitated materials from the oropharynx. One or more laryngoscope handles with charged batteries and at least two laryngoscope blades (Miller 2 and Macintosh 3 are recommended), as well as multiple sizes of ETTs should be at the bedside. At least one ETT should have a semirigid stylet inserted. A method for delivering positive-pressure ventilation must be at hand before intubating the patient (e.g., bag-valve-mask). A patent intravenous (IV) line is imperative, and all appropriate medications should be immediately available.

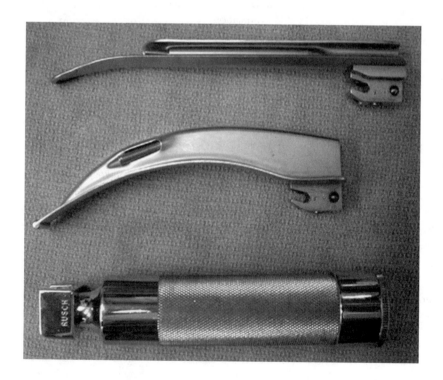

Common Endotracheal Tube Sizes

AGE AND SEX	APPROPRIATE SIZES	MOST COMMON SIZE	DEPTH OF INSERTION AS MEASURED AT TEETH
Children	Age + $\dfrac{16}{4}$ (age = 4 + 4)	Variable	Age + 10 cm
Adult men	7.5-8.5	8.0	23 cm
Adult women	6.5-7.5	7.0	21 cm

Common Medications Used in Rapid Sequence Intubation

MEDICATIONS	USES	DOSES (mg/kg)	ADVANTAGES	CONSIDERATIONS
Sodium thiopental (Pentothal)	Induction of anesthesia	4-6	Rapid onset, short duration	Hypotension, apnea
Etomidate (Amidate)	Induction of anesthesia	0.2-0.3	Rapid onset, short duration Cardiovascular stable May allow spontaneous ventilations	Myoclonus
Propofol (Diprivan)	Induction of anesthesia	2.0-2.5	Rapid onset, short duration	Hypotension, apnea
Ketamine (Ketalar)	Induction of anesthesia	1.0-2.0	Increased sympathetic tone bronchodilation	Tachycardia, increased sympathetic tone, salivation
Succinylcholine (Anectine)	Depolarizing neuromuscular blockade	1.0-1.5	Rapid onset, 5-7 min duration Gold standard for RSI	Muscular fasciculations Hyperkalemia, bradycardia, and dysrhythmias
Rocuronium (Zemuron)	Nondepolarizing neuromuscular blockade	0.9-1.2	Rapid onset; no risk of hyperkalemia	Extended duration (45-90 min) Potential for IV precipitation
Vecuronium (Norcuron)	Nondepolarizing neuromuscular blockade	0.2	Cardiovascular stable	"Slow" onset (>2-3 min) Extended duration (60+ min)

RSI, Rapid sequence intubation; *IV,* intravenous.

If the patient is alert and cooperative, then 30 ml of sodium citrate (Bicitra) can be administered to decrease the acidity of the stomach contents. If time permits, 50 mg of IV ranitidine (Zantac) or 10 mg of IV metoclopramide (Reglan) may be administered to decrease the risks involved with regurgitation and aspiration. However, most RSIs are attempted in emergent conditions, precluding the use of many premedications.

Preoxygenation is recommended before attempting intubation of any patient. Despite differences in how preoxygenation is performed, its use is universal. Traditional methods include spontaneous ventilation of 100% oxygen for 3 to 5 minutes or three to five vital capacity breaths of 100% oxygen. The latter method demands a cooperative patient. Preoxygenation allows the patient's FRC to be filled with oxygen. FRC is that portion of the total lung volume that is not normally expired during spontaneous ventilation. By filling these areas of the lung with oxygen, the patient is provided with a *reserve* (albeit sometimes small) of oxygen. In a young, healthy man, filling the FRC with 100% oxygen allows up to a 5- to 7-minute reserve of oxygen if the patient becomes apneic. Significantly, the duration of apnea caused by an induction dose of succinylcholine (Anectine) (1.0 to 1.5 mg/kg) is close to 5 to 7 minutes. Both obesity and pregnancy can significantly reduce the physical volume of the FRC, whereas tachycardia, sepsis, and other hyperdynamic states cause a more rapid use of the oxygen in the FRC. Additionally, both obesity and pregnancy increase the cephalad movement of the diaphragm on induction of anesthesia, further decreasing the FRC considerably.

When the oropharynx is filled with blood, secretions, or foreign material, these should be suctioned and an attempt should be made at preoxygenation in all but the most dire situations. Unconscious and trauma patients that have lost their normal protective airway reflexes and are not spontaneously ventilating pose a unique problem. Any positive pressure breaths administered via a bag-valve-mask increase the chances for regurgitation and aspiration of gastric contents. Many practitioners choose to skip preoxygenation and establish a controlled airway via immediate tracheal intubation in such cases.

The next distinguishing technique in RSI is the use of cricoid pressure or the Sellick maneuver. The cricoid cartilage is the first tracheal cartilage ring below the larynx. More importantly, the cricoid cartilage is the **only** continuous cartilaginous ring below the larynx.

Application of pressure (from 0.5 to 8.0 lb/ft) to this cartilage ring results in compression of the esophagus, which lies immediately posterior to the trachea. Firm pressure helps prevent the chances of gastric content regurgitation, but excessive pressure can actually hinder intubation attempts.

An acronym that has been used to aid those applying cricoid pressure is B-U-R-P. **B** stands for *backward* or posterior displacement; **U** stands for a slightly *upward* or cephalad movement; **R** stands for a slight *right* displacement of the larynx; and **P** stands for the *pressure* used to occlude the esophagus. The person assisting with the intubation must correctly identify the cricoid cartilage before applying pressure. From the prominence of the *Adam's apple* (thyroid cartilage),

TAKE HOME POINTS

Vital capacity is defined as a maximum inspiration immediately after a maximum expiration.

Many disease states can significantly alter both the physical amount of the FRC and the amount of time the body takes to use this oxygen reserve.

TAKE HOME POINTS

Suction should always be available when intubating a patient.

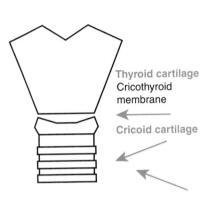

Thyroid cartilage
Cricothyroid
membrane

Cricoid cartilage

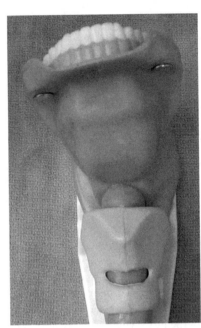

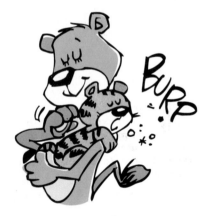

TAKE HOME POINTS

To apply cricoid pressure, remember
B-U-R-P:
Backward
Upward (slight)
Right displacement (slight)
Pressure to occlude the esophagus

the nurse slides the fingers down the anterior aspect of the patient's neck until the first depression is felt, which marks the *cricothyroid membrane*. The next cartilage ring is the cricoid cartilage. Pressure is applied by the use of the thumb and first two fingers on opposite sides of the cricoid cartilage. The assistant's hand should not be on the larynx or thyroid cartilage (see Color Plate 3).

It is also important to note that the application of cricoid pressure is not without risks. Complications range from interference with tracheal intubation, to esophageal rupture, to fracturing the cricoid cartilage. Once pressure to the cricoid cartilage has been applied, it is not removed until placement of the ETT has been confirmed by end-tidal carbon dioxide ($ETCO_2$) and bilateral breath sounds (BBS). Cricoid pressure may be lessened if it interferes with endotracheal intubation, therefore anyone assisting with an RSI must remain attentive to the needs of the person performing laryngoscopy.

Practitioners are split in their opinions of the best time to apply cricoid pressure. Slight pressure may be applied before administering any medications, increasing the pressure as the patient loses consciousness. Alternatively, cricoid pressure may be applied just as or immediately after the patient loses consciousness. Excessive pressure is quite uncomfortable in an awake patient; however, patients lose their protective airway reflexes within one *arm-brain* circulation (10 to 15 seconds), predisposing them to regurgitation and aspiration. Informing conscious patients of the actions and goals before applying any pressure may be one more reassuring step in an emergency situation.

As previously stated, an RSI does not allow for a test-breath ventilation after the patient is induced. Once preoxygenation is completed and cricoid pressure is applied, an appropriate induction drug is administered, which is followed by a neuromuscular-blocking agent that is almost immediately administered. Succinylcholine (Anectine) is the "gold standard" for RSI because of its rapid onset and short duration of action. However, succinylcholine causes an increase in serum potassium levels of up to 0.5 to 1.0 mEq/L, making it contraindicated in patients with, most notably, burns and neurologic disorders (e.g., denervation injuries, spinal cord injuries, stroke, Guillain-Barré syndrome). These patient groups are potentially susceptible to cardiac-arresting hyperkalemia induced by succinylcholine (Anectine).

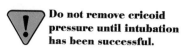

Do not remove cricoid pressure until intubation has been successful.

In search of a safe alternative for RSI in the patient who cannot take succinylcholine (Anectine), practitioners have traditionally used higher doses of a nondepolarizing neuromuscular-blocking agent such as vecuronium (Norcuron) or the rapid onset nondepolarizer rocuronium (Zemuron). Both drugs may be given in doses that allow for rapid tracheal intubation; however, their duration of action is significantly increased (see Table titled, "Common Medications Used in Rapid Sequence Intubation" on page 44). This increased duration can prove disastrous in cases where the trachea cannot be intubated and the patient cannot then be ventilated with a mask. Again, no test-breath procedure can assess the ability to mask ventilate a patient during an RSI.

A long-acting neuromuscular-blocking agent should be administered with extreme caution and in consideration of the potential consequences.

Practitioners should also be aware that administering rocuronium (Zemuron) too rapidly after giving sodium thiopental (Pentothal) could lead to remarkable precipitation in the IV line, rendering it unusable. Precipitation can also occur in and adjacent to injection ports of *needleless* systems.

Unconscious patients may be safely intubated without the use of a neuromuscular-blocking agent. In emergency situations and in some elective intubations requiring RSI in which succinylcholine (Anectine) is or may be contraindicated, the use of etomidate (Amidate) may allow successful intubation without the risks involved with the nondepolarizing neuromuscular-blocking agents. A key benefit of etomidate (Amidate) is that many patients continue to ventilate spontaneously, even after receiving an induction dose. Before deciding to skip paralyzation, the person performing an RSI should assess the need for some form of muscle relaxation. Patients with tightly clenched jaws may not be able to be intubated without some form of pharmacologic relaxation. However, only personnel skilled in intubating patients in all conditions should attempt to intubate a patient without some form of neuromuscular blockade.

The delay between the administration of induction medications and the direct laryngoscopy allows for the medications to circulate and have a therapeutic effect. Oxygen should be applied via a mask, whether or not preoxygenation took place before induction. Although no positive pressure ventilation is applied during this time, the high concentration of oxygen at the mask allows for diffusion.

Most induction medications have an onset of one arm-brain circulation, or about 15 to 20 seconds in patients with normal cardiac outputs. Patients already receiving external cardiac compressions may have extended onset times. Different practitioners administer the neuromuscular-blocking agent (if used) at varying times for RSI. Many will wait until the induction agent has had an effect (i.e., loss of eyelid reflex), whereas others will administer the paralytic agent immediately after inducing the drug. Still others give the neuromuscular-blocking agent before administering the induction agent to reduce the time delay of an unconscious, apneic patient. This last method may result in an awake but paralyzed patient.

Usually patients may be safely intubated approximately 1 minute after administering neuromuscular-blocking agents in RSI. Alternatively, the patient may be intubated once muscle fasciculations have ceased if succinylcholine (Anectine) is used. Suction must be immediately available because direct vocal cord visualization can be dramatically hindered by even small amounts of foreign matter in the oropharynx.

Either BBS or ETCO$_2$, or a combination of the two, must verify the placement of the ETT. The definitive standard for ETT placement is an anteroposterior chest x-ray, which should be obtained as soon as possible.

Cricoid pressure may be released only after the ETT placement has been verified. Although the laryngoscopist may ask for changes in the manner of cricoid pressure, it should never be completely removed.

Prognosis

Up to 40% of emergent intubations are unsuccessful on the first attempt. Any repeated attempts at intubation require some change in technique or current situation. The oropharynx may require deep suctioning, a different laryngoscope blade may be used, or the patient's airway may need to be repositioned. Although cricoid pressure may need to be lessened, it should never be completely removed.

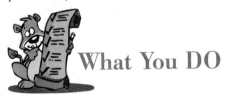

What You DO

The ability to secure a patent airway in an emergency depends in large part on being prepared. The immediate availability of the following items is imperative:
- Laryngoscope handles with fresh batteries or a working light source if fiberoptic
- Multiple laryngoscope blades of various types and lengths with working light bulbs if not fiberoptic
- ETTs of various diameters; at least one ETT with an inserted semirigid stylet
- Suction oropharynx secretions
- Induction and paralytic medications
- ETCO$_2$ monitor if required at institution
- Gloves

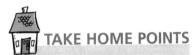
TAKE HOME POINTS
It is crucial to verify the placement of the ETT.

Meticulous attention to detail, including the proper labeling of the medications used in the induction and intubation of patients, is essential.

The nurse's role may also involve moving the patient and applying cricoid pressure. If the professional performing the intubation uses a flexible stylet in the ETT, then he or she may ask the nurse to remove the stylet once the ETT is past the vocal cords. Only the stylet should be grasped and removed. Too vigorous removal or grasping the ETT may result in accidental extubation.

FIRST-LINE AND INITIAL TREATMENT FOR RSI

- Preoxygenate the patient (may be omitted if airway reflexes are lost or foreign material is observed in the oropharynx).
- Apply cricoid pressure.
- Administer medications (induction without ventilation).
- Provide intubation.
- Check placement of ETT.
- Release cricoid pressure (only after proof of endotracheal intubation [via BBS or $ETCO_2$]).

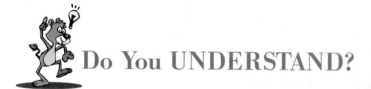

Do You UNDERSTAND?

DIRECTIONS: Fill in the blanks to complete the following statements.

1. The cricoid cartilage lies _____ the thyroid cartilage.

2. Aspiration of as little as _____ ml of gastric contents may result in

   significant injury to the patient.

3. Mrs. Smith is coming to the labor and delivery department for a scheduled

   full-term Cesarean delivery. She has ingested nothing by mouth for

   9 hours. Will she still require an RSI? _____

   Why? _____

   _____

Answers: 1. below; 2. 25; 3. Yes, All obstetric deliveries require an RSI.

DIRECTIONS: **Select the best answer, and place the appropriate letter in the space provided.**

_____ 4. One of the critical dangers of an RSI is:
   a. Increased chance of gastric content aspiration
   b. Inability to preoxygenate conscious patient
   c. Use of fiberoptic scopes
   d. Lack of a test-breath to assess airway patency

_____ 5. Nurses administrating the medications for RSI should watch for which possible problem(s)?
   a. Bovine plasma reactions from administration of succinylcholine (Anectine)
   b. Precipitation in the IV line with the use of certain combinations of induction and neuromuscular-blocking agents
   c. Ultrashort duration of action of drugs such as rocuronium (Zemuron) and vecuronium (Norcuron)
   d. Rapid-eye movements resulting in corneal abrasions

What IS Increased Intracranial Pressure?

Intracranial pressure (ICP) is a dynamic state that reflects the pressure of cerebrospinal fluid (CSF) within the skull. Increased ICP is described as pressures ≥20 mm Hg.

Normal ICP ranges according to age:
- Adults and older children: <10 to 15 mm Hg
- Young children: 3 to 7 mm Hg
- Infants: 1.5 to 6.0 mm Hg

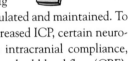

ICP is a dynamic physiologic process that is well regulated and maintained. To understand the pathophysiologic characteristics of increased ICP, certain neurologic concepts must become familiar. These include intracranial compliance, intracranial elastance, the Monro-Kellie hypothesis, cerebral blood flow (CBF), and cerebral perfusion pressure (CPP).

Intracranial compliance is the ability of the brain to tolerate increases in intracranial volume without adversely increasing ICP.

Intracranial compliance:

$$\text{Compliance} = \frac{\text{Volume}}{\text{Pressure}}$$

The ability of the brain to respond to intracranial volume changes with no increase in ICP indicates normal and adequate compliance. In contrast, a low compliance indicates that a small volume increase exists, which will cause an elevation in ICP.

Intracranial elastance is the ability of the brain to tolerate and compensate for an increase in intracranial volume through distention or displacement.

Intracranial elastance:

$$\text{Elastance} = \frac{\text{Pressure}}{\text{Volume}}$$

High elastance means that the brain is tight because the intracranial volume and the ability to distend and displace intracranial components is at its limit, thus resulting in a significant elevation of ICP.

The *Monro-Kellie hypothesis* states that the skull acts as a closed, rigid vault containing the intracranial components of brain tissue (84%), blood (4%), and CSF (12%) under which the total brain volume remains fixed.

When any one of the three components increases in volume, another must decrease to maintain the overall volume.

Normal intracranial values:

Normal Intracranial Values = 1700 to 1900 ml Intracranial Contents

CBF delivers oxygen to the tissues in the brain and maintains cerebral perfusion through the compensatory mechanism of autoregulation. When changes in the blood pressure (BP) occur, cerebral blood vessels automatically constrict or dilate to maintain perfusion and deliver oxygen to the tissues. Autoregulation is maintained with a mean arterial pressure (MAP) of 50 to 70 mm Hg.

CPP is defined as a pressure gradient across the brain and is the difference between the arterial blood entering and the return of venous blood exiting the neurovascular system. It is viewed as an estimated pressure and is calculated as the difference between the incoming MAP and the opposing ICP on the arteries, affected of course by the ability of the venous volume to exit.

Cerebral perfusion pressure:

$$\text{CPP} = \text{MAP} - \text{ICP}$$

$$\text{MAP} = \frac{\text{Systolic BP (SBP)} + 2(\text{Diastolic BP [DPB]})}{3}$$

What You NEED TO KNOW

Monitoring ICP and recognizing increased ICP is crucial when caring for patients with neurologic diseases. ICP is a dynamic physiologic process. In the uninjured brain, mild transient elevations and fluctuations occur in everyday activities such as coughing or sneezing. During these periods of mild elevations, the process of autoregulation makes adjustments to accommodate the transient elevation in ICP. However, with the loss of autoregulation (i.e., an injured brain), the mild, transient increases in ICP will cause the cell membrane to become more permeable, which disrupts the normal sodium and potassium pump. This loss also allows for the leakage of proteins and fluids into the brain tissue, which causes cerebral edema. Cerebral edema increases the tissue volume of the brain, which increases ICP and decreases CPP. Patients who are considered to be at risk for increased ICP include those with:

- Head injury
- Intracranial hematoma
- Glasgow Coma Scale (GCS) score £8
- Decorticate or decerebrate (or both) posturing
- Space-occupying lesion (tumor, abscess, infection)
- Hypoxia
- Hypercarbia
- Cerebral edema (secondary to surgery, trauma, hemorrhage)

Elevations in ICP produce changes in the patient's neurologic assessment. These changes may be subtle or occur rapidly.

EARLY SIGNS AND SYMPTOMS OF INCREASED INTRACRANIAL PRESSURE

- Changes in level of consciousness
- Restlessness
- Irritability
- Mild confusion
- Decreased Glasgow Coma Scale score
- Changes in personality
- Changes in pupil size or reactivity
- Motor or sensory deficits (e.g., paresthesia, weakness of extremities)
- Changes in speech (slurred, inappropriate, aphasia)
- Headache (early morning, especially upon waking)
- Vomiting (frequently without nausea)

LATE SIGNS AND SYMPTOMS OF INCREASED INTRACRANIAL PRESSURE

- Abnormal posturing
- Absent Babinski reflex
- Arm drift
- Changes in level of consciousness
  - Decreased level of arousal
  - Decreased GCS score
- Changes in respiratory patterns (irregular to apnea)
- Changes in speech (slurred, inappropriate, none)
- Changes in vital signs (Cushing triad: bradycardia, hypertension, irregular respirations)
- Cranial nerve dysfunction (cough, gag, corneal reflexes)
- Decreased reaction or no response to painful stimuli
- Flaccidity of extremities
- Hemiparesis
- Hemiplegia on opposite side of brain affected
- Loss of protective reflexes
- Motor deficits
- Possible seizure activity
- Pupil changes (unilateral or bilateral dilation)
- Weakness

TAKE HOME POINTS

In the injured brain, the compliance is low and the degree of elastance is high, thus the brain is unable to accommodate the fluctuations in the volume (fluid, blood, tissue) that can cause dangerous elevations of ICP.

Dangerous, sustained elevations in ICP can lead to brainstem compression and herniation of brain tissue, resulting in coma and ultimately death.

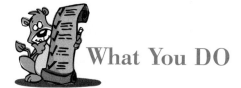

What You DO

Monitoring and identifying increased ICP is achieved through the use of various ICP monitoring devices: ventricular catheters, subarachnoid screws and bolts, parenchymal implanted devices, and epidural sensors. Each device has its own advantages and disadvantages. The monitoring device of choice is often dependent on the type of injury or the anticipated intervention or both.

Continuous ICP monitoring is routine in evaluating and managing intracranial disorders. The process of monitoring ICP requires a monitoring device sensor that may be inserted in the operating department or at the patient's bedside. Once the sensor is in place, the device is connected to a transducer cable, which goes to the bedside monitor. The pressure signal is conducted through the transducer, which translates the pressure to a visual image (waveform) and a numeric value.

The purposes of ICP and CPP monitoring are to diagnose increased ICP, enable interventions, and provide a tool for predicting the level of injury and patient outcome. The goals of monitoring ICP and CPP are to (1) restore them to normal values, (2) prevent serious and prolonged elevations in ICP, (3) prevent serious and prolonged decreases in CPP, (4) provide a means to reduce ICP, and (5) provide a means to maintain CPP.

Although ICP is monitored with a transducer, a fluid-coupled system is not connected to heparinized or saline-flush solution. Nothing should be infused into intracranial contents.

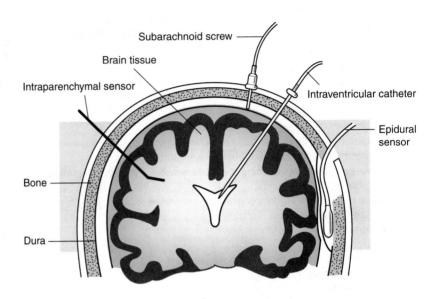

ICP Monitoring Devices: Advantages and Disadvantages

ICP MONITORING DEVICE	ADVANTAGES	DISADVANTAGES
Subarachnoid bolt and screw	Less invasive	Unable to drain CSF
Parenchymal sensor	Decreased infection Not dependent on ventricular placement Provides wave and numeric value Does not require setup and maintenance of fluid-coupled system	Can be unreliable with excessive (high) values Risk for leaks Risk for hemorrhage Risk for hematoma
Intraventricular catheter	Most reliable Ability to drain CSF Ability to sample and observe CSF Ability to administer intrathecal medications	Increases chance of infection (indwelling device) May become clogged with debris (tissue, blood) Difficult to place (especially with swollen brain) Values and drainage are level-dependent (depending on positioning and calibration)
Epidural	Lowest risk of infection Easy to insert Can be used in the neonate	Unable to drain or sample CSF May provide false readings

CSF, Cerebrospinal fluid.

Interventions used in the treatment of increased ICP and the manipulation of ICP and CPP include the following:

- Body positioning (head in straight alignment—care should be taken to avoid slight flexion caused by pillows)
- Elevation of head of bed ≤30 degrees
- Prone position and extreme flexion of hips, avoiding the Trendelenburg position
- Staggered timing and sequence of nursing care
- Controlled environmental conditions (quiet, darkened room)
- Temperature controlled to maintain normal or mild hypothermia (≤37° C [≤98.6° F])
- BP control, maintaining CBF and CPP
- CSF drainage
- Fluid restriction
- Ventilation and airway management
- Medications: osmotic diuretics, steroids, anticonvulsants, barbiturates, vasoactive drugs (to increase or decrease BP), sedatives, analgesics

Because of its potent effects on cerebral blood vessels, the ability to control and manipulate ventilation management is an important intervention in an attempt to decrease and maintain ICP. Preventing hypoxia and monitoring oxygen and carbon dioxide (CO_2) levels are critical skills. Preventing hypoxia (oxygen tension in the arterial blood [PaO_2] at <60 mm Hg) is achieved through administering oxygen and monitoring pulse oximetry readings and blood gas values. Monitoring arterial CO_2 is vital because of its potent vasoconstrictive properties with cerebral blood vessels. Hyperventilation works by decreasing the arterial level of CO_2 ($PaCO_2$), which causes vasoconstriction of the cerebral arteries that result in reducing CBF and decreasing ICP. Controlled hyperventilation means that the $PaCO_2$ is kept at the low-to-normal range. To control acute ICP elevations, hyperventilation is an immediate and key intervention that should be instituted by manually hyperventilating the patient for a brief period.

The use of positive end–expiratory pressure (PEEP) should be used with caution because of its possible effect on decreasing venous drainage and outflow, which results in increasing ICP and CPP.

Monitoring and maintaining BP within desired limits is critical to maintaining ICP, CPP, and CBF. Physicians designate MAPs and systolic parameters that are to be maintained. MAP and CPP values can be manipulated through the use of various IV vasoactive agents such as dopamine (Intropin) and sodium nitroprusside (Nipride).

Osmotic diuretics such as mannitol (Osmitrol) are also an effective management strategy for reducing ICP. Mannitol (Osmitrol) has a rapid effect on ICP, and its onset is 10 to 15 minutes.

The placement of a ventricular catheter allows for CSF to be drained. Physician orders and protocols usually allow for the drainage of CSF to maintain certain ICP levels.

Increased ICP and the understanding of intracranial dynamics are important concepts to comprehend to assess adequately, monitor, and provide appropriate interventions and management strategies to optimize patient outcomes.

⚠ Prolonged hyperventilation can reduce cerebral perfusion, cause shifts in the intracranial dynamics, and result in cerebral ischemia or infarction.

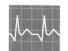

Intracranial dynamic monitoring levels:
Desired CPP levels:
60 to 70 mm Hg
Desired MAP levels: >60 mm Hg

⚠ Osmotic diuretics can cause hypotension and tachycardia, which can compromise CBF and CPP. In addition, rapid fluid shifts from healthy to injured brain tissue can result in increased swelling and increased ICP.

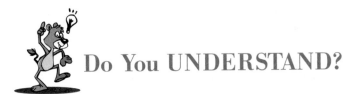

Do You UNDERSTAND?

DIRECTIONS: Fill in the blanks to complete each of the following statements with the appropriate words provided in the list below.

aphasia
blood pressure
cerebral blood flow
cerebral edema
cerebral perfusion pressure
cerebral spinal fluid
compliance

decorticate
elastance
epidural
hyperventilation
intraventricular catheter
Monro-Kellie hypothesis
parenchymal sensor

pressure
pupil changes
restlessness
Trendelenburg
vasoconstriction
vasodilation
volume

1. Intracranial _____ is the ability of the

    brain to tolerate intracranial volume increases without increasing ICP.

2. _____ _____

    _____ is calculated by subtracting the ICP read-

    ing from the MAP and estimating the pressure gradient across the brain.

3. _____ _____ are a late sign of increased ICP.

4. Using a(n) _____ _____ is the

    most reliable means of monitoring ICP.

5. _____ is an early sign of increased ICP.

6. The _____ position should

    be avoided because it can actually increase ICP.

7. _____ is used to keep $PaCO_2$ low, which causes

    _____ of the cerebral arteries and decreases CBF and ICP.

8. To maintain ICP, CPP, and CBF, the patient's _____

    _____ must be frequently monitored.

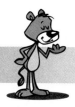

What IS Traumatic Brain Injury?

Traumatic brain injury (TBI) is a collective term describing a wide range of pathologic conditions and types of trauma involving the brain. TBI occurs when a substantial force strikes the skull, which can be blunt, penetrating, or a combination of the two. The result is a brain injury. TBI is one of the leading causes of trauma death; in fact, it is responsible for nearly 50% of the 150,000 injury-related deaths in the United States each year. Not only is TBI the most lethal of all trauma-related injuries, but its survivors also suffer the greatest disability with long-term effects and deficits.

The contributory causes of TBI are customarily associated with motor vehicle crashes (MVCs), falls, and violence. Head trauma occurs when the generated force is greater than the cranial vault can absorb, transferring the kinetic injury to the delicate neural tissues beneath. The specific categories of TBI are discussed later in this chapter.

The understanding of basic anatomy, physiology, types of injury, and effects of trauma on the brain, as well as the rapid recognition of these signs and symptoms, are imperative in treating patients with brain trauma. Even a basic comprehension of TBI and its mechanisms can assist in the delivery of quality nursing care. The study and management of the central nervous system (CNS) can be intimidating and complex; however, it can be easily learned with the knowledge of a few simple facts and treatment principles.

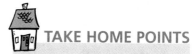

TAKE HOME POINTS

The extent of the injury—its effects and survivability—has many factors and is ultimately unique to each individual patient.

Initial assessment may be deceiving. For example, in the patient with a closed-head injury, brain damage may not be obvious because of an absence of external blood.

What You NEED TO KNOW

Types of Trauma Brain Injury

Five major types of primary TBI have been established: (1) skull fractures, (2) concussion, (3) contusion, (4) diffuse axonal injury, and (5) hematomas.

When a patient suffers a *skull fracture*, approximately two out of every three patients acquire a mild-to-severe brain injury. A single blunt strike, which usually fractures along a fissure line in the cranium, is called a *linear fracture*. The linear fracture is most common, accounting for 75% to 80% of all skull fractures. The linear fracture is highly associated with subdural and epidural bleeds. A backward fall that is significant enough to cause a fracture to the skull usually involves the occiput, which is a *basal skull fracture*. These fractures can involve a shifting of bone articulations (e.g., break away or opening of the occipitosphenoidal fissure). These fractures are not usually life threatening but may disrupt the meningeal layers and allow leakage of CSF and blood from the ears and nose. A closer assessment

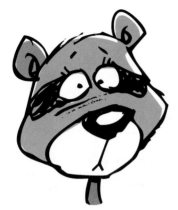

TAKE HOME POINTS

CO and peripheral vascular resistance directly affects BP. If a patient's BP decreases, then either the flow (CO) or the resistance (SVR) has changed.

 The edema and extent of the bleeding from a contusion are an immediate clinical concern.

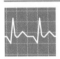 The degree and progression of the injury requires close monitoring and frequent neurologic testing to track the onset or change of symptoms that indicate increased ICP.

Symptoms of TBI may be progressive, which requires vigilant monitoring of neurologic functions, ensuring the patient's subtle changes are appropriately tracked.

finding of a basal skull fracture includes ecchymosis at the site of the mastoid process (battle signs) or around the periorbital area (raccoon eyes) or both.

This injury often exposes the brain to the exterior environment with disruption of the *cribriform plate*, which is a small, thin bone that is separated by tissue in the nasal cavity. The patient with this type of fracture is at risk for encephalitis and meningitis. Another type of cranial bone injury is a *depressed skull fracture*, which may cause contusion or laceration to the brain tissue. If a fracture with a perforated scalp is observed, then it is an *open fracture*. The patient with this type of fracture is at risk for developing an infection. The disruption of bones can damage brain, vessels, and cranial nerves as they pass through the skull, requiring diligent and ongoing neurologic assessments.

A *concussion* is a direct brain injury involving neural tissue (parenchyma); it is generally mild but may have underlying pathologic consequences such as slow subdural bleed that is not observed until days after the injury. The MOI involving concussion is usually associated with a blunt trauma from a blow to the head or from a fall. The injury is traditionally diagnosed by the patient's manifestation of symptoms because obvious physical injury is not always present. In cases of concussion, a complete recovery usually occurs; however, many patients suffer amnesia involving events surrounding the trauma. In moderate-to-severe concussions, the symptoms may include a loss of consciousness, a diminished or complete loss of deep tendon reflexes (DTRs), and an apneic episode in some patients. The energy absorbed through the cranium is believed to stun the brain to the point of momentarily ceasing neurologic function.

Contusions occur when the head suffers a direct impact with a rigid object. The MOI is similar to that of a concussion but more severe. When the tissue damage occurs directly at the site of impact, it is categorized as a *coup injury*. A more involved contusion is often a result of an acceleration-deceleration event. This MOI causes the brain to shift rapidly and strike one side and then the opposing side of the cranium, causing lesions in two areas of the brain, known as a *coup-contrecoup injury*. The cerebral contusion is most often seen in temporal and frontal lobes of the brain. The contusion produces tissue edema and capillary hemorrhage.

Diffuse axonal injury describes extensive damage involving a wide area of neural tissues throughout the cerebrum and brainstem. Up to this point, the injuries discussed primarily involve localized lesions involving the outer neural gray matter. Diffuse axonal injury refers to damage that involves the innermost centroaxial areas of the neural white matter. These injuries disrupt the neural network fibers and tracts that facilitate communication among the brainstem, cerebellum, and hemispheres of the cerebrum. This type injury is associated with MOI involving mechanical sheering forces generated by an MVC or other similar events. Diffuse axonal injuries occur in approximately one half of all trauma-related comas and are responsible for long-term neural deficits in the recovering patient with a TBI.

An *epidural hematoma* develops under the arterial pressure of the bleed, which tears the periosteal layer (a part of the dura mater) from the cranium as the hematoma expands, resulting in the compression of brain tissue. The symptoms may involve a rapid onset of neurologic signs, or the patient may remain lucid many hours after the TBI and then suddenly deteriorate. An epidural hematoma is an emergency condition that requires the hematoma to be drained quickly to prevent permanent brain damage.

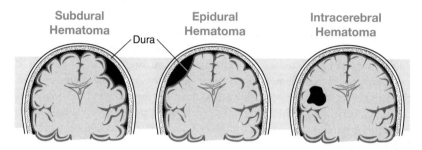

A *subdural hematoma* is an intracranial bleed involving the space between the dura's meningeal layer and the arachnoid layer. A subdural hematoma often involves the bridging veins that transverse the dura mater, occurring commonly on the lateral aspects of the cerebrum's hemispheres. Subdural hematomas expand as a result of venous bleeding (low pressure bleed), and the onset of symptoms are slow in developing—an average of 48 hours. The characteristic symptoms include increased drowsiness, confusion, and a nonlocalizing headache directly related to the increase of ICP. A minor head injury can initially cause similar signs and symptoms observed in the subdural bleed.

Other traumatic intracranial hematomas that may occur include bleeding into the ventricles, subarachnoid space, and superior sagittal sinus. Any of these bleeds can occur together and may involve any combination of the previously mentioned TBIs. Patients with an intracranial hemorrhage quickly lose their ability to physiologically compensate, and this development can occur with less than 100 ml of blood.

A catastrophic brain injury is a severe injury that includes the cranium being exposed to extraordinary force involving MVCs, falls from significant heights, mechanical crushing, and missile penetration. The brain's direct or indirect absorption of this momentous kinetic energy (KE) lacerates or tears the parenchymal tissue, causing a disruption of the meninges, neural tissue, nerve tracts, and blood vessels. A TBI caused by a projectile that forcefully enters the cranium creates a cavitation that displaces tissue in the brain, delivering direct and extensive damage as it travels through the cranium and possibly exiting the skull. This patient often has a terminal prognosis; if only the brain is involved, then the patient becomes a prime candidate for organ donation.

TAKE HOME POINTS

An epidural hematoma is an arterial bleed and develops quickly; a subdural hematoma is a venous bleed and develops slowly.

 Without a solid knowledge base and understanding of TBI, a serious injury could be easily overlooked.

TAKE HOME POINTS

Survivability is low in the patient with a catastrophic brain injury.

Secondary Brain Injuries

A *secondary brain injury* consists of neurologic tissue damage that occurs after the initial injury and increases the morbidity and mortality of the patient as a result of altered ability of the brain to maintain a homeostatic environment. Most often, MAP, CBF, ICP, and CPP are adversely affected. As the symptoms and damage progresses, acid-base issues become evident as a result of hypoventilation and hypoperfusion states and causes the accumulation of cellular toxins and decreases the autoregulation ability. Once the blood flow to the brain becomes compromised, then the brain tissue does not receive oxygen or the essential nutrients that are carried in the blood, which results in further injury. A late sign of severe cerebral ischemia is the *Cushing response*, a feedback mechanism that attempts to reduce the ischemia by increasing CBF. If the rising ICP is not treated, then ultimately death occurs as the brainstem herniates through the foramen magnum, ceasing all cardiopulmonary function and causing brain death. Understanding the intracranial perfusion principles is paramount in managing complications caused by TBI. (Refer to the discussion on increased ICP on page 50.)

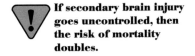

If secondary brain injury goes uncontrolled, then the risk of mortality doubles.

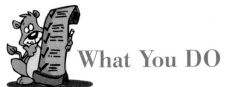

What You DO

When the patient arrives in the emergency department or trauma center, basic standardized steps are taken to stabilize an acutely impaired patient. Without a uniform approach, patients with horrific wounds can easily distract care team members and crucial resuscitative steps can be omitted with deleterious patient outcomes. The operational tenet of the ABC algorithm is to "keep it simple," which allows the care team to function in an orchestrated manner during stressful, time-compressed events involving TBI.

The first and most important step is airway evaluation. Patients with extensive brain injury usually arrive at the hospital via the emergency medical service (EMS), often with initial airway measures accomplished. In TBI cases, other than obvious foreign body obstruction or traumatic injury to the oral pharynx, an accepted threshold for initiating RSI is based on the patient's GCS score and the ability to protect his or her airway. Ensuring that cervical spine precautions are adhered to at all times is imperative because of the increased risk of cervical spine fracture, which is four to six times more likely when involving a patient with a TBI. As the assessment begins, key questions are asked to treat and anticipate the immediate needs of the patient (refer to the discussion on RSI on page 42).

Assessment Question 1

Is the patient's GCS score at 9 or above?

YES	NO
Use supplemental oxygen. Continue assessment.	Prepare to implement RSI protocol. Intubate. Securely fasten ETT. Set up appropriate oxygen delivery system. Limit ETT movement (manipulation can irritate the vagus nerve and therefore increase ICP). Suction equipment available (increased ICP can cause projectile emesis and posttraumatic seizures).

When evaluating the respiratory status of a patient with a TBI, hypoxia along with the TBI can further increase the ICP, decreasing both MAP and CBF and further injuring the brain by increasing ischemia. Aggressive hyperventilation is not recommended; however, maintaining a $PaCO_2$ of approximately 35 mm Hg should be the therapeutic goal for ventilation management.

Assessment Question 2

Is the patient able to ventilate adequately with a spontaneous regular rate and effort?

YES	NO
Continue assessment: • Rate and depth of respirations • Saturations (pulse oximeter >97%) • Satisfactory ABG results	Assist with breathing (high-flow oxygen and airway delivery systems). Consider intubation, if not already intubated. Maintain normocapnia ($PaCO_2$ of ~35 mm Hg); may require hyperventilation of patient.

The degree of brain injury and its ability to compensate are reflected in the circulatory system's response. Assessing the patient's circulatory status involves distinguishing the rate, rhythm, and intensity of the pulse. Next, secondary signs of hypoxia, such as cool clammy skin and cyanosis of the nail beds and oral membranes, must be observed. Hypotension is a priority over other interventions for the brain injury and must be corrected early in an attempt to maintain CBF and CPP. Hemodynamic monitoring protocols must be initiated and therapeutic modalities need to be used to help keep the patient's circulation within normal or acceptable parameters.

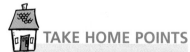

TAKE HOME POINTS

The identification of low BP and rapid reversal of this deficit provides positive outcomes in managing TBI.

If a nasogastric (NG) tube is needed, extreme caution must be taken during placement. An undiagnosed skull fracture could allow the NG tube to perforate into the parenchyma of the brain.

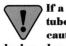

TAKE HOME POINTS

The early hours of brain injury are very tenuous, making continuous monitoring of the vital signs and the neurologic status an essential task for the nurse.

Assessment Question 3

Is the patient's SBP above 90 mm Hg, and are there strong peripheral pulses?

YES	NO
Obtain 1 or 2 IV sites (preferably 18-gauge).	Obtain two large-bore (16-gauge) IV sites; may need to assist in central-line placement.
Continue assessment.	Prepare to deliver crystalloid rapidly or other colloid IV fluids.
Await fluid and medication orders.	Obtain rapid fluid infuser.
	Closely monitor cardiovascular status.
	Anticipate the use of emergency medications.
	Place urinary catheter.
	Closely monitor fluid status (intake and output).

The ABCs (airway, breathing, circulation) of trauma resuscitation are the primary life-saving measures used in stabilizing the patient, but **D** for *disability* is the treatment step that collectively takes the brain injury into account. This step incorporates ABC management to help reduce secondary brain injury and thus improves the patient's chance of recovery. The "tools of the trade" are used to obtain a baseline neurologic examination to help determine the primary injury, anticipate urgent care needs, and further monitor the stabilization process. In addition, the nurse needs to anticipate using therapeutic medications to assist in stabilizing the patient with TBI.

The nursing objective in caring for the patient with TBI is vigilant, accurate, and objective monitoring. This caring objective is achieved with a strong knowledge base of applied anatomy and physiology and keen observational skills. Regardless of the skill level, a standardized tool or instrument needs to be used properly to quantify the patient's recordings and observations and to make comparative assessments.

The most prominent and widely used tool for tracking a patient's neurologic baseline and injury progression is the GCS. The GCS uses a number system to describe the LOC of patients with TBI. The GCS ranges from 3 (poor, no response) to 15 (normal). The GCS rates (1) eye opening, (2) motor movement of the arms and legs, and (3) verbal response. Adding the scores from the three parts of the scale produces an overall score. Importantly, the GCS is not a tool used to determine or predict the patient's final outcome.

A complete neurologic examination requires assessment of the pupils and extremities. These assessment components are completed in the mental status, motor movement, and cranial nerve assessments. Neurologic changes and trends are best observed by conducting serial assessments, using a standardized format, and ensuring that all elements are approached in the similar manner. These standardized serial assessments ensure that each examiner has a lesser degree of variation and provides a more objective clinical record.

GLASGOW COMA SCALE

Eye Opening
4 = Spontaneous
3 = Response to voice
2 = Response to pain
1 = No response

Best Motor Response
6 = Follows commands
5 = Localizes to pain
4 = Withdrawal to pain
3 = Decorticate (flexion to pain)
2 = Decerebrate (extension to pain)
1 = No response

Best Verbal Response
5 = Oriented and converses
4 = Disoriented and converses
3 = Inappropriate words
2 = Incomprehensible sounds
1 = No response

Note: Best score is 15; the lowest score is 3.

COMPONENTS OF NEUROLOGIC ASSESSMENT

Mental Status
- Level of consciousness (GCS score)
- Orientation (time, person, place)
- Memory (ability to recall three items)
- Judgment (process of forming an opinion that is accurate and reasonable)
- Cognition (serial 7s)

Motor Testing
- Flex and extend all extremity joints against resistance
- Grading:
    5/5: Movement against gravity with full resistance
    4/5: Movement against gravity with some resistance
    3/5: Movement against gravity only
    2/5: Movement with gravity eliminated
    1/5: Visible and palpable muscle contraction; no movement
    0/5: No contraction

Cranial Nerves
- Olfactory—assessment of ability to smell
- Optic—assessment of vision; document pupils—equal, round, reactive to light and accommodation (PERRLA)
- Oculomotor—assessment of eye movement and tracking
- Trochlear—assessment of eye movement
- Trigeminal—assessment of bilateral facial sensation and ability to chew
- Abducens—assessment of lateral eye movement
- Facial—assessment of whether smile is symmetric
- Auditory—assessment of hearing and balance
- Glossopharyngeal—assessment of gag reflex and ability to feel ears
- Vagus—observe the soft palate and check to see whether arch is symmetric (the "aahh" test)
- Accessory—assessment of shoulder muscle resistance as patient shrugs shoulders
- Hypoglossal—assessment of tongue position

GCS, Glasgow Coma Scale.

The reoccurring theme in managing the patient with TBI involves monitoring and managing the ICP. The immediate treatment goal in the acute phase of brain injury is to keep the patient quiet to avoid agitating the patient further and inadvertently increasing the ICP. Equally important in reducing elevated ICP are medications designed to manage and reduce the fluid (blood or obstructed CSF) and edema collecting on the brain. Only a few medications are available for use in the treatment of TBI; when these agents fail or require augmentation, invasive procedures are then used to relieve pressure on the brain. (Refer to the discussion on increased ICP on page 50.)

The pharmacologic agents discussed in this chapter and the box that follows offer a brief overview of the pharmacologic treatments in managing TBI. The dosing information provided is only an example, and an approved drug reference should always be consulted when administering medications to patients.

 TAKE HOME POINTS

The GCS provides a common language and quickly communicates the patient's neurologic status to other health care providers.

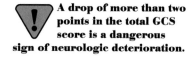 **A drop of more than two points in the total GCS score is a dangerous sign of neurologic deterioration.**

TAKE HOME POINTS

Pupil changes will be on the same side (ipsilateral) as the brain injury; extremity symptoms (weakness) will be in the opposite side (contralateral).

Corticosteroid therapy—current research indicates that the use of steroids is not beneficial in the treatment of ICP. In addition, they suppress immune response, placing the patient at increased risk for infection. The drug is not contraindicated and may still be used in some hospital settings.

Brain Injury Association
www.biausa.org
Brain Trauma Foundation
www.braintrauma.org
American Association of Neuroscience Nurses
www.aann.org

PHARMACOLOGIC TREATMENTS

Modality 1: Sedation
Benzodiazepines
- Midazolam (versed)—used most often
  Adults: Titrate slowly to achieve desired effect. Usual dose range is between 1-5 mg IV administered over 2-minute period
Opiates
- Morphine
  Adults: 4-10 mg IV; with appropriate dose titration, there is no maximum dose of morphine

Modality 2: Fluid Reduction
Osmotic diuretics
- Mannitol (Osmitrol)—predominate drug used in the United States*
  Adults: Initially, 1.0-2.0 g/kg IV, followed by 0.25-1.00 g/kg IV q4h

*The mechanism of action mannitol (Osmitrol) remains unclear; however, it reduces ICP, draws water off the brain, can affect cardiac preload, and, in turn, increases CBF.

At this point in the patient's treatment, assessment and reassessment continues with a goal toward obtaining radiologic studies (e.g., computed tomography [CT], x-ray series, and possibly a magnetic resonance image [MRI], [depending on availability and condition of the patient]). Baseline blood work is prescribed with close attention to ABG results, hemoglobin, hematocrit, and other values based on the complete patient history. The extent of the patient's TBI and resultant deficits is determined during the first hours or days after the initial care is received.

Although TBI is usually presented as a singular injury, approximately 75% of patients with brain trauma involve significant injuries to other body systems. The actual resuscitation is more complex, but the rudimentary basics for the resuscitation are the same.

Do You UNDERSTAND?

DIRECTIONS: **Provide the spelled out meaning of each of the following acronyms.**

1. MOI: _____

2. ICP: _____

3. LOC: _____

4. GCS: _____

Answers: 1. mechanism of injury; 2. intracranial pressure; 3. level of consciousness; 4. Glasgow Coma Scale.

DIRECTIONS: Identify the following statements as *true* (T) or *false* (F).

_____ 5. TBI is just under 30% of trauma related injuries in the United States.

_____ 6. TBIs are associated with MVCs, falls, and violence.

DIRECTIONS: Match the types of TBIs in Column A with the most appropriate descriptions in Column B.

Column A

Column B

_____ 7. Diffuse axonal injury

a. Localized lesion on the brain; predominantly limited to the area of impact on the skull

_____ 8. Epidural hematoma

b. Diffuse cerebral injury involving only the gray matter, deep within the cerebrum

_____ 9. Subdural hematoma

c. Venous bleed under the dura mater

d. Deep-tissue injury in the brain, disrupting neural paths and involving white matter

e. Arterial bleed between the cranium and dura mater

DIRECTIONS: Provide short answers to the following questions.

10. What is the drug of choice to remove edema and fluid from brain?

_____

11. What GCS score is used as the threshold to initiate RSI?

_____

12. Which cranial nerve effects pupil constriction when compressed?

_____

What IS Brain Attack?

Brain attack (acute ischemic stroke) is a sudden neurologic impairment caused by a decrease in the blood flow to any vascular territory in the brain; it is considered a medical emergency. When blood flow is impeded in the brain, the patient may have a gradual or rapid onset of symptoms that might resolve quickly (transient ischemic attack) (TIA) or last longer (cerebrovascular accident) (CVA). The goals of the management of the patient who has had a brain attack are to maximize neurologic function and prevent the development of complications or the extension of the stroke.

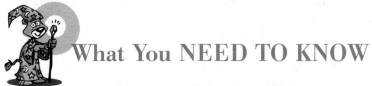

What You NEED TO KNOW

Acute ischemic stroke is the most prevalent disease of the CNS and is the third leading cause of death and the leading cause of disability in the United States. Acute ischemic stroke accounts for 80% to 85% of all strokes. More than 700,000 new strokes occur each year with an estimated cost of more than $40 billion. Currently, the medical approach is aimed at stroke prevention through the identification of risk factors, modification of any risk factors, pharmacologic therapy, surgical intervention, and patient and family education.

Brain Attack Risk Factors

NONMODIFIABLE	MODIFIABLE	OTHER
Age	Hypertension	Obesity
Gender	Heart disease (atrial fibrilla-	Migraine headaches
Race	tion, MI, heart failure, CAD)	Oral contraceptive use
Prior stroke	Hyperlipidemia	Bleeding disorders
(brain attack)	Diabetes mellitus	(hypercoagulopathy,
Heredity	Cigarette smoking	sickle cell anemia)
	Excessive alcohol intake	
	Drug abuse	

MI, Myocardial infarction; *CAD,* coronary artery disease.

TAKE HOME POINTS

- If neurologic and retinal symptoms clear completely in less than 24 hours, the patient has had what is known as a TIA.
- If neurologic and retinal symptoms last for 24 hours or more, he or she has had a CVA.

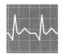 **Cerebral edema may cause neurologic demise (herniation) if ignored.**

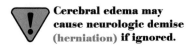 One of the earliest signs of neurologic dysfunction is an altered LOC or a patient who is confused or disoriented.

Brain attack is caused by a decrease in blood flow to any vascular territory. When blood flow is impeded, ischemia occurs, which leads to infarction and necrosis of neuronal cells. When neuronal cells become infarcted or necrotic, they are nonfunctional.

Although neuronal cells are nonfunctional, an important point to remember is that they may still be viable and the ischemia may be possibly reversed with pharmacologic agents if brain attack symptoms are identified in a timely manner. If the time frame has lapsed for possible reversal, then secondary cellular injury to the neuronal cells occurs from the depletion of oxygen to the cells and thus leads to the development of lactic acid. Cerebral edema can develop within minutes of the insult to the neuronal cells; it can peak within 2 to 4 days and contribute to the patient's neurologic dysfunction.

The signs and symptoms of brain attack depend on the location and severity of the insult to the brain. Brain attacks usually have no warning signs, although a TIA is a warning sign. The signs and symptoms of a brain attack and its effects according to the hemisphere and cerebral circulation are outlined in the tables on the following page.

Signs and Symptoms of Acute Ischemic Stroke According to Hemisphere

LEFT-SIDED STROKE	RIGHT-SIDED STROKE
Right-sided hemiplegia	Left-sided hemiplegia
Expressive aphasia	Spatial-perceptual deficits
Receptive aphasia	Denial
Global aphasia	Tendency for distractibility
Intellectual impairment	Impulsive behavior
Slow and cautious behavior	Poor judgment
Defects in the right visual fields	Defects in left visual fields

Signs and Symptoms of Acute Ischemic Stroke According to Cerebral Circulation

ANTERIOR (CAROTID) CIRCULATION	POSTERIOR (VERTEBROBASILAR) CIRCULATION
Contralateral paralysis	Vertigo
Numbness	Blurred vision
Aphasia	Diplopia
Dysarthria	Paralysis
Blurred vision	Numbness
Monocular blindness	Dysarthria
	Ataxia

Identification of the patient who is having a brain attack is crucial in determining treatment strategies. In 1996 the American Heart Association recommended thrombolytic therapy for use on selected patients who have had a brain attack; this treatment has since been added to the *Emergency Cardiovascular Care Guidelines*. The *Cincinnati Prehospital Stroke Scale* is a valid assessment tool that assists the professional in identifying the patient who has had a brain attack by using three physical findings: (1) facial droop, (2) motor arm drift, and (3) speech difficulties. The *Cincinnati Prehospital Stroke Scale* is easy to perform, can be completed in less than 1 minute, and is a strong predictor of probability that stroke is present. To assess facial droop, the patient is asked to smile or show his or her teeth. Facial droop is considered abnormal if one side of the patient's face does not move as well as the other. To assess motor-arm drift, the patient is asked to close his or her eyes and hold both arms straight out in front for 10 seconds. Motor arm-drift is considered abnormal if one arm drifts down when compared with the other. To assess speech difficulties, the patient is asked to repeat a phrase such as, "No ifs, ands, or buts" or "You can't teach an old dog new tricks." If the patient slurs the words, uses the wrong words, or is unable to speak, then he or she is considered to have difficulties with speech. If a patient is abnormal in just one of these findings, he or she is considered to have a 72% chance of having a brain attack. If the patient is abnormal in all three findings, he or she is considered to have greater than an 85% chance of having a brain attack.

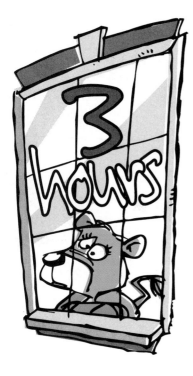

If a brain attack is suspected, the patient must seek immediate emergency care. The onset of signs and symptoms of a stroke must be established to determine whether the patient falls within the 3-hour window for thrombolytic administration such as alteplase (recombinant tissue plasminogen activator [rt-PA]).

Once the patient with a suspected brain attack is admitted to the emergency department, he or she must be tended to in a timely fashion. A CT scan without contrast is performed to determine whether brain pathologic conditions such as a tumor or hemorrhage are present and to make the initial diagnosis. Next, a complete medical history, a physical examination, and a neurologic examination are obtained. The patient also undergoes laboratory studies that include complete blood counts (CBCs), platelets, chemistry, prothrombin time (PT), partial thromboplastin time (PTT), and pregnancy testing.

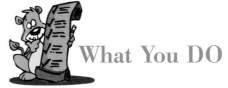

What You DO

The goal of the management of a patient with a brain attack is to maximize neurologic function. The patient will need to be placed on a cardiac monitor and will need frequent assessment and monitoring of his or her neurologic status and vital signs, especially BP. Treatment of hypertension should be carefully approached to avoid causing a rapid decline in BP, which would compromise CBF.

TAKE HOME POINTS

Time is critical. Initial recognition of brain attack symptoms is crucial for the possible treatment with thrombolytic agents. Only a 3-hour window for treatment exists.

Recommended Emergency Antihypertensive Therapy for Brain Attack

BLOOD PRESSURE	TREATMENT
NONTHROMBOLYTIC CANDIDATE	
DBP >140 mm Hg	Sodium nitroprusside (Nipride): titrated for prescribed effect
SBP >220 mm Hg	Goal: 10%-20% reduction in DBP
DBP >120 mm Hg or MAP >130 mm Hg	Labetalol (Normodyne): 10-20 mg IV push
	May repeat or double the dose every 20 minutes to a maximum dose of 150 mg
SBP <220 mm Hg DBP <120 mm Hg or MAP >130 mm Hg	Emergency antihypertensive treatment is deferred
THROMBOLYTIC CANDIDATE	
Pretreatment	
SBP >185 mm Hg or DBP >110 mm Hg	Nitroglycerin topical paste (NitroBid): 1-2 inches Labetalol (Normodyne): 0-20 mg IV

SBP, Systolic blood pressure; *DBP,* diastolic blood pressure; *MAP,* mean arterial pressure; *IV,* intravenous.

Recommended Emergency Antihypertensive Therapy for Brain Attack—cont'd

BLOOD PRESSURE	TREATMENT
THROMBOLYTIC CANDIDATE—cont'd	
During and after treatment	
DBP >140 mm Hg	Sodium nitroprusside (Nipride): 0.5 mcg/kg/min
DBP >230 mm Hg or	Labetalol (Normodyne): 10 mg IV
DBP 121-140 mm Hg	May repeat or double dose every 10 minutes to a maximum dose of 150 mg, or give bolus and then initiate a drip at 2-8 mg/min
	If not controlled by labetalol (Normodyne), then consider sodium nitroprusside (Nipride): titrated for prescribed effect
SBP 180-230 mm Hg or	Labetalol (Normodyne): 10 mg IV
DBP 105-120 mm Hg	May repeat or double dose every 10 minutes to a maximum dose of 150 mg, or give bolus and then initiate a drip at 2-8 mg/min

SBP, Systolic blood pressure; *DBP,* diastolic blood pressure; *MAP,* mean arterial pressure; *IV,* intravenous.

The advent of thrombolytic therapy has made it possible to dissolve an occlusion and reestablish blood flow to the ischemic brain tissue before infarction, providing that the patient meets the inclusion and exclusion criteria that have been established. The thrombolytic drug that has been approved for treatment of brain attack is rt-PA (alteplase). The dose of rt-PA is dependent on the patient's weight:

rt-PA formula:

$$\text{Patient's Weight (kg)} \times 0.9 \text{ mg} = \frac{\text{Dose of rt-PA to be Given}}{\text{(not to exceed 90 mg)}}$$

Of the total rt-PA (alteplase) dose, 10% is given as an IV bolus over 1 to 2 minutes; the remainder is infused over 1 hour. If the patient is outside the time frame (3 hours) for receiving rt-PA or does not meet the criteria for rt-PA administration, then the patient is medically managed. Before administering thrombolytic therapy, the patient should have invasive catheters and tubes (e.g., central-line IV; arterial catheter, bladder catheter, NG tube) placed, otherwise the introduction of these devices after the thrombolytic has been administered could result in uncontrolled bleeding. If such devices are needed, then they should be placed 24 hours after the administration of the thrombolytic medication (except bladder catheters; they can be placed 30 minutes after the infusion is complete).

During the administration of thrombolytic therapy, if the patient begins to deteriorate and the cause is suspected to be bleeding, then the infusion should be immediately stopped and the physician should be notified. The patient will likely

Importantly, the patient's actual weight must be obtained because thrombolytic dose is calculated according to weight.

Thrombolytic Inclusion and Exclusion Criteria

INCLUSION CRITERIA	EXCLUSION CRITERIA
Symptom onset <3 hours	Stroke or serious head trauma within past 3 mo
	SBP >185 mm Hg
Clinical diagnosis of ischemic stroke	DBP >110 mm Hg
	BP levels that require aggressive treatment
Measurable neurologic deficit	Subarachnoid or intracerebral hemorrhage
	Recent MI (within last month)
>18 years of age	Major surgery within past 2 weeks
	GI bleed within past 3 weeks
	Arterial puncture at a noncompressible site within past 1 week
	Lumbar puncture within past 1 week
	Blood glucose <50 mg/dl; >400 mg/dl
	INR >1.7
	Platelet count <100,000/mm^3
	Rapidly improving or minor neurologic symptoms
	Deteriorating neurologic symptoms
	Seizure at onset
	Heparin within past 48 hours
	Pregnant

SBP, Systolic blood pressure; *DBP,* diastolic blood pressure; *BP,* blood pressure; *MI,* myocardial infarction; *GI,* gastrointestinal; *INR,* international normalized ratio.

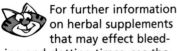

Different herbal supplements such as vitamin E, ginkgo biloba, and garlic have been found to prolong bleeding and clotting times.

For further information on herbal supplements that may effect bleeding and clotting times, see the *Real World Nursing Survival Guide: Complementary & Alternative Therapies.*

receive a CT scan to rule out hemorrhage. In addition, CBC, platelet count, PTT and PT levels, and fibrinogen are prescribed and drawn. Depending on the laboratory results and the patient's condition, the decision to transfuse blood, cryoprecipitate, FFP, or platelets (or any combination thereof) may be made.

After the patient has received rt-PA (alteplase), he or she will likely be admitted to the critical care unit to ensure close monitoring of neurologic status, bleeding, vital signs (especially BP), and laboratory tests. To decrease the likelihood of possible bleeding, the patient should not receive heparin, warfarin sodium (Coumadin), or antiplatelet agents (aspirin, nonsteroidal antiinflammatory drugs [NSAIDs]) for 24 hours after thrombolytic administration.

The desired outcome of thrombolytic therapy is to dissolve the occlusion and reperfuse the ischemic brain tissue. If thrombolytic therapy is successful, then the signs and symptoms of the patient's brain attack should improve and have a 30% likelihood of minimal or no disability.

Brain attack does have the potential to affect and influence multiple body systems. Possible clinical problems and interventions related to brain attack are discussed in the Table "Common Problems and Interventions for the Patient with Brain Attack" on the following page. The focus of nursing care must be early rehabilitation to maximize the patient's recovery from his or her brain attack.

Common Problems and Interventions for the Patient with Brain Attack

PROBLEM	INTERVENTION
Increased ICP	• Provide ongoing neurologic assessment. • Measure ICP and CPP. • Space patient care activities to prevent prolonged periods of increased ICP. • Keep neck in neutral position. • Adjust head of bed to minimize ICP and maximize CPP. • Assess and manage ventriculostomy drain.
Sensorimotor disability and immobility	• Assess and perform range of motion. • Ensure correct positioning of flaccid extremity. • Use support hose and sequential inflation devices. • Assess for DVT and signs and symptoms of pulmonary embolus. • Administer low-dose heparin. • Assess skin integrity for evidence of breakdown (especially pressure points—heels, elbows, occiput). • Provide specialty bed and mattress, if needed. • Provide physical and occupational therapy consultations. • Involve family in care. • Ensure adequate nutrition and hydration.
Dysphagia	• Assess swallowing ability and presence of a gag reflex. • Implement aspiration precautions. • Maintain a patent airway. • Assess respiratory status and signs and symptoms for aspiration pneumonia. • Consult with a speech therapist and dietitian. • Ensure adequate nutrition (possible feeding tube). • Monitor intake and output levels. • Educate patient or family or both.
Incontinence	• Assess for the appropriateness of urinary catheter (use only if necessary or for short periods to prevent occurrence of UTI). • Implement bladder and bowel-training program. • Assess for the presence of a UTI, drug- or diet-related problem (diarrhea), fecal impaction.
Unilateral neglect	• Provide safe environment. • Implement falls protocol. • Provide occupational therapy. • Involve patient in care. • Provide patient and family education.

ICP, Intracranial pressure; *CPP,* cerebral perfusion pressure; *DVT,* deep venous thrombosis; *UTI,* urinary tract infection.

National Stroke Association
www.stroke.org
National Aphasia Association
www.aphasia.org
American Stroke Association
www.strokeassociation.org
American Heart Association
www.americanheart.org
National Institutes of Neurological Disorders and Stroke
www.ninds.nih.gov

Continued

Common Problems and Interventions for the Patient with Brain Attack—cont'd

PROBLEM	INTERVENTION
Communication deficit	• Assess for the presence of aphasias or dysarthria or both. • Consult a speech therapist. • Use alternative communication methods. • Use prescribed exercises. • Provide patient and family education.
Poststroke depression	• Assess for signs and symptoms of depression. • Use therapeutic communication techniques, including good listening skills. • Administer antidepressant, if prescribed. • Provide patient and family education.
Cognitive dysfunction	• Assess for short- and long-term memory loss. • Assess for altered insight, judgment, and reasoning skills. • Provide an evaluation from a speech therapist. • Provide neuropsychologic evaluation .

ICP, Intracranial pressure; *CPP,* cerebral perfusion pressure; *DVT,* deep venous thrombosis; *UTI,* urinary tract infection.

Do You UNDERSTAND?

DIRECTIONS: **Select the best response to complete a statement or answer a question. Place the appropriate letter in the space provided.**

_____ 1. Stroke is defined as:

a. A heterogenous, neurologic syndrome with a gradual or rapid onset of neurologic deficits that corresponds to a cerebrovascular area that dissipates in less than 24 hours

b. A heterogenous, neurologic syndrome with a gradual or rapid onset of neurologic deficits that corresponds to a cerebrovascular area that remains for 24 hours or more

_____ 2. Hypertension is what kind of stroke risk factor?

a. Nonmodifiable

b. Modifiable

c. Hypertension is not a risk factor.

_____ 3. Age is what kind of stroke risk factor?

a. Nonmodifiable

b. Modifiable

c. Age is not a risk factor.

Answers: 1. b; 2. b; 3. a.

_____ 4. Diabetes mellitus is what kind of stroke risk factor?
   a. Nonmodifiable
   b. Modifiable
   c. Diabetes mellitus is not a risk factor.

_____ 5. Denial, spatial perceptual deficits, and impulsive behavior are signs and symptoms of what sided stroke?
   a. Left
   b. Right

_____ 6. Which of the following diagnostic tests is most beneficial and timely in determining the presence of brain pathologic condition, blood, or fluid?
   a. Carotid duplex
   b. Cerebral angiogram
   c. CT scan
   d. Transcranial Doppler

_____ 7. Time of symptom onset is especially important with an acute ischemic stroke because the patient may be a candidate for:
   a. Immediate rehabilitation placement
   b. Admission to the ICU
   c. Thrombolytic therapy

_____ 8. Which thrombolytic agent has been approved for the treatment of acute ischemic stroke?
   a. rt-PA (alteplase)
   b. Warfarin (Coumadin)
   c. Heparin
   d. Aspirin

_____ 9. The dose for rt-PA is determined according to the patient's:
   a. Eye and hair color
   b. Weight
   c. Fat percentage
   d. Body surface area

_____10. Between 80% and 85% of all strokes are what type?
   a. Hemorrhagic
   b. Ischemic

_____11. The management goal of any patient who has had a stroke is to maximize neurologic function.
   a. True
   b. False

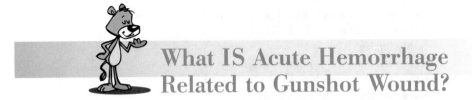

What IS Acute Hemorrhage Related to Gunshot Wound?

Penetrating trauma is one of the leading causes of hemorrhage, and gunshot wounds are the leading source of high-velocity penetrating trauma. These injuries are often treatment challenges, particularly because only a small hole may be observed externally; however, internal injuries may be massive and life threatening.

What You NEED TO KNOW

TAKE HOME POINTS

KE, which is carried by the bullet and subsequently transferred into the tissues, causes the damage in a gunshot victim.

⚠ • **Contamination of the wound may result from the debris and bacteria that has been pulled into the wound.**
• **The bullet easily lodges or travels through organs with the end result being organ or hemodynamic compromise (or both), dysfunction, or even death.**

TAKE HOME POINTS

Tissues that are elastic sustain less damage.

Once a bullet penetrates the skin, it meets resistance as it travels at a high velocity through the tissues, creating an enlarged cone-shaped path that results in significant damage to tissues. The bullet either exits or comes to rest within the body. The amount of destruction is directly related to the caliber of the gun, type of bullet, and proximity of the muzzle to the victim. According to the American Trauma Life Support (ATLS) Manual, the important indicators for determining the extent of injuries include the gun's caliber, the presumed path and velocity of the bullet, and the distance from the weapon to the victim's entrance point.

Many sources describe the entrance wound (inlet velocity) (V_1) as the maximal point of energy. If the bullet never exits the body, the exit wound (outlet velocity) (V_2) is said to be zero. One bullet can cause tremendous damage by deflecting off bone and traveling across the body, damaging many structures in its path. As the projectile of the bullet travels, it meets resistance of the tissues, which is known as *retardation*. The high V_1 creates an inward path along which the bullet travels, but a negative pressure also exists behind the bullet, which pulls debris and bacteria into the wound.

The path subsequently collapses as all energy is expended into the tissues. The bullet and its path is nondiscriminatory and destroys or damages muscle, vascular tissue, nerves, and bone tissue. Different tissues have varying degrees of specific gravities or densities that allow for the prediction of how much energy can be transferred from the bullet to the tissues.

Tissue that is dense has a tendency to take up more energy, resulting in greater damage. For example, ribs have a specific gravity of 1.11 and lungs have a specific gravity of only 0.5 to 0.4. As expected, if a bullet strikes a rib, the rib shatters, creating more projectiles and the possibility of significant damage to surrounding structures and tissues. In contrast, if a bullet strikes a lung, although the damage to the lung may cause tremendous detriment to the patient secondary to oxygenation issues, the damage to the surrounding tissues is not directly affected by the damage to lung tissue.

Physics offers a description of a gunshot injury for consideration. Handguns shoot a single bullet that contains powder encased in metal, whereas shotgun shells are metal encasements containing multiple smaller pellets—as few as 6 or as many as 200, depending on the gauge of the shotgun. In addition, a small piece of material, usually paper, separates the pellets from the gun powder. The mechanisms and extent of injury vary because of these differences. Overall, the basic concept includes a dart-shaped projectile (bullet) launched at significant speed through the bore of a gun. The bullet may deviate slightly from its path and begin to slow, secondary to the air force encountered once it leaves the gun and enters the atmosphere. The speed at which the bullet meets the skin is V_1, where most of the energy is expended into the tissues. It may penetrate as a direct hit or on an angle, which affects how the bullet will travel as it progresses through the layers of tissue and results in retardation. Some bullets travel in a slightly upward and downward motion as they push forward; this is known as *yawing*. Other bullets tumble end-over-end through the tissues. Either way, the extent of damage is directly related to the transference of energy from the bullet into the tissues. Some manufacturers manipulate bullets to create more devastation on impact; the hollow-point bullet is an example. Hollow-point bullets tend to flatten on impact and transfer a great amount of KE. In contrast, smaller diameter or lower caliber bullets tend to produce less damage.

V_2 is the velocity at which the bullet exits the body. As previously mentioned, if the bullet fails to exit the body, V_2 is equal to zero. The calculation describing this concept is the "law of energy" output.

Calculation of KE:

$$KE = \tfrac{1}{2}\, mv^2 \text{ or } KE = \frac{Mass \times (V_1^2 - V_2^2)}{2 \times g}$$

An increased V_1 and decreased V_2 result in significant internal damage. In addition, if the mass is doubled, then the energy is doubled; however, if the velocity is doubled, then the energy is quadrupled.

Some degree of hemorrhage is frequently involved with the victim of a gunshot wound. *Hemorrhage* refers to a rapid loss of circulating intravascular volume. Various stages of hemorrhage are characterized by the amount of blood lost, in relation to the total blood volume and the signs and symptoms expected at that particular level of depletion. Unfortunately, no one at the scene can collect the blood that has been lost and then inform the emergency department personnel of the need for fluid resuscitation or blood transfusion or both. Another concern is that the patient may be primarily bleeding internally. Although a significant amount of blood is not identified at the scene, the patient may exhibit symptoms of intravascular depletion, which may indicate that they are hemorrhaging internally.

The abdomen, chest, and thighs are quite capacious and may retain large amounts of blood volume. In some cases, the skin may become very taut, distended, and shiny or the patient may exhibit signs and symptoms of compromise from organs in the body compartment involved. However, sometimes the bleed

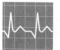

TAKE HOME POINTS

The average person weighs 70 kg and has approximately 5000 ml of total blood volume.

The attending nurse must be alert for signs of internal bleeding and remember that certain body compartments are capable of holding significant amounts of blood.

is more insidious and therefore more difficult to detect. A retroperitoneal bleed is an example. The methods of estimating fluid loss in the next section may be very helpful in treating the trauma patient. However, aggressive resuscitative measures should be implemented the minute that blood loss is apparent.

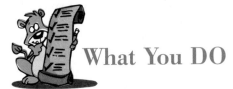 What You DO

Patients with Class I and II blood loss can be managed with crystalloid replacement at a rate of 3 ml for every 1 ml of blood loss. Patients with Class III and IV blood lost, however, require blood replacement therapy in addition to crystalloids. Patients with Class IV hemorrhage usually die if immediate emergency intervention is not implemented because compensatory mechanisms are short term and inadequate to handle a blood loss of this volume.

Classification of Fluid and Blood Losses*

	CLASS I	CLASS II	CLASS III	CLASS IV
Blood loss (ml)	≤750	750-1500	1500-2000	>2000
Blood loss (% blood volume)	≤15%	15%-30%	30%-40%	>40%
Pulse rate	<100	>100	>120	>140
Blood pressure	Normal	Normal	Decreased	Decreased
Capillary refill	Normal	Delayed	Delayed	Delayed
Respiratory rate	14-20	20-30	30-40	>35
Urine output (ml/hr)	>30	20-30	5-15	Negligible
Mental status	Slightly anxious	Mildly anxious	Anxious and confused	Confused, lethargic
Fluid replacement (3:1 rule)	Crystalloid	Crystalloid	Crystalloid and blood	Crystalloid and blood

*Amounts are based on the patient's initial presentation.
From American College of Surgeons Committee on Trauma: *The advanced trauma life support student manual,* Chicago, 1993, American College of Surgeons.

Identifying the classification of blood loss and administering the appropriate treatment needed to stabilize the patient are important.

The main treatment goals are to decrease blood loss and increase intravascular volume. These goals can be accomplished by instituting specific interventions to control bleeding and to replenish intravascular volume with crystalloids and/or blood products. If the patient continues to bleed despite resuscitative measures, surgical intervention may be necessary.

FIRST-LINE AND INITIAL TREATMENTS FOR ACUTE HEMORRHAGING

- Secure or support a patent airway (cervical spine precautions).
- Optimize breathing.
- Maintain circulation.
- Establish intravascular access.
- Replace intravascular volume (blood products or crystalloids).
- Manage bleeding by applying direct pressure on a compressible site.

TAKE HOME POINTS

The patient who is hemorrhaging—internally or externally—exhibits the pathophysiologic signs and symptoms of hypovolemic shock. (Refer to the discussion on hypovolemic shock in Chapter 2.)

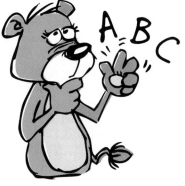

The usual ABCs should be followed in the management of the patient with hemorrhage. The airway should be assessed, oxygen should be applied, and, if necessary, the patient should be intubated. The goal is to maintain tissue perfusion. The patient has already lost some oxygen-carrying capacity secondary to the bleeding; therefore it is important to saturate the hemoglobin that remains with as much oxygen as possible to enhance tissue perfusion.

 Vasopressors, steroids, and sodium bicarbonate should not be considered in the initial treatment of the bleeding patient. The patient must have their intravascular volume replenished first.

Careful assessment of the breathing and assisting or managing ventilation as necessary are required. Circulation should be assessed by both physical examination and vital signs. Estimating the patient's SBP is accomplished by palpating the pulses and assessing the pulse characteristics (i.e., rate, rhythm, strength).

Pulse Site	Approximate SBP Value
Radial	80 mm Hg
Femoral	70 mm Hg
Carotid	60 mm Hg

TAKE HOME POINTS

Cervical spine precautions are included in the A of the ABCs of all trauma patients. Without proper stabilization, securing a patent airway may not be possible without compromising the integrity of the cervical spine.

At this time, two IV accesses should be obtained with large-bore (16- or 18-gauge) IV catheters, preferably in the upper extremities; antecubital is preferred. The prudent practitioner should also collect blood to be sent for baseline testing that include CBC, basic metabolic panel, PT, PTT with international normalized ratio (INR), type and cross match, ABGs, and beta human chorionic gonadotropin (hCG) in women of childbearing age to determine whether the patient is pregnant. Fluid resuscitation should be initiated with crystalloid solutions, normal saline (NS), or lactated Ringer's solution.

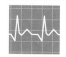 A urinary catheter should also be placed to assess the patient's fluid status and the adequacy of renal perfusion.

FIRST-LINE AND INITIAL TREATMENT FOR BLOOD LOSS

- Infuse lactated Ringer's solution.

Crystalloids are administered at a rate of 3 ml for every 1 ml of blood loss. All fluids should be warmed, and a rapid infusing device may be necessary.

TAKE HOME POINTS

It is reasonable to have lactated Ringer's solution infusing on one side and NS infusing on the other side in preparation for possible blood transfusion.

The American College of Surgeons recommends fluid replacement with 1 to 2 L of fluid administered rapidly for the adult patient and 20 ml/kg for the pediatric patient.

TAKE HOME POINTS

O-negative blood is usually transfused in the emergent patient without a type and cross match. O-positive blood may be substituted in life-threatening situations if O-negative blood is not available.

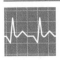

The patient should be continuously reevaluated for hemorrhage that is not totally visible.

TAKE HOME POINTS

Ongoing, careful assessments of the patient and response to interventions is crucial.

Blood transfusions should be considered when the intravascular requirements are not being met by crystalloid infusion. Initially, O-negative packed red blood cells (PRBCs) may be given; however, once the type and cross have been completed, patient-specific blood should be transfused. Whole blood is rarely administered, although it would provide all the blood components that the patient has lost and decrease the exposure to the number of donors.

Whole blood is not usually given because most patients do not need all the components. Further, most blood banks cannot store whole blood cost effectively. Autotransfusion is another option; however, certain restrictions and contraindications apply. Injuries that result in the contamination of blood at the site of injury (e.g., perforation of the colon) are usually not ideal for the use of the cell-saver device. The reason for this is that bacteria from the colon is now present in the blood; this same blood would be subsequently transfused to the patient and could result in the development of sepsis. In addition, certain chemicals used during orthopedic surgery, such as methylmethacrylate, may not be appropriate for autotransfusion.

When the patient's blood volume has become significantly depleted, additional transfusions with other blood components may be indicated.

Devices may be used to assist in attaining hemostasis from an actively bleeding wound in addition to increasing venous return. One such device is the pneumatic antishock garment (PASG), formerly known as medical antishock trousers (MAST). Current indications for the use of PASG or MAST devices include the treatment of hypotension (SBP <80 or <100 mm Hg if symptoms of shock are present) to help stabilize lower extremity or pelvic fractures and to control bleeding anywhere under the device. The current use of these devices is sometimes controversial. Absolute contraindications include pulmonary edema, left ventricular dysfunction, or known diaphragmatic rupture. Controversial uses include injuries to the head, thorax, and cardiac tamponade. Relative contraindications are pregnancy (regarding inflation of the abdominal apparatus), abdominal evisceration, impalement of the abdomen, compartment syndrome, lumbar spine instability, or inability to control bleeding outside of the garment. Tourniquets are no longer indicated in the treatment of hemorrhage because they cause ischemia to tissues distal to the injury. The only time the application of tourniquets is used is in the event of traumatic amputation.

Prevention of hypothermia in the hemorrhaging patient is another very important intervention. Although it is important to expose the patient to assess for injuries, maintenance of body temperature is critical and all fluids and blood should be warmed either before or during administration. Patients with hypothermia who are bleeding have less ability to tolerate the loss in blood volume.

The end result of massive blood loss is hypovolemic shock. Rapid and aggressive intervention is critical in the hemorrhaging patient to prevent the deterioration and possible hemodynamic instability of the patient. The nurses' role in the management of the patient who is hemorrhaging from a gunshot wound is of utmost importance, and the information gathered or missed can significantly influence patient outcome.

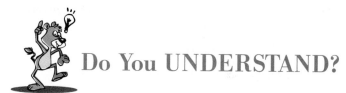

Do You UNDERSTAND?

DIRECTIONS: Fill in the blanks to complete each of the following statements.

1. One of the most common causes of high-velocity penetrating trauma is a

   _____ _____.

2. V_1 refers to energy transferred from bullet to tissue when

   _____ the wound.

3. V_2 refers to energy transferred from bullet to tissue when

   _____ the wound.

4. The loss of 15% of the blood volume describes Class _____ hemorrhage.

5. Class II hemorrhage is the loss of _____ to _____ ml of blood.

6. The patient with a Class III hemorrhage has a(n) _____

   BP and a(n) _____ heart rate.

7. The patient with a Class IV hemorrhage has a(n) _____

   pulse pressure.

8. The patient with a Class IV hemorrhage usually requires

   _____ _____ _____ and

   _____ _____ to survive.

9. Blood is replaced with crystalloids at a rate of _____ ml for every

   _____ ml of blood loss.

10. Palpation of a radial pulse usually indicates the patient's systolic pressure is

at least _____ mm Hg.

11. Palpation of a femoral pulse usually indicates the SBP to be about

_____ mm Hg.

12. Palpation of the carotid pulse usually indicates the SBP is

_____ mm Hg.

13. Primary goals for treating the victim with a hemorrhaging gunshot wound

include control of _____ and _____ replacement.

DIRECTIONS: **Identify the following statements as *true* (T) or *false* (F).**

_____ 14. Vasopressors are beneficial as initial treatment for the hypotensive
patient with a gunshot wound.

_____ 15. Tourniquets are routinely used to control bleeding in most
patients with trauma.

_____ 16. $D_5\frac{1}{2}$ NS is the intravascular fluid (IVF) of choice and is rapidly
transfused into the patient with trauma on arrival to the emergency
department.

_____ 17. MAST or PASG devices are beneficial to patients with pulmonary
edema, left ventricular dysfunction, or diaphragmatic rupture.

What IS Cardiac Tamponade?

Cardiac tamponade is a life-threatening condition requiring immediate intervention. Cardiac tamponade is defined as major compression of all four chambers of the heart caused by an accumulation of one or more of the following: blood, clots, pus, other fluid, or gas. The fluid accumulates in the pericardial sac that surrounds the heart, causing hypotension and jugular venous distention. The amount of fluid necessary to cause cardiac tamponade in an adult varies. As little as 150 ml of rapidly accumulating fluid to 1 L of slowly accumulating fluid in the pericardial sac can cause cardiac tamponade.

This fluid accumulation increases the pressure in the pericardial sac. This rising pressure results in an equalization of the diastolic pressure in all four chambers of the heart. This change in pressure leads to a decrease in cardiac filling, resulting in a decrease in stroke volume. Cardiac tamponade becomes fatal when the pericardial pressure increases to the point that the heart cannot effectively pump to maintain circulation.

Many diseases may result in cardiac tamponade. These diseases include acute and chronic pericarditis, cancer, renal disease, and systemic lupus erythematosus. Cardiac tamponade may also occur as the result of certain procedures: cardiac catheterization, balloon angioplasty, pacemaker insertion, central-line insertion, transmyocardial revascularization, fine-needle biopsy of the chest, coronary artery bypass surgery, and heart transplantation. Certain medications also predispose patients to tamponade. These medications include anticoagulants and thrombolytic agents. Acute cardiac tamponade may also occur as the result of chest trauma or rupture of the heart after a myocardial infarction (MI).

- Premature infants are at the greatest risk of tamponade associated with central lines. Central lines can be in place as long as 48 hours before causing tamponade in premature infants.
- Women and older adults are at the greatest risk for tamponade after revascularization procedures.

What You NEED TO KNOW

The clinical manifestations of cardiac tamponade vary. The signs and symptoms can be similar to the signs and symptoms of other conditions such as heart failure and pulmonary embolism. The patient may report chest tightness, dizziness, shortness of breath, vague discomfort or uneasiness, and dysphagia. Clinical signs include tachycardia, rising central venous pressure, a decrease in the difference between the SBP and DBP (narrowing of the pulse pressure), shocklike symptoms, and pulsus paradoxus. *Pulsus paradoxus* is defined as a >10 mm Hg drop in SBP occurring on inspiration. Pulsus paradoxus can be observed on arterial line tracing or measured using a sphygmomanometer.

 A patient with dehydration will quickly develop cardiac tamponade with less fluid accumulation.

TAKE HOME POINTS

Cardiac tamponade is a serious, life-threatening condition requiring immediate intervention.

HOW TO MEASURE PULSUS PARADOXUS

1. Inflate the BP cuff 15 mm Hg above the highest systolic measurement.
2. Deflate the BP cuff slowly until the first Korotkoff sounds are heard. Initially, the sounds will only be heard during expiration in the presence of cardiac tamponade.
3. Continue to deflate the BP cuff until the Korotkoff sounds are heard throughout the respiratory cycle (i.e., inspiratory and expiratory).
4. The difference between the first measurement obtained (Step 1) and the last measurement is the pulsus paradoxus.

An electrocardiographic (ECG) tracing may show a decrease in the amplitude of the QRS complex, an alternating high and low voltage (electrical alternans), and other T-wave abnormalities. However, ECG changes are observed in only about 20% of patients with tamponade.

V_3 V_6

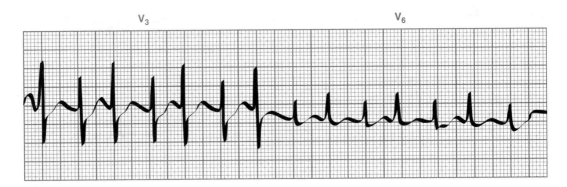

Hypotension, muffled heart tones, and severe jugular vein distention (JVD) are considered classic signs of cardiac tamponade and are referred to as Beck's triad.

When an underlying disease is causing the tamponade, the symptoms reported by the patient may be similar to the disease.

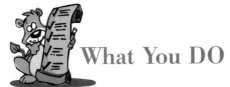

What You DO

Heart catheterization and echocardiography can confirm cardiac tamponade. An echocardiogram is the safest method for detecting cardiac tamponade and is used more frequently because of the time required to prepare the client for a heart catheterization. An echocardiogram shows increasing tricuspid and pulmonary flow velocities and decreasing mitral and aortic valve flow velocities during inspiration. A heart catheterization shows that the right atrial, pulmonary capillary wedge, and pulmonary artery DBPs are elevated and are all equal to each other (within 5 mm Hg). Cardiac output is also decreased, whereas systemic vascular resistance is elevated. A chest x-ray film shows an enlarged heart, which can be indicative of tamponade when compared with recent x-ray studies.

Once the diagnosis of tamponade has been confirmed, a physician needs to remove the excess fluid in the pericardial space. This fluid can be removed by needle aspiration, needle pericardiocentesis, or open-surgical drainage. Needle pericardiocentesis can be performed at the bedside using a local anesthetic; it involves the insertion of a needle through the chest wall into the pericardial sac. The fluid is gently aspirated.

The characteristics of the fluid aspirated will vary with the cause of the tamponade. For example, the fluid appears bloody if the tamponade is the result of bleeding, but it may appear purulent if the cause is infection. A sample of the fluid should be sent to the laboratory for smear, culture, and cytologic studies. Open-surgical drainage may be performed when the cause of the tamponade is unknown.

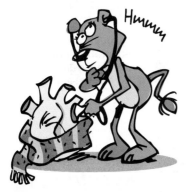

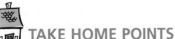

TAKE HOME POINTS

Beck's triad consists of hypotension, muffled heart sounds, and JVD.

Although many of the symptoms in infants and children are similar to those in adults, infants develop bradycardia instead of tachycardia. Cardiac tamponade should be ruled out in any infant who has a central-line catheter and who develops bradycardia and hypotension.

Although Beck's triad is a classical sign of cardiac tamponade, it is frequently a late development; other symptoms may occur earlier.

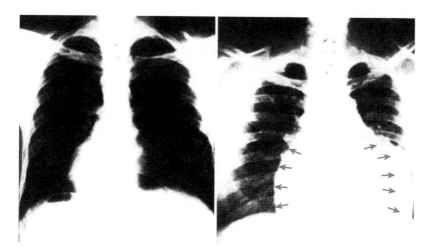

Normal Chest X-Ray   Enlarged Cardiac Silhouette

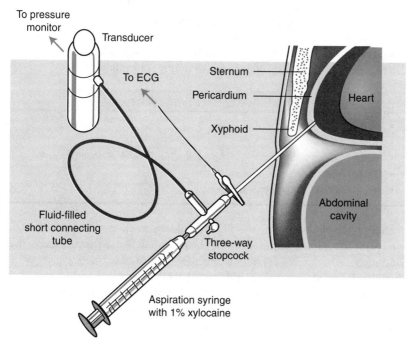

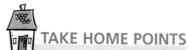

TAKE HOME POINTS

Pericardiocentesis is safer when guided by a two-dimensional echocardiogram.

The removal of as little as 10 ml of pericardial fluid can mean the difference between life and death for the patient.

The use of nitroglycerin should be avoided because the patient's preload is already reduced.

While the patient is awaiting drainage of the pericardial fluid, IV fluids may be given to expand the intravascular blood volume. Dobutamine, dopamine, or nitroprusside may be administered to increase cardiac output and maintain BP; these are only temporary measures.

The goal of most nursing interventions is early detection of cardiac tamponade. Any patient undergoing a procedure that places him or her at high risk for cardiac tamponade should be closely monitored for at least 24 hours after the

For further information on hemodynamic monitoring, see the *Real World Nursing Survival Guide: Hemodynamic Monitoring.*

For further information on the electrical conduction system and ECG interpretation, see the *Real World Nursing Survival Guide: ECGs & the Heart.*

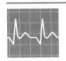

TAKE HOME POINTS

Cardiac tamponade can be detected early with careful assessment.

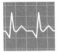

Signs and symptoms of cardiac tamponade can be similar to other conditions, making additional careful assessment necessary.

Continuous ECG monitoring for arrhythmias and frequent assessment of vital signs are necessary during pericardiocentesis.

procedure. The patient is observed for symptoms associated with cardiac tamponade (e.g., shortness of breath, vague discomfort, anxiety, dizziness, JVD, chest tightness or discomfort). Heart tones and breath sounds are assessed, paying particular attention for muffled heart tones (possibly indicative of cardiac tamponade) or adventitious breath sounds (possibly indicative of other problems). Vital signs are monitored for tachycardia (adults) or bradycardia (infants), for changes in BP, and for narrowing of pulse pressures and pulsus alternans.

If the patient has a pulmonary artery catheter in place, central venous pressure, pulmonary capillary wedge pressure, and cardiac output are monitored. An ECG is assessed for changes in voltage and alternating patterns of high and low voltage. Laboratory values are monitored for signs of dehydration and hypokalemia. Hypokalemia can precipitate arrhythmias during pericardiocentesis. Intake and output levels are monitored to assess for dehydration. Chest tube drainage of a patient who has had open-heart surgery is closely monitored because blocked or kinked chest tubes can result in cardiac tamponade. A sudden decrease in chest tube drainage should be investigated.

When cardiac tamponade is suggested, oxygen is administered. The physician is immediately notified, and an immediate request for a chest x-ray, 12-lead ECG, and echocardiogram is made. If the patient does not already have an IV in place, one should be started. If time allows, a blood sample is sent to the laboratory for type and cross match and for an assessment of the potassium level. Hypokalemia can increase the occurrence of arrhythmias during pericardiocentesis.

FIRST-LINE AND INITIAL TREATMENT FOR CARDIAC TAMPONADE

- Provide oxygen.
- Notify physician.
- Request an immediate chest x-ray, 12-lead ECG, and echocardiogram.
- Obtain IV access.
- Prepare for pericardiocentesis

During pericardiocentesis, the ECG should be monitored for arrhythmias; vital signs should be monitored during the procedure. After the procedure, the vital signs are monitored every 15 minutes for the first hour, then agency policy should be followed for frequent vital signs. After the procedure, the dressing over the needle insertion site should be monitored. Any excessive drainage should be reported to the physician.

Emotional support and patient teaching are necessary to help decrease anxiety. A calm and consistent demeanor can also help decrease anxiety. The patient should be encouraged to report all symptoms. Diagnostic tests such as echocardiogram should be provided. If needle pericardiocentesis is to be performed, the patient should be provided with information. Staying with the patient before the procedure should also provide reassurance and emotional support. If possible, the nurse should stay with the patient during the needle pericardiocentesis. Preoperative teaching should be provided to the patient having open-surgical drainage.

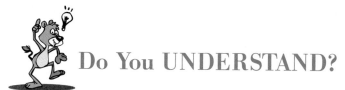 Do You UNDERSTAND?

DIRECTIONS: **Fill in the blanks to complete each of the following statements.**

1. Cardiac tamponade occurs when _____ accumulates

   in the _____ _____ around the heart.

2. The fluid accumulation in the pericardial causes the pressure in the sac to

   _____; this leads to a _____

   in cardiac filling.

3. _____ _____ are at

   the greatest risk for tamponade resulting from central-line placement.

DIRECTIONS: **Provide a short answer to each of the following questions.**

4. What is pulsus paradoxus?

   _____

   _____

5. What are the signs of cardiac tamponade that are referred to as Beck's triad?

   _____

   _____

6. What sign of cardiac tamponade is different in infants?

   _____

   _____

Answers: 1. fluid, pericardial sac; 2. increase, decrease; 3. premature infants; 4. >10 mm Hg drop in BP occurring on inspiration; 5. hypotension, muffled heart tones, and severe JVD; 6. they develop bradycardia.

DIRECTIONS: **Identify the following statements as** *true* **(T) or** *false* **(F).**

_____ 7. A cardiac catheterization is the safest method for diagnosing cardiac tamponade.

_____ 8. If possible, a potassium level should be checked before performing pericardiocentesis.

_____ 9. An ECG tracing can be used to detect pulsus paradoxus.

_____ 10. If cardiac tamponade is suspected, the nurse should notify the physician immediately.

What IS Spinal Cord Compression?

Spinal cord compression (SCC) is a disorder of sensory and motor dysfunction caused by direct pressure or compromised vascular supply to the spinal cord or cauda equina. Patients rarely die from SCC; however, it is considered a medical emergency because delay in treatment can result in irreversible paralysis and a loss of voluntary and involuntary sphincter control.

What You NEED TO KNOW

Cord ischemia or necrosis with neurologic impairment occurs by three processes. The most common pathophysiologic mechanism for cord compression is vertebral collapse or pathologic fracture. Vertebral bodies shift and occlude the spinal canal where the cord runs the length of the spine.

Although less common, SCC can also occur as a result of direct compression of the spinal cord or cauda equina or because of interference in the vascular supply to the spine. Regardless of the precise causal mechanism, spinal cord ischemia results in neuronal damage and a severing of communications between the peripheral sensory and motor nerves and the brain. This pathophysiologic damage is clinically represented as a loss of sensation and paresis or paralysis.

At-Risk Populations

Patients who are at greatest risk of developing SCC are those with diseases involving the vertebrae. These include spinal degenerative disease, malignant bone metastases, radiation-induced myelopathy, multiple sclerosis, osteoporosis, syringomyelia, and cervical sprain (whiplash). Interruption of blood flow to the

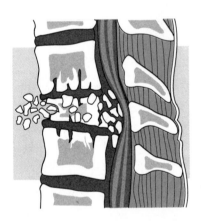

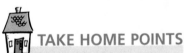
TAKE HOME POINTS

Communication of the sensory and motor nerve impulses are damaged or lost with spinal cord ischemia.

spinal cord can also occur from traumatic injury, aortic aneurysm repair, or tumor compression. The most common cause for all mechanisms is malignant disease because more than one mechanism may cause SCC. The most prevalent malignant associations are breast cancer, multiple myeloma, lung cancer, prostate cancer, and renal cell cancer as a result of the propensity for these malignancies to infiltrate the bones.

Clinical Manifestations

SCC can occur anywhere along the spinal cord, and symptoms are related to the location and extent of the spinal cord nerve injury, although SCC is always characterized by sensory and motor defects below the level of the spinal cord lesion. A summary of clinical manifestations according to the location of spinal injury is outlined in the following table.

Overview of Spinal Cord Compression

LOCATION OF LESION	RISK FACTORS	PHYSICAL SYMPTOMS	AUTONOMIC SYMPTOMS
Cervical spine	• Degenerative arthritis • Cervical spondylosis • Multiple sclerosis • Rheumatoid arthritis • Syringomyelia • Cervical sprain • Late effect of spinal cord injury • Head and neck or esophageal cancer	• Radicular pain in the neck, occipital region, and shoulders, brachial area (pain may be provoked by neck movement) • Quadriplegia • Upper extremity weakness (may be spastic or atrophic) • Sensory loss in area of weakness • Weakness or paralysis of the diaphragm may occur with lesion at or above C4 (may be unilateral or bilateral)	• Hypotension • Bradycardia • Loss of temperature autoregulation • Autonomic hyper-reflexia • Gastric hypersecretion and paralytic ileus • Reflex bowel, bladder, and erection • Hoffman's sign (flicking of the middle finger induces flexion of the ipsilateral thumb or index finger)
Thoracic spine	• Osteoporitic vertebral compression fractures • Late effect of spinal cord injury • Spinal aneurysmal bone cyst • Spinal epidural abscess • Breast cancer	• Pain (local, radicular, or both) • Paraplegia • Sensory loss below the level of lesion • Reflex abnormalities distal to lesion	• Venous stasis and associated complications • Reflex bowel, bladder, and penile erection
Lumbar spine	• Osteoporitic vertebral compression fractures • Late effect of spinal cord injury • Spinal epidural abscess • Ruptured or herniated disks	• Bowel and bladder dysfunction • Extensor plantar response	• Venous stasis and associated complications • Reflex bowel, bladder, and penile erection

Continued

Overview of Spinal Cord Compression—cont'd

LOCATION OF LESION	RISK FACTORS	PHYSICAL SYMPTOMS	AUTONOMIC SYMPTOMS
Cauda equina	• Prostate cancer	• Pain (may be local, referred, or radicular) • Sphincter disturbances • Loss of buttock and leg sensation • Lower extremity weakness or paralysis	• Areflexic bowel, bladder, and erection

TAKE HOME POINTS

Back pain is the first and most common symptom.

TAKE HOME POINTS

Along with numbness and paresthesias, patients will often complain of a sensation of "heaviness" in the affected extremities.

Once motor deficits are present, treatment is unlikely to improve functional motor ability.

TAKE HOME POINTS

Patients who have bowel or bladder dysfunction at the time of diagnosis have a poor prognosis.

The severity of symptoms may also be affected by the time of onset of the etiologic mechanism. Most patients can expect some improvement of neurologic function from the symptoms they exhibited when they first presented for evaluation and treatment. The exception to this statement is in the case of complete paresis, which is rarely reversible.

Back pain is the earliest and most common symptom, often preceding other clinical findings by several months. The onset of pain is usually gradual, progressive, and unremitting. It can be localized, radicular, or referred. Radicular pain is a type of radiating pain that follows a specific dermatome and is considered a symptom indicative of compression of the nerve root. Radicular pain can be elicited by having the patient flex the neck or raise the legs straight while in a supine position. Back pain associated with SCC is also unique because it can be exacerbated by manual palpation of the area.

The most prevalent sensory deficits are numbness and paresthesias. Patients complain of numbness and tingling or feelings of coldness in the affected area. Numbness typically begins in the toes and gradually ascends to the level of spinal cord involvement. Most patients experience weakness by the time SCC is diagnosed, although it chronologically occurs after sensory changes. Because most cord compression is at or below the thoracic area, lower extremity weakness is most common. Motor weakness may exhibit in the form of an unsteady gait, ataxia, or a favoring of the affected extremity.

Approximately one half of patients exhibit autonomic dysfunction, such as bowel or bladder difficulties at diagnosis. Constipation occurs as a result of decreased peristalsis and is an early indication of neurologic impairment. Loss of sphincter control with intractable constipation occurs as cord compression worsens. Diminished urge to defecate and an inability to bear down are initial signs of autonomic dysfunction involving the bowel, which contributes to constipation, obstipation, and finally incontinence. Urinary dysfunction begins with hesitancy and incomplete voiding and progresses to urinary retention and finally incontinence; eventually, the bladder is filled to capacity and unable to empty. Increased postvoid volume on catheterization may be an indication of early autonomic dysfunction. SCC can also affect the nerves controlling penile erection or ejaculation, causing altered sexual function in many patients.

Diagnostics

Spinal x-ray studies show bone deformities (e.g., necrotic bone lesions from metastatic tumor). MRI is used to identify precisely the location of all lesions. MRI is sensitive to neurologic tissue and has the ability to distinguish extradural, intradural, and extramedullary lesions. The disadvantage of this diagnostic test is that it requires the patient to remain motionless for approximately 1 hour in a small, confined space. If the patient moves during the examination, poor imaging is the result.

A myelogram of the spine could be selected as the imaging diagnostic tool of choice. An injection of dye into the epidural space permits visualization of compressed areas of the spine. The flow of dye and obstructions encountered show on a nuclear scan of the area. However, MRI has generally replaced this diagnostic test for the diagnosis of SCC because MRI: (a) is noninvasive, (b) is diagnostically more sensitive, (c) shows the entire spine, and (d) indicates the presence of SCC and paraspinal masses. The benefits of a myelogram are that CSF sampling can occur, enabling meningeal carcinomatosis to be ruled out.

TAKE HOME POINTS

- Spinal x-ray films are used to validate a potential etiologic factor in the presence of suspicious symptoms.
- Myelogram can be used when MRI assessment cannot explain neurologic deficits.

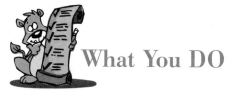

What You DO

For some patients with malignant bone metastases, the risk of developing SCC can be reduced by systemic treatment with bisphosphonates such as pamidronate sodium (Aredia) and zoledronate. These agents block osteoclast activity in the bone matrix, reducing bone demineralization and the risk of vertebral collapse. The incidence of SCC occurring from other causes can be minimized by prompt definitive and effective treatment of its primary disorder. No established adjunctive or complementary therapies are known to be effective in reducing bone disease or enhancing neurologic recovery when SCC occurs.

The immediate treatment of suggested SCC is IV administration of corticosteroids to reduce inflammation and edema. Dexamethasone (Decadron) 16 to 100 mg is administered as an initial bolus, followed by 4 mg qid for about 14 days. A comparable steroid potency dose of hydrocortisone (Cortef) may used as an alternative to dexamethasone (Decadron).

Radiation therapy is the best definitive treatment for malignancy-related SCC because response rates are equivalent to those with surgery but with less morbidity. Treatment must be immediately implemented for optimal reversal of neurologic deficits. The maximal tolerated lifetime radiation exposure of the spine is 6000 Cy, and each treatment for an episode of SCC uses about 2000 to 3000 Cy. Patients often develop recurrent SCC that can no longer be treated with radiation. Radiation is ineffective in the treatment of SCC caused by nonmalignant causes.

Surgical decompression (e.g., partial resection of the tumor or laminectomy) with or without Harrington rod stabilization is performed in patients who are in otherwise good health and have slow-growing tumors or nonmalignant diseases.

Surgical decompression is used for patients with rapidly progressing neurologic dysfunction and for those who have had previous maximal radiation to the involved area. Because most vertebral lesions are positioned on the anterior surface, the anterior surgical approach may be necessary to achieve vertebroplasty or laminectomy. The posterior (back) approach is less invasive and preferred whenever feasible. Newer posterolateral thoracoscopic approaches have been used with reduced morbidity and enhanced recovery.

Nursing Responsibilities

Patients with SCC are faced with a number of physiologic and psychologic challenges. Nurses caring for these patients must be skilled in pain management, rehabilitation strategies, and physical maintenance of immobile patients. Multidisciplinary management commonly involves neurosurgeons, oncologists, radiation oncologists, pain experts, and rehabilitation medicine. The role of the nurse in coordination of these efforts is essential because of the involvement of various subspecialty clinicians. Nursing care is planned around the degree of physical deficit that is apparent or anticipated.

The nurse is at times involved with patients at high risk for developing SCC, not patients who have actually experienced it. It is important to teach the patient and family the importance of early reporting of sensory changes (especially in the lower extremities) or a worsening of his or her symptoms throughout the day. Patients must realize that back pain is an important early symptom that should be investigated when unresolved with rest. Some patients experience mild or incomplete compression of the spinal cord and may implement interventions such as pain medication or peristaltic stimulants. These patients must have frequent medical follow-up for detection of worsening symptoms.

Pain and other sensory changes are common and neuropathic in origin, making management more complex that the usual somatic pain. Patients often require nontraditional therapies such as a surgical sympathectomy or antidepressant medications. Chronic pain and its management add to the existing safety risk that exists as a result of potential sensory and motor impairment.

The patients' altered mobility necessitates several nursing interventions. Nurses are involved in planning for specialized skin care for immobilized patients and assist in applying supportive devices such as splints or braces. Some patients may require assistance in purchasing mobility devices (e.g., wheelchair), modifying the home, and scheduling rehabilitation training for the patient and family. Patients and family need to be taught unique safety interventions that are based on their defined neurologic deficits.

In severe SCC with autonomic dysfunction, modifications must be made for visceral organ dysfunction, which may initially mean insertion of a urinary catheter and periodic enemas to manage bladder and bowel dysfunction. However, the ultimate goal is for patients and families to perform intermittent self-catheterization and enemas. When the upper spine is involved, breathing may be weak and shallow and swallowing may be impaired. Supportive therapies may include the use of a cuirass ventilator or the insertion of a jejunal feeding tube.

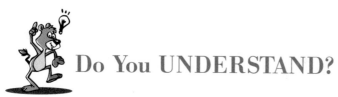

Do You UNDERSTAND?

DIRECTIONS: **Fill in the blanks to complete each of the following statements.**

1. SCC can occur from vertebral collapse, pathologic fractures, or

   _____ _____.

2. When compressed, the spinal cord becomes _____

   or _____, which results in neurologic impairment.

3. A lesion in the _____ region will result

   in quadriplegia and possible breathing difficulties.

4. Numbness and _____ are the

   most prevalent sensory deficits for a patient with SCC.

5. _____ is the most sensitive diagnostic test that precisely

   identifies the lesion location.

6. Immediate treatment of a patient with suspected SCC consists of

   administering a _____.

7. The complaints of _____ makes the management

   of the SCC complex and may require nontraditional therapies.

Answers: 1. cauda equina; 2. ischemic, necrotic; 3. cervical; 4. paresthesias; 5. MRI; 6. corticosteroid; 7. pain.

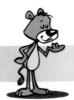

What IS Hypothermia?

Hypothermia can be defined as a fall in the core body temperature below 35° C (95° F). The temperature reading must be obtained from a source that measures core temperature and from preferably two such sources. Hypothermia can be classified as primary (accidental) or secondary (deliberate).

Environmental exposure or prolonged surgical tissue exposure, especially during surgery of the thoracic or abdominal cavities, are the causes of primary or accidental hypothermia. Deliberate, mild hypothermia is used during neurosurgical procedures to provide protection of the brain and spinal cord during periods of interrupted perfusion. Profound hypothermia (as low as 28° C) is often used during cardiopulmonary bypass.

Primary or accidental hypothermia occurs as a result of cold exposure. Secondary or deliberate hypothermia may be observed in patients with decreased heat production, such as hypoadrenalism and hypothyroidism, or abnormal temperature regulation, such as brain injuries involving the hypothalamus. Many mental or physical disease states or medications may interfere with the body's heat-balancing mechanisms. Some of the risk factors for developing hypothermia are listed in the following box.

RISK FACTORS FOR HYPOTHERMIA

- Extremes of age
- Trauma, especially CNS trauma
- CVA
- Hypothyroidism
- Hypoadrenalism
- Parkinson's disease
- Multiple sclerosis
- Burns
- Extensive skin diseases
- Vasodilation induced by alcohol or prescription or "street" drugs
- Malnutrition
- Sepsis
- Shock
- Renal or hepatic failure
- Alzheimer's disease and psychiatric problems that alter ability to respond to hypothermia
- Paraplegia or quadriplegia
- Trauma

CNS, Central nervous system; *CVA,* cerebrovascular accident.

In the United States, hypothermia is responsible for more than 700 deaths per year, and half of these deaths occur in patients who are 65 years old and older. The older patient has age-related impairment of homeostatic mechanisms affecting thermoregulation, cultural and economic factors that increase the likelihood of exposure to cold, and diseases and drugs that can impair thermoregulation, interfere with heat generation, or impair conservation of body heat. With advanced age comes a progressive weakening of the shivering response; the vaso-constrictor response develops, and a progressive reduction in the ability to detect and respond to changes in environmental temperature occurs.

What You NEED TO KNOW

The physiologic effects of hypothermia are summarized in the following table.

Physiologic Effects of Hypothermia

HYPOTHERMIA STAGE	CORE TEMPERATURE	SIGNS AND SYMPTOMS
Impending hypothermia	36° C	• Skin: pale, numb, waxy • Shivering • Fatigue • Weakness
Mild hypothermia	32°-35° C	• Uncontrolled, intense shivering • Movement less coordinated • Coldness creates pain and discomfort • Tachycardia • Vasoconstriction • Increase BP • Increase CO • Increase CVP (from shivering) • Increase in oxygen consumption • Myocardial ischemia, pulmonary edema, CHF (in patients with impaired cardiac function) • Metabolic acidosis
Moderate hypothermia	28°-32° C	• Absence of shivering (stops below 32° C) • Muscles stiffen • Mental confusion • Apathy • Slowed, vague, slurred speech • Slow, shallow breathing • Drowsiness • Strange behavior • No complaints of being cold (occurs below 35° C)

BP, Blood pressure; *CO,* cardiac output; *CVP,* central venous pressure; *CHF,* congestive heart failure.

Continued

• With advanced age, impairment of the compensatory mechanisms occurs, and the older adult has a decreased ability to detect and respond to changes in temperature.
• Neonates can generate heat, but they have a small body size, a greater ratio of body surface–to–body weight than adults do, and a thin layer of subcutaneous fat; consequently, they become hypothermic more easily than adults do.

In the United States, most cases of hypothermia occur in urban areas and are caused by environmental exposure and alcohol abuse, street drug abuse, mental illness, or homelessness. However, some cases are a result of outdoor work or recreation.

Physiologic Effects of Hypothermia—cont'd

HYPOTHERMIA STAGE	CORE TEMPERATURE	SIGNS AND SYMPTOMS
Moderate hypothermia— cont'd	28°-32° C	• Decreased heart rate • Decreased cardiac output • Increased risk of atrial and ventricular arrhythmias • "J" or Osborne wave (hypo-thermia hump) may appear on ECG • Decreased respiratory rate • 50% reduction in oxygen consumption • Impaired insulin action • Hyperglycemia
Severe hypothermia	28°-30° C	• Skin cold, bluish-gray in color • Weak • Lack of coordination • Decreased level of consciousness to coma • Absent tendon reflexes • Rigid extremities (may appear dead) • Decreased or absent respirations • Pupils dilated • Nonreactive pupils (29°-30° C) • Loss of cerebral autoregulation • Decrease cerebral blood flow • Decrease cardiac output • Decrease renal blood flow (oliguria)

BP, Blood pressure; *CO,* cardiac output; *CVP,* central venous pressure; *CHF,* congestive heart failure.

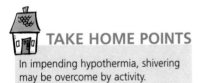

Bradycardia is due to slowed depolarization of pacemaker cells. A *J* or Osborne wave may appear on the downstroke of the QRS.

TAKE HOME POINTS

In impending hypothermia, shivering may be overcome by activity.

- **Bradycardia during hypothermia may be unresponsive to atropine or pacing.**
- **A high risk of aspiration exists that is due to altered mental status and ileus.**
- **If core body temperature falls below 26° C and is not corrected, then respirations stop and asystole occurs.**

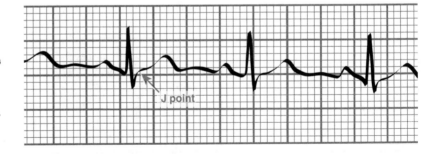

J point

In addition, hypothermia impairs platelet function, the coagulation cascade, and fibrinolysis, all of which lead to increased bleeding, which is of great significance during trauma resuscitation and surgery. The immune system is involved with impaired neutrophil and macrophage function. Vasoconstriction and increased blood viscosity and decreased tissue partial pressure for oxygen occur, all of which increase the risk of wound infection. Hypothermia impairs the response to catecholamines. Hypothermia also impairs drug metabolism by decreasing hepatic and renal blood flow. Hypothermia causes a "cold diuresis" that is due to impaired renal tubular function, leading to increased urinary loss of sodium, potassium, and water. Hypothermia causes depletion of high-energy phosphates such as adenosine triphosphate (ATP). Hypothermia shifts the oxyhemoglobin dissociation cure to the left, which impairs tissue oxygen delivery. Hypothermia can also cause hypokalemia because of a depression of the sodium-potassium-adenosinetriphosphatase (Na-K-ATPase) pump, as well as hyperglycemia because of the decreased release of insulin and peripheral use of glucose.

Heat Balance

In humans, an internal thermoregulatory system maintains core body temperature within a narrow range, coordinating heat loss, heat production, and heat conservation. Many of the chemical processes necessary to maintain life can only take place within a specific temperature range.

Humans have both core and peripheral thermal compartments. The *core* is defined as the well-perfused central tissues; they include the brain, thorax, and abdomen. The temperature in the core compartment is kept constant within a narrow range. Heat is rapidly distributed, and most of the metabolic processes, which require energy and produce heat, take place in the core compartment. Heat generated by metabolic processes in the core must get to the external environment. The *peripheral* compartment consists of the extremities and skin.

Temperature in the peripheral compartment may be 1° to 3° C lower than the temperature in the core, depending on the thermal environment. Temperature gradients may occur between the superficial and deep structures within the compartment. Contraction of voluntary muscles, either by normal muscle activity or shivering, produces heat in the peripheral compartment.

Heat moves from the core to the peripheral compartment by both convection and conduction of heat within the blood vessels and is influenced by the amount of blood flow to the peripheral tissues. (Conduction and convection is discussed in the section on heat loss mechanisms later in this chapter.)

The hypothalamus is the body's temperature regulation control center. The hypothalamus has both heat and cold sensitive neurons and receives afferent input from temperature sensors in the skin, spinal cord, abdominal viscera, and in or near the great vessels in the thorax. The sensory data are transmitted via the anterior spinothalamic tracts to the preoptic nuclei of the hypothalamus. The hypothalamus continuously maintains the core body temperature at the set point of approximately 37° C. If the core temperature falls, then heat production increases to maintain the core body temperature at this set point. The efferent component of this temperature control system is the sympathetic nervous system, which initiates shivering to produce heat and vasoconstriction to conserve heat.

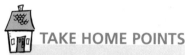

TAKE HOME POINTS

- The body's core compartment makes up approximately 50% to 60% of body mass.
- Approximately 90% of heat leaves the body through the skin and 10% leaves through the respiratory tract.

TAKE HOME POINTS

A normal white blood cell (WBC) count is necessary for hypothalamus temperature regulation.

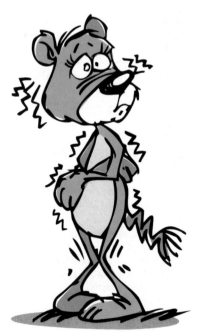

Mechanisms of Heat Production and Loss

The body increases heat production by increasing muscle tone and by shivering. Shivering is a fairly effective method for heat production because most of the energy produced is retained as heat. Shivering can increase body heat production four to five times above normal levels. Shivering requires increased muscle blood flow, which reduces the effectiveness of vasoconstriction to maintain the core temperature.

Epinephrine is released and causes vasoconstriction, which shunts blood to the core compartment where heat cannot be lost by the usual mechanisms. Epinephrine also generates chemical thermogenesis by increasing the basal metabolic rate on a short-term basis. Prolonged cold exposure also stimulates the release of thyroxine, which also increases the metabolic rate.

The body loses heat by four mechanisms: radiation, conduction, convection, and evaporation. *Radiation* is heat loss or gain in the form of infrared rays, which are a type of electromagnetic energy. Radiation is the most important source of heat loss, making up approximately 60% of total heat loss. All objects with a temperature above absolute zero radiate heat waves. The warmth sensed when standing in direct sunlight or next to a hot stove is produced by radiation. If body temperature is higher than surrounding air or objects, then more heat is radiated away from the body than toward the body.

Conduction is the transfer of heat to a solid object directly in contact with the skin, such as an operating room table, and is responsible for only about 3% of body heat loss. Hypothermia that results from administering cold IV fluids is an example of conduction because the fluids are warmed to body temperature by conduction from blood and tissues.

Convection is responsible for about 15% of body heat loss. In convection, conduction of heat occurs into the air that surrounds the body; once that same air reaches body temperature, no more heat is lost until the air molecules move away from the body and are replaced with other molecules at a lower temperature. Convection is an important source of heat loss in operating rooms, where air-flow should be 10 full-room air exchanges per hour and even higher in laminar-flow rooms. Convection is the basis for the well-known "wind-chill" factor.

Evaporation is heat lost during evaporation of water from the respiratory tract and skin and accounts for 22% of body heat loss. Even when there is no diaphoresis, 450 to 600 ml of water is lost per day from evaporation. This heat loss cannot be controlled because of the continuous loss of water by diffusion through the skin and respiratory mucosa. Heat loss is increased if more fluids are available at the skin surface, and fluid is then actively secreted through the sweat glands. Evaporative cooling occurs in response to sympathetic nervous system stimulation, and the amount of heat lost by sweating is dependent on the difference between the temperature of the body and the environment and the relative humidity of the air.

Clothing traps air next to the skin, creating a private air zone. Clothing decreases conductive, convective, and radiation heat losses. A typical suit of clothes can decrease heat loss by one half when compared with a nude body. Arctic-type or thermal-insulated clothing can also decrease the heat loss to one sixth. Clothing does not assist in maintaining body temperature when it is wet, even with perspiration. Water has a high thermal conductivity—32 times greater than air. Concrete has an even higher thermal conductivity than water, contributing to hypothermia in the older patient who falls on a concrete surface, becomes immobilized, and is not found for hours.

Alcohol increases a patient's risk of becoming hypothermic because it causes vasodilation, suppresses the hypothalamic temperature regulating center, impairs shivering, and decreases the patient's awareness of and response to a cold environment.

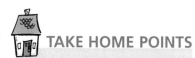

TAKE HOME POINTS

The body adapts over time to warm environments and high altitudes, but no significant physiologic adaptation to cold is apparent in the body.

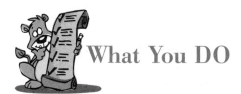

What You DO

Diagnosis and Treatment of the Patient with Hypothermia

Early recognition of hypothermia is critical. A treatment facility must have thermometers able to measure core temperatures of 25° C or less, and temperature must be measured at two core sites.

Laboratory tests should include the following:

- **Blood glucose.** Both hyperglycemia and hypoglycemia (with prolonged hypothermia) can be observed.
- **Potassium.** Both hyperkalemia and hypokalemia can exist. Hyperkalemia is usually indicative of extensive tissue damage.
- **ABGs.** ABGs should not be corrected for temperature. Patients with hypothermia have a higher level of oxygen and CO_2 and a lower pH than normothermic patients.
- **Hemoglobin.** Hemoglobin rises 2% for each 1° C fall in temperature as a result of cold diuresis and subsequent hypovolemia.
- **Coagulation studies.** Hypothermia interferes with the enzymes needed to activate the coagulation process. Platelet function is also inhibited because platelet production of thromboxane B2 is impaired by cold. Transfused platelets also functions poorly. However, the coagulation studies may not reflect these changes because the tests are performed at 37° C and the enzymes have been reactivated by warming the test tube.

TREATMENT

Airway and breathing. Supplemental oxygen is indicated for the hypothermic patient because of the leftward shift of the oxyhemoglobin dissociation curve. Oxygen should be heated to 40° to 45° C and humidified to return heat to the core compartment. If the patient's protective airway reflexes are impaired as a result of an altered mental status, then the patient should be given oxygen before intubation and intubated as gently as possible to avoid triggering ventricular arrhythmias.

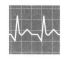

MONITORING: Temperature must be measured at two core sites.

- **The cold heart is very irritable, and diagnostic maneuvers such as central-line insertion (which may be necessary because of peripheral vasoconstriction), intubation, or even patient movement may precipitate ventricular fibrillation.**
- **The very cold heart (core temperature of 30° C or less) is not responsive to vasoactive drugs, defibrillation, or pacemaker activation to increase the heart rate.**

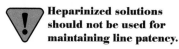

Heparinized solutions should not be used for maintaining line patency.

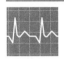

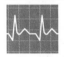

Circulation. Hypothermic patients are usually volume depleted and need infusion of warm saline. The hypothermic liver cannot metabolize the lactate from lactated Ringer's solution. The saline solution should be heated between 40° and 42° C, but it may not contribute significantly to core rewarming unless large volumes of crystalloid solution are used. Central lines may be needed not only to monitor intravascular volume but also because peripheral access is difficult as a result of peripheral vasoconstriction. If the patient is hypotensive and his or her BP remains low despite volume and rewarming, IV dopamine (Intropin) 2 to 5 μg/kg/min may be considered. The patient should be carefully monitored for any cardiac arrhythmias. Atrial arrhythmias can usually be watched until rewarming because the ventricular rate will be slow as a result of hypothermia. If ventricular arrhythmias occur, then they must be treated. The patient having ventricular arrhythmias may not respond to conventional therapy, and resuscitation must continue until core temperature reaches at least 30° C.

Methods of rewarming. Three methods of rewarming can be used: (1) passive, (2) active external rewarming, and (3) active internal rewarming.

Methods of Rewarming with Interventions

METHODS OF REWARMING	INTERVENTIONS
Passive	Remove wet clothing and items. Cover with blankets. Prevent convective loss from wind chill.
Active external	Provide: • Water baths (Hubbard tank) • Heat lamps • Circulating water blankets • Forced-air systems (Bair Hugger)
Active internal	Provide: • Lavage of numerous body cavities with warm saline (gastric, colonic, bladder, thoracic through chest tube) 　• Gastric 　• Colonic 　• Bladder 　• Thoracic • Hemodialysis with potassium-free dialysate (warmed 40°-45° C) • Extracorporeal venovenous rewarming • Cardiopulmonary bypass

Care must be taken with warming extremities of moderate-to-severe hypothermic patients, especially patients who have been hypothermic for prolonged periods. Peripheral vasodilation from application of external heat can cause cold, acidotic blood to return to the core compartment. The patient can develop hypotension, which can progress to shock, ventricular arrhythmias, and a sudden fall in core temperature called an *afterdrop*. Application of forced-air rewarming methods to the trunk alone may prevent afterdrop.

Active internal methods of rewarming will likely be needed for moderate-to-severe hypothermia and are definitely needed if the patient is in cardiac arrest because heat must be added to the core compartment.

Complications subsequent to rewarming the severely hypothermic patient include rewarming shock because of a dilated vascular bed, a depressed myocardium, and hypovolemia. Complications also include pneumonia, gastrointestinal bleeding, cardiac arrhythmias, pulmonary edema, gangrene, myoglobinuria and rhabdomyolysis, intravascular thrombosis, and compartment syndrome.

Cardiopulmonary resuscitation (CPR) in the patient with hypothermia. CPR should begin unless the patient has a documented "Do not resuscitate" order, a fatal injury, or a chest wall that is frozen, making external cardiac massage not possible. A history of cardiac arrest before the onset of hypothermia most likely indicates a poor prognosis because the hypothermia probably had no protective effect on the brain before cardiac arrest. The American Heart Association's *Advanced Cardiac Life Support Provider Manual* (2001) states that severe hypothermia with a core temperature below 30° C reduces blood flow to the heart, brain, and all other vital organs and reduces BP. The patient needs to be kept horizontal because of impaired cardiovascular reflexes and resultant hypotension. In addition, the pulse and respiratory effort may be hard to detect. At least 30 to 45 seconds should be allowed to detect a pulse or respirations before starting chest compressions; if available, Doppler may be useful in detecting the pulse.

FIRST-LINE AND INITIAL TREATMENT FOR HYPOTHERMIA

- Maintain the patient's ABCs.
- Apply rewarming therapy.
- Consider underlying causes, and correct them.

TAKE HOME POINTS

Forced-air rewarming systems (Bair Hugger) are practical and efficient and can be used together with warmed IV fluids and warmed, humidified oxygen.

Hypotension may be worsened by catecholamine depletion from prolonged shivering and cold diuresis.

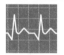

Continuous temperature monitoring is needed if active internal rewarming methods are used.

Vasoactive drugs are not effective in the presence of hypothermia and are poorly metabolized by the cold liver. If repeated doses are given during the time the patient is hypothermic, drug toxicity from these repeated doses can occur during rewarming.

TAKE HOME POINTS

A serum potassium level of more than 10 mEq/L indicates extensive cell destruction and a poor prognosis.

Vasoconstricting medications should be avoided because they will probably have minimal effect on the vasculature as a result of the ongoing vasoconstriction from the hypothermia.

• **The hypothermic heart
is very irritable and
prone to ventricular
fibrillation. The patient should
be given three shocks, per the
basic life support (BLS) protocol, but the cold heart may not
respond to defibrillation, and
further shocks should not be
given until the patient's core
temperature is warmed above
30° C.**
• **Rewarming therapy should
continue until the patient's
core temperature is at least
32° C before any decision is
made to terminate life support
efforts.**

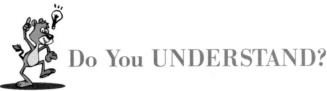

Do You UNDERSTAND?

DIRECTIONS: **Fill in the blanks to complete each of the following
statements.**

1. Hypothermia is caused by exposure to a cold environment, but it can also

   be the result of medical illnesses such as _____

   and _____.

2. The very _____ and _____ are

   especially susceptible to hypothermia.

3. With severe hypothermia, the patient may be _____,

   with a fall in _____ blood flow, _____

   blood flow, and _____ output.

4. Body temperature is regulated by the _____ and

   is carefully regulated to a _____ _____ of approximately 37° C.

5. The body is divided into _____ and _____

   thermal compartments.

6. The four mechanisms of heat loss are _____,

   _____, _____,

   and _____.

7. _____ accounts for most of the body's heat loss.

8. Mechanisms for heat production and conservation include

   _____ and _____.

9. "Wind chill" is a form of _____ heat loss.

10. Both water exposure and alcohol consumption increase the risk for

    hypothermia. Water can absorb body heat much faster and better than

    _____, and alcohol _____ reduces the

    effectiveness of the _____ and decreases

    _____ of the cold environment.

11. When treating the patient with hypothermia, gentle movement is neces-

    sary; great care must be exercised when placing central lines to prevent

    triggering _____ arrhythmias.

12. Laboratory abnormalities seen in hypothermia may include elevated

    _____ and _____ _____

    _____ as a result of hemoconcentration and

    either high or low _____ and _____.

13. Active external rewarming includes forced-air _____,

    which can add heat to both _____ and

    _____ compartments.

14. Airway assessment is always the first intervention, and supplemental

    _____ heated to _____ should be

    provided even to the mildly hypothermic patient because the oxyhe-

    moglobin dissociation curve is shifted to the _____.

Answers: 8. shivering, vasoconstriction; **9.** convective; **10.** air, vasodilates, hypothalamus, awareness;
11. ventricular; **12.** hematocrit, blood urea nitrogen, potassium, glucose; **13.** rewarming, peripheral,
core; **14.** oxygen, 40° C, left.

15. Active external rewarming may include _____ via a

    Foley catheter, NG tube, and chest tubes.

16. _____ bypass may also be needed,

    especially if the patient is in cardiac arrest as a result of hypothermia.

17. Warming of _____ fluids and administering _____

    is important to help prevent heat loss from the core compartment.

18. Complications of rewarming may include rewarming _____,

    pulmonary _____, and myo-_____.

19. CPR for the patient with hypothermia requires _____ initial

    defibrillations, but further shocks should wait until _____

    _____ is above 30° C.

20. The hypothermic patient in arrest may not respond to vasoactive

    _____. On successful resuscitation, blood levels of

    those _____ given during resuscitation can become

    _____ after rewarming because of _____

    and because a cold _____ metabolizes drugs poorly.

What IS Near Drowning?

Drowning is the third-leading cause of accidental death with 40% of victims 5 years or younger. **Drowning** is the death of a victim from suffocation by asphyxiating immersion or submersion in any fluid or liquid medium when the cause of death cannot be attributed to other lethal disorders. Over 140,000 drowning deaths occur worldwide each year with more than 8000 reported in the United States alone. Risk factors include hypothermia (refer to the discussion on hypothermia earlier in this chapter), the inability to swim, diving accidents, alcohol and drug ingestion, and exhaustion.

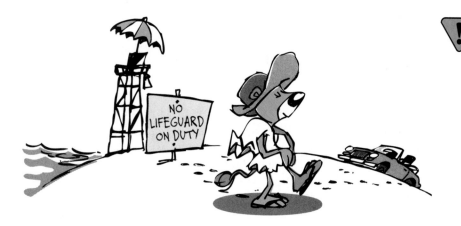

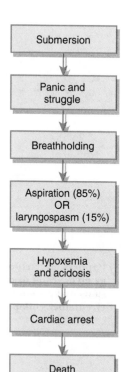

Submersion rapidly leads to hypothermia.

Submersion
↓
Panic and struggle
↓
Breathholding
↓
Aspiration (85%) OR laryngospasm (15%)
↓
Hypoxemia and acidosis
↓
Cardiac arrest
↓
Death

When the victim recovers spontaneously or is successfully resuscitated (at least temporarily) **near drowning** is said to occur. These incidences account for 50,000 annually reported cases. When cardiac BLS is initiated early, many victims of cold water immersion have a good chance of survival. After submersion in water, near drowning results from one of two main mechanisms: *dry* drowning or *wet* drowning. Dry drowning occurs after immersion in cold water; the cold water causes laryngospasm and vagal stimulation, which leads to asphyxiation, hypoxia, and cardiac arrest. Drowning and near drowning more commonly occur as a result of wet drowning. After a period of breath holding while immersed in water, the individual is forced to inhale by a reflex mechanism. Water is aspirated into the lungs along with large volumes of water that have been swallowed. Adequate gas exchange is prevented as the inhaled water obstructs the lower airways. The individual quickly becomes hypoxic, leading to unconsciousness and cardiac arrest. Immediate CPR on the victim after removal from the water is a significant factor in survival.

Difference between Near Drowning and Secondary Near Drowning

Near drowning occurs when the victim recovers spontaneously or is successfully resuscitated—at least temporarily (submersion with recovery).

Secondary near drowning is the delayed onset of respiratory insufficiency from submersion. It can occur up to 72 hours after the initial insult; therefore the victim should be taken to the hospital for observation, regardless of how he or she appears immediately after the event. Inflammatory reactions in the lung injure the alveolocapillary membrane and surfactant function. Approximately 10% to 15% of deaths associated with drowning is due to secondary drowning. Unconscious at the scene, a history of cyanosis, apnea, or the requirement of CPR are all strong markers for later deterioration. Near-drowning victims should be observed for at least 24 hours.

Vasoconstricting medications should be avoided because they will probably have minimal effect on the vasculature as a result of the ongoing vasoconstriction from the hypothermia.

TAKE HOME POINTS

- In dry drowning, little or no water enters the lower airways or lungs.
- The actual cause of death in drowning is hypoxia, secondary to asphyxiation.

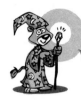

What You NEED TO KNOW

Physiologic Responses Stimulated with Drowning

Near-drowning victims exhibit symptoms that vary, depending on the length of submersion, water temperature, quality of water, associated injuries, onset of CPR, and the patient's resuscitative response.

Infrequently, near-drowning victims may be asymptomatic. Conversely, most exhibit mild dyspnea, a deathlike appearance with blue or gray coloring, apnea or tachypnea, hypotension, a heart rate as slow as four to five beats per minute or pulselessness, cold skin, dilated pupils (known as fish eyes), hypothermia, and vomiting.

Significant neurologic impairment occurs in up to 25% of near-drowning patients. Neurologic injury results from hypoxia and can lead to cerebral edema and brainstem herniation. Hypothermia is an important clinical feature in determining the outcome because it decreases the metabolic demands of the body, thereby delaying or even preventing severe cerebral hypoxia.

A common finding in near-drowning patients is acidosis. Metabolic acidosis is primarily due to tissue hypoxia, but a respiratory component may present itself after aspiration.

 Hypoxia and acidosis act as myocardial depressants and precipitate circulatory collapse.

Near Drowning Survival

Factors that increase survival include:
- Immediate, quality CPR
- Cold water 24° C (<76° F)
- Clean water
- Short immersion time
- Less struggle
- No associated injuries

Field resuscitation of the near-drowning victim is critical for survival. A significant factor in the survival of the victim after his or her removal from the water is the immediate performance of CPR.

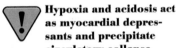 **TAKE HOME POINTS**

Excellent, prompt, field-initiated CPR, regardless of the availability of advanced life support knowledge, increases the chances for survival.

Signs and Symptoms of Pulmonary Failure

Pulmonary failure is common after drowning unless aspiration is prevented by laryngospasms. Two mechanisms that may cause pulmonary failure are fresh-water and salt-water aspiration. Fresh-water aspiration causes pulmonary damage because of washout of surfactant and reflex mechanisms that cause increased airway resistance. Salt-water aspiration causes pulmonary damage via an osmotic gradient, leading to shifts of protein-rich fluid into the alveoli. The fluid shifts caused by both types of aspiration generally do not cause significant severe electrolyte imbalances. Water contaminates add to the damage from either type of aspiration. Particulate material such as sand or mud, gastric contents, chemical irritants, or microorganisms may be aspirated along with water and result in pneumonia.

CNS damage caused by cerebral hypoxia occurs in 12% to 27% of survivors. Cold water temperatures can lower brain temperatures to protective levels before cardiac arrest occurs. No adjuvant therapies have been proven to be effective. Victims of cold water immersion may appear dead. If the victim has been submersed for less than 1 hour, resuscitation is indicated until the core temperature is >30° C.

FIRST-LINE AND INITIAL TREATMENT FOR THE NEAR-DROWNING PATIENT

- Maintain the patient's ABCs.
- Assess for possible ventilator support (even when the chest x-ray film is clear).

Near-Drowning Problems and Potential Problems

SYSTEM	PROBLEM
Cardiac	Primary cardiac problems (unusual) Myocardial depression Arrhythmias (bradycardia or atrial fibrillation)
Neurologic	Neuronal tissue damage Cerebral hypoxia or brain tissue acidosis Cerebral edema
Renal	Acute tubular necrosis Renal failure Hemoglobinuria Myoglobinuria
Gastrointestinal	Distended abdomen Vomiting during resuscitation
Metabolic	Acidosis Rare electrolyte changes
Hematologic	Rarely affected

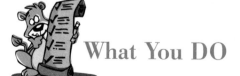

What You DO

Prompt resuscitation is the key. The following identifies the treatment for the near-drowning victim.

For a more detailed listing of the management of the near-drowning victim see the table on page 106.

Complications associated with near drowning are the direct cause of the hypoxic event. Primary complications affect the pulmonary, cerebral, and cardiovascular systems, including pulmonary edema, pneumonitis, ARDS, anoxic

TAKE HOME POINTS

Laryngospasms occur in 10% to 20% of drowning victims.

Cervical spinal cord injuries from diving accidents are common and should be assessed.

TAKE HOME POINTS

- Shock is uncommon in near drowning; if present, a prompt search for other causes should be initiated.
- No preventative prophylactic antibiotics are needed.

TAKE HOME POINTS

- Cardiac arrhythmias are usually secondary to hypothermia, acidosis, or hypoxemia.
- Cerebral hypoxia causes the neurologic damage.
- Renal function is usually normal after a submersion event. However, problems can arise.

encephalopathy, and cardiopulmonary arrest. Later complications include cerebral edema, disseminated intravascular coagulation (DIC), acute tubular necrosis, and renal failure.

TREATMENT FOR THE NEAR-DROWNING VICTIM

Before the Emergency Department
- Monitor the patient's ABCs (cervical spine precautions).
- Initiate CPR.
- Establish IV access.
- Correct hypoxia.
- Correct acidosis.
- Correct hypotension.
- Transport victim to nearest hospital.

In the Emergency Department
- Monitor the patient's ABCs (cervical spine precautions).
- Initiate monitoring (cardiac and pulse oximeter).
- Provide rewarming therapy.
- Determine duration of submersion.
- Remove wet clothing; wrap in dry blankets.
- Provide aggressive rewarming efforts if core temperatures fall below 32° C (90° F).
- Gently handle patient to prevent arrhythmias.
- Anticipate profound neurologic changes.
- Monitor ICP (hyperventilation, administer diuretics and barbiturates.
- Monitor hypoxic seizures (oxygen, ventilation, administer diazepam, phenytoin).

ABCs, Airway, breathing, circulation; *CPR,* cardiopulmonary resuscitation; *IV,* intravenous; *ICP,* intracranial pressure.

TAKE HOME POINTS

Early rewarming is fundamental to the prevention of ventricular fibrillation.

⚠ • **Do not attempt to rewarm the victim at the scene unless the hospital is less than 15 minutes away.**
• **The heart is resistant to drug therapy and electroconversion when the core temperature is lower than 30° C (86° F).**

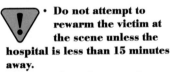

Do You UNDERSTAND?

DIRECTIONS: **Fill in the blanks to complete the following statements.**

1. When the victim is submersed but has been recovered and resuscitated, it

   is said that he or she has experienced _____ drowning.

2. In determining the outcome of the victim, _____ is an

   important finding and indicates that the metabolic demands of the body

   have been lowered and that possibly cerebral hypoxia has been prevented.

Answers: 1. near; 2. hypothermia.

3. Unless aspiration of water is prevented by laryngospasms, _____ failure is common.

4. Usually _____ is not a symptom of near drowning; if present, the cause must be identified and promptly treated.

5. Prompt _____ is the key when treating a near-drowning victim.

6. _____ changes should be anticipated when resuscitating and treating a near-drowning victim.

What IS Overdose?

Various situations require emergent and critical care for patients. Among these is the presentation of a patient with a drug overdose. Intentional drug overdoses are the most common reported method for attempted suicide. Treatment for these patients includes stabilization, reducing further drug absorption, eliminating the drugs from the body, and ongoing monitoring as conditions warrant.

A drug overdose can be a life-threatening situation, resulting in serious long-term consequences and even death. Overdose is defined as the accidental or intentional use of an illegal drug or legal medicine in an amount that is higher than prescribed. Any drug or medication has the potential to cause an overdose. The legally, as well as the illegally, obtained drugs can be lethal when improperly used. The patient with a possible drug overdose requires emergent care and can be a challenge for the health care provider. A drug overdose can result in multisystem involvement that dictates the need for immediate attention to avoid further complications.

Of additional concern when dealing with an overdose is determining whether the consumption was accidental or an attempt to commit suicide. Until this issue is resolved, patients must be closely monitored to ensure no further attempts at self harm are made, if indeed this was the intention. Stabilizing the patient's physical condition is the first and most crucial treatment step.

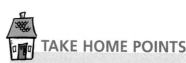

TAKE HOME POINTS

All drugs, whether prescribed by a physician, purchased over the counter, or purchased "on the street," have the potential for detrimental outcomes.

Answers: 3. pulmonary; 4. shock; 5. resuscitation; 6. Neurologic.

What You NEED TO KNOW

The initial evaluation of a patient with a possible drug overdose includes obtaining a complete and reliable history. The goal is to identify the drug or drugs taken alone or in combination with other drugs or substances. It is important to find out what drug has been taken, what amount has been taken, and the time of the intake. Any medical and psychiatric history, current medications, allergies, and any history of drug overdose should also be obtained. Next, a thorough physical examination is performed, which provides baseline information and identifies any physical symptoms. This examination must be completed as quickly as possible because time is of the essence. The initial physical evaluation must determine whether the patient's life is in immediate danger and to identify any additional medical conditions or injuries that might become a concern while providing the necessary care for the overdose.

Obtaining a complete history may be difficult because the patient may be in a state of confusion, unconscious, or unable to provide information. In such cases, family members may be the main source for information. In other cases, the patient and family may find it embarrassing to provide information related to the addiction, or the patient may be found alone or he or she has been brought to the hospital for emergent care. In these cases, the emergency medical technicians may become the main source of information. Those providing patient information should be questioned about the circumstances in which the patient was found by asking the following questions:

- Was the patient conscious? Could he or she provide any information when initially found, including location and time?
- Were any prescription bottles present—with or without pills?
- Was any drug paraphernalia found?

As previously mentioned, a physical evaluation must be completed as quickly as possible. If the history of the patient is unattainable, the physical evaluation becomes the only means of obtaining vital information in the search to identify the drugs of the overdose and to make decisions regarding appropriate care. The initial physical evaluation should include the review of vital signs, skin, breath (odor), ears, nose, throat, lungs, heart, abdomen, extremities, and neurologic (seizures) status. Each assessment finding will help identify the actual and possible systems affected by the drug overdose and will also provide clues as to the type of drug or drugs used and how each was introduced into the system. For example, the inspection of the skin may reveal fresh needle marks.

As an additional adjunct, laboratory tests can provide valuable information. Blood can be screened for drugs in the system, and ongoing monitoring can determine how fast the drug is being eliminated from the body. Urine tests can also be used to screen for some drugs and to detect changes in body chemistry. In addition,

The older adult is at greater risk for inadvertently overdosing or underdosing medications because of diminished eyesight.

TAKE HOME POINTS

Questions help identify the drug, how much was taken, and when it was taken.

TAKE HOME POINTS

- An extensive physical examination is required because various drugs produce various symptoms.
- Common sites of IV drug entry include the arms, in between the toes, and the lower leg.

kidney and liver damage can be detected with blood and urine tests. If the evaluation eliminates the need for advanced life support efforts, supportive care becomes the choice of medical management for the patient who has overdosed.

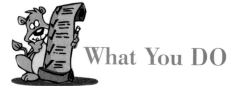

What You DO

The ideal first step is to obtain a complete history and physical evaluation; however, a critical patient requires immediate medical interventions. Assessment of the LOC is necessary to determine whether the patient is alert, arousable, or unresponsive. Sufficient ventilation and perfusion must be priorities. Airway and breathing assessment is performed to ascertain whether the patient's trachea is blocked. Correct positioning of the head (head tilt–chin lift or jaw thrust) prevents the posterior of the tongue from occluding the airway. This positioning may be all that is required to ensure that the patient can resume breathing on his or her own. Intubation may be necessary in the patient who is comatose, has lost the gag reflex, or is having seizures. Oropharyngeal airways can also assist. These airways are used in the patient who is spontaneously breathing but remains unconscious. These prevent the tongue from blocking the airway and provide for suction of secretions. Oxygen should be administered after ABGs are obtained if possible (refer to the discussion on RSI on page 42).

FIRST-LINE AND INITIAL TREATMENT FOR THE PATIENT WHO HAS OVERDOSED

- Assess responsiveness.
- Establish an airway (head tilt–chin lift position, jaw thrust, oropharyngeal airway, intubation).
- Provide oxygen.
- Check pulse. If no pulse, initiate CPR.
- Initiate cardiac monitoring.
- Establish IV access (20- or 18-gauge for an adult).
- Provide fluid replacement.
- Determine substance taken; give appropriate reversal agent.

IV lines need to be initiated as soon as possible. Fluid replacement is necessary for patients who experience drug-induced hypotension. In addition, an IV is the preferable route for administering medications. For the patient with cardiac compromise, a central venous line may also be indicated and an ECG may be ordered to assist in determining the presence of any cardiac injury. The patient's cardiac status needs to be monitored until medically cleared.

If the patient exhibits an altered mental status, a trial dose of a therapeutic reversal agent may be administered. Naloxone (Narcan), dextrose, Thiamine, and oxygen are all considered safe and innocuous agents. Glucose and Thiamine may be life-saving measures to the patient who has hypoglycemia. Thiamine is also effective in preventing Wernicke-Korsakoff syndrome, which is associated with alcohol withdrawal.

FOCUS AREAS FOR THE MANAGEMENT OF THE PATIENT EXPERIENCING AN OVERDOSE

Supportive care
Prevention of absorption
Enhancement of excretion (if possible)
Administration of an antidote (if available)

One of the more important elements in the management of the patient who has ingested an overdose is supportive care. This includes frequent monitoring of vital signs with particular focus on the temperature, which assists in identifying hypothermia or hyperthermia. It is necessary to monitor multiple systems as indicated to identify any system failure. Acute and subtle changes to the LOC must be detected quickly to avoid further complications such as aspiration. IV fluids are given for fluid maintenance and replacement or to provide forced diuresis. Frequent monitoring of ABGs are needed when using alkaline therapy or when the patient is on a ventilator. Lastly, the management of hypotension requires care based on patient needs and the drug ingested.

Most overdoses occur by way of the gastrointestinal tract. In these situations it is most important that further gastrointestinal absorption is stopped. Several methods are available to remove the drug from the gastrointestinal tract. These include emesis, gastric lavage, cathartics, and absorbents.

To induce emesis in the alert patient, the drug of choice is ipecac syrup. Ipecac is the dried root or rhizome of *Cephaelis ipecacuanha* and *C. acuminata*, plants found in Brazil and Central America. Ipecac induces emesis by acting locally in the stomach, as well as a delayed action in which stimulation of the chemoreceptor trigger zone of the CNS occurs. The adult dose of ipecac is 30 ml and should produce emesis in 20 minutes. Fluids should be encouraged after the initial dose to promote further gastric emptying. Any fluids except milk are recommended.

Gastric lavage is another method for removing gastric contents. This procedure calls for the passage of the largest tube passable through the patient's oropharynx. A 32 to 40 French orogastric tube is used for an adult. The patient is placed in a left lateral decubitus, Trendelenburg position with knees flexed. This position allows for the greatest abdominal relaxation and gastric emptying, as well as reduces the risk for aspiration should emesis occur. Gastric lavage is used when the patient is comatose, seizing, or the gag reflex is lost. In these situations the patient requires protection of the airway via intubation with a cuffed ETT. Intubation is not required if the patient demonstrates the presence of the gag reflex. Confirmation of proper tube placement is obtained before lavage and via an x-ray film. Tap water or saline, typically 10 to 20 L, is induced into the stomach. The solution may be warmed, which hastens the dissolution of pills that remain in the stomach. The solution is then emptied from the stomach by

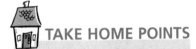

TAKE HOME POINTS

Milk causes a delay of emesis when ipecac has been administered.

⚠ Ipecac should not be given to patients who have overdosed on tricyclic antidepressants, theophylline, or drugs that cause major changes in mental status. Ipecac should never be given to the unconscious patient because of the risk of choking and aspiration.

way of lowering the tube to the floor and siphoning off the fluid or suctioning, which is known as *stomach pumping*. The patient is lavaged until the return is clear. The ingestion of a large number of pills or capsules in a short period can result in the formation of concretions, which provide ongoing absorption of the drug. Massaging the left upper quadrant may be used to remove existing or potential concretions. Gastric lavage is generally most effective if administered within 1 hour of ingestion. However, because of the delayed gastric emptying of some drugs, it can be effective hours after ingestion.

The use of ipecac and lavage is not without complications. These include laryngospasm, cyanosis, gastric erosion, esophageal tears, and worst of all, mediastinitis. Although rare, these possible complications cause concern. The use of ipecac and lavage are contraindicated when a caustic substance is ingested.

Ipecac and lavage are typically not used alone because of the low return and may not totally clear the stomach. As a means to decrease further drug absorption, activated charcoal and a cathartic are administered. Absorbents provide the means for decreasing any further absorption of the involved overdose drug into the system. Activated charcoal and cathartics are used for this purpose. Activated charcoal plays a major role in the treatment of the overdose patient. Activated charcoal is a residue of destructive distillation of burned organic materials such as wood, pulp, paper, bone, and sawdust—just to name a few. Heating with CO_2, which increases the surface binding area and in turn increases the absorption ability of the materials, activates the charcoal. Activated charcoal is a fine, black powder with a gritty consistency that is tasteless and odorless. It is mixed with 60 to 90 ml water to make a slurry mixture. Between 30 to 100 g for an adult is then induced into the stomach by way of an NG or lavage tube. It can be administered orally if the patient is alert and cooperative. The recommended dose for an adult is 50 to 100 mg mixed in 8 ounces of water. Major prevention of further drug absorption occurs the sooner the activated charcoal is given after ingestion of the drug. No identifiable contraindications exist, but patients with ileus who have repeated charcoal doses are predisposed to vomiting. Vomiting has been documented in 10% to 15% of patients who are given charcoal alone.

Cathartics are administered as a means of eliminating drugs from the gastrointestinal tract, as well as assisting with the passage of charcoal. They decrease the gastrointestinal transit time of the drug, thus decreasing the possibility for absorption. The cathartics include the following agents: sorbitol, magnesium sulfate (Epsom salt), magnesium citrate, sodium sulfate (Glauber's solution), and disodium phosphate (Fleet enema). The fastest and most potent cathartic is the osmotic agent, sorbitol. Magnesium sulfate and magnesium citrate and hypertonic saline agents are slower acting, and magnesium levels need to be monitored. These agents should be avoided in patients with salt-intake restrictions and in those with a history of heart failure.

Multiple methods can be used to enhance the excretion of drugs from the body. These methods include forced diuresis, alteration of urine pH, hemodialysis and hemoperfusion. Each has limited use and is instituted when an antidote is not available.

Disodium phosphate (Fleet enema) must be used cautiously in children because of anatomic and physiologic factors. Absorption of the drug is dependent on the anatomic care of the rectum. Medications administered in the lower portion of the rectum will bypass the liver circulation and metabolism. In addition, caution must be taken regarding possible fluid and electrolyte shifts that occur when an enema is administered.

TAKE HOME POINTS

- Peritoneal dialysis should not be used as the mode of dialysis because it is inefficient, and most overdose substances bind to plasma proteins.
- Hemodialysis is effective and essential in overdose cases with methanol, ethylene glycol, and salicylates.

Forced diuresis involves the flow of urine at the rate of 3 to 5 ml/kg/hr, which may require a diuretic. This process should only be used when specifically indicated, such as an overdose with phenobarbital, bromides, lithium, salicylate, and amphetamines. It is not used frequently because of complications such as volume overload or electrolyte disturbances.

Alteration in urine pH involves the concept of ion trapping. Rapid movement across membranes is enhanced with low degrees of ionization and high-lipid solubility. Weak acids will be ionized in a more alkaline medium, and weak bases will be ionized in a more acidic medium. If a pH difference exists across the membrane, then ion trapping occurs. More total drug will exist in the compartment where ionization is greater because the nonionized form crosses the lipid cellular membrane more readily than does the ionized form.

Hemodialysis and *hemoperfusion* can be valuable adjuncts to treatment, though many drugs such as diazepam (Valium), digoxin (Lanoxin), and phenytoin (Dilantin) are not well removed with these invasive and complicated procedures. Similarities between hemoperfusion and hemodialysis exist. Both call for an extracorporeal means through which blood is passed. Hemoperfusion requires the blood to be delivered through a cartridge that contains an absorbent such as activated charcoal. The blood is then returned to venous circulation. Hemodialysis is similar except the blood is sent through a dialyzer, which helps separate diffusible substances from other less diffusible substances.

It is important to know that some patients that come to the emergency department with an overdose may respond to the administration of an antidote. Antidotes are divided into physiologic and specific. General or supportive antidotes are also available. General or supportive antidotes are not true antidotes but assist in treating overdose symptoms and include activated charcoal and sodium bicarbonate. Although numerous treatments are available, the following table lists the basic rules of supportive care that need to be instituted for all patients with a possible overdose.

Drug Antidotes and Antagonists

DRUG	ANTAGONIST	DOSE
Acetaminophen (Tylenol)	Acetylcysteine (N-acetylcysteine)	Oral solution (5%) Adult loading dose 140 mg/kg, followed by maintenance dose 70 mg/kg, q4h, for 17 additional doses
Opioids	Nalmefene (Revex)	Administered IV, IM, SQ, titrated individually
	Naloxone (Narcan)	Administered IV, IM, SQ Adults 0.4-2.0 mg
	Naltrexone (Revia)	Administered orally 50 mg/day or 100 qod

IV, Intravenously; *IM*, intramuscularly; *SQ*, subcutaneously; *q4h*, every 4 hours; *qod*, every other day.

Common Overdose Drugs and their Symptoms

As previously mentioned, all drugs have the potential to be an agent of overdose. Accidental or intentional drug overdoses can result from drugs commonly prescribed, bought over the counter, or purchased on the street. Various symptoms of overdose are present, depending on the type of drug ingested. The following table lists some drugs commonly seen in overdose situations.

Common Drugs and the Symptoms of Overdose and Treatment

DRUG	SYMPTOMS OF OVERDOSE	TREATMENT
Anticholinergics (Atropine, scopolamine, belladonna, antihistamine, antidepressants, antipsychotics, OTC cough and cold medicines)	• Increased respirations • Increased or decreased BP • Increased heart rate (dysrhythmias) • Dry, hot skin and membranes • Dilated pupils • Decreased bowel sounds • Urinary retention • Seizures	Supportive care
Acetaminophen (Tylenol)	• Immediate symptoms: nausea, vomiting, diaphoresis, anorexia, fatigue, paleness • Advanced symptoms: nausea, vomiting, jaundice, right upper quadrant pain, lethargy, coma, bleeding, hypoglycemia, renal failure	Gastric lavage Administration of antidote (N-Acetylcysteine, Naloxone, Nalmefene, methadone) Supportive care
Salicylates (aspirin, muscle and joint pain creams)	• Increased respirations, respiratory alkalosis, hyperventilation • Nausea, vomiting, diaphoresis, gastrointestinal discomfort • Confusion, lethargy, seizures, tinnitus, irritability • Cardiovascular failure, increased heart rate, metabolic acidosis	Gastric lavage Activated charcoal Forced diuresis Supportive care
CNS stimulants (amphetamines, cocaine, methylphenidate)	• Increased heart rate, dysrhythmias, myocardial infarction, cardiac arrest, increased BP • Stroke, seizures, behavioral changes, headache	Gastric lavage Activated charcoal Supportive care

OTC, Over the counter; *CNS,* central nervous system; *LSD,* lysergic acid diethylamide; *MCMA,* methylenedioxymethamphetamine; *PCP,* phencyclidine; *BP,* blood pressure.

Continued

Common Drugs and the Symptoms of Overdose and Treatment—cont'd

DRUG	SYMPTOMS OF OVERDOSE	TREATMENT
CNS depressants (sedatives, Choral hydrate, Meprobamate) hypnotics) Benzodiazepines (Xanax, Ativan, Valium, Klonopin)	• Decreased BP, decreased heart rate, cardiac arrest • Decreased respirations, respiratory arrest • Drowsiness, stupor, coma	Gastric lavage Activated charcoal Forced diuresis Dialysis Hemoperfusion Supportive care
Barbiturates (phenobarbital, Nembutal, secobarbital)	• Decreased heart rate, decreased BP • Decreased respirations, respiratory depression, pulmonary edema	Gastric lavage Administration of antidote (Naloxone) Supportive care
Narcotics and opioids (morphine, codeine, heroin, Percocet, methadone, clonidine, Lomotil)	• Decreased level of consciousness, pinpoint pupils	
Hallucinogens (LSD, MDMA [also known as Ecstasy], PCP)	• Increased heart rate, increased BP • Hyperreflexia • Stupor, coma (PCP)	Gastric lavage Activated charcoal Supportive care
Alcohol (Ethanol)	• Neurologic—visual impairment, headache, poor coordination, stupor • Cardiac—increased heart rate, cardiac collapse • Respirations—decreased respirations • Gastrointestinal—nausea, vomiting, abdominal pain, hypoglycemia	Gastric lavage Supportive care

OTC, Over the counter; *CNS,* central nervous system; *LSD,* lysergic acid diethylamide; *MCMA,* methylenedioxymethamphetamine; *PCP,* phencyclidine; *BP,* blood pressure.

Special Considerations

Once the overdose patient has been medically stabilized, the decision must be made whether ongoing observation is needed. Complications from treatments may require ongoing observation. The patient who experiences a drug overdose may require hospitalization for numerous reasons. In addition, those who have additional medical problems outside of the overdose may also require continued hospitalization. Finally, some drugs such as acetaminophen have a latent phase. In 24 to 72 hours, the patient who appears to be doing well may begin to decompensate.

Drug withdrawal may necessitate the need for ongoing hospital observation. Withdrawal from some drugs can be life threatening and require medical management (see the following table for a listing of drugs and signs of withdrawal). Once the patient has been through withdrawal, follow-up care such as rehabilitation should be obtained.

Patients who intentionally overdose will require close monitoring while in the emergency department. Suicide precautions such as active listening and effective communication should be initiated to avoid further attempts. Depressed patients, those who have suicidal thoughts, and those who have attempted suicide in the past are at high risk for overdose. All patients who have overdosed should receive a psychiatric clearance before being discharged from the hospital.

Drug Withdrawal Syndromes

DRUGS	WITHDRAWAL SIGNS AND SYMPTOMS
CNS stimulants	Muscular aches, abdominal pain, chills, tremors, hunger, anxiety, prolonged sleep, lack of energy, profound depression, suicidal, exhaustion
CNS depressants	Dilated pupils, rapid pulse, gooseflesh, lacrimation, abdominal cramps, muscle jerks, "flu" syndrome, vomiting, diarrhea, tremors, yawning, anxiety

CNS, Central nervous system.

Do You UNDERSTAND?

DIRECTIONS: **Identify the following statements as *true* (T) or *false* (F).**

_____ 1. Physician-prescribed medications cannot produce drug overdoses.

_____ 2. The primary goal when dealing with an overdose patient is physical stabilization.

_____ 3. The four areas of focus for managing the overdose patient is providing supportive care, preventing absorption, enhancing excretion, and administering antidotes.

_____ 4. Activated charcoal and cathartics are used to enhance excretion.

_____ 5. Drug withdrawal may require ongoing hospitalization for the patient treated for a drug overdose.

Cardiovascular System

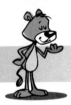

What IS Angina?

Angina pectoris literally translates as pain in the chest. This symptom occurs as a result of myocardial ischemia. Anginal chest pain is transient, lasting only 3 to 5 minutes and is usually relieved whenever the precipitating event is discontinued or nitroglycerin is administered. The most common cause of angina is preexisting cardiovascular disease, which narrows or occludes the arteries that feed the heart muscle. Numerous disorders occur along the pathophysiologic continuum of cardiovascular disease; these include atherosclerosis, angina, cerebrovascular accident, myocardial infarction (MI), and heart failure.

What You NEED TO KNOW

TAKE HOME POINTS

The four major risk factors for CAD are hyperlipidemia, hypertension, smoking, and physical inactivity.

Atherosclerosis and *coronary artery disease* (CAD) are synonymous terms used to describe fatty deposits that harden in the arteries over time. Because CAD is the primary cause of angina pectoris, the risk factors for both are thus inextricably intertwined. A long list of risk factors has been identified and categorized as either modifiable or unmodifiable. Although modifiable risks can be altered by individuals attempting to decrease their risk of CAD, unmodifiable risks cannot.

Atherosclerosis

Atherosclerosis is the primary cause of angina. Atherosclerosis describes plaque formation within the intimal (innermost) lining of the artery, which occurs as a result of complex interactions among various components in the blood and the vascular wall itself. Initially, the endothelial lining of the artery becomes injured either by chemical irritation, such as hyperlipidemia (nondenuding), or by

Coronary Artery Disease Risk Factors

UNMODIFIABLE	MODIFIABLE
• Age • Gender • Race • Genetic inheritance	• Elevated serum lipids • Hypertension • Smoking • Sedentary lifestyle • Diabetes • Obesity • Heavy alcohol consumption • Psychologic factors

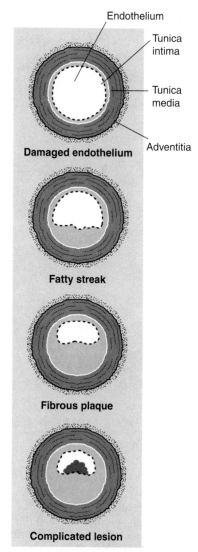

Damaged endothelium

Endothelium
Tunica intima
Tunica media
Adventitia

Fatty streak

Fibrous plaque

Complicated lesion

mechanical irritation, such as hypertension (denuding). This tissue injury activates platelets, causing the release of a substance called *growth factor*, which in turn stimulates smooth muscle, fibroblasts, and collagen proliferation at the site. Lipids, cholesterol, leukocytes, and other cellular waste products accumulate at these injury sites and become calcified over time. Eventually, the raised, damaged site causes a narrowing of the arterial lumen. Further, platelets easily adhere to the lesion because the area is rough with jagged edges, which can further decrease the lumen size, leading to partial or even complete arterial obstruction. The following illustration shows the progression of atherosclerosis from damaged endothelium through to the development of a complicated lesion.

Angina Pectoris

The coronary arteries, which arise from the ascending aorta immediately on exiting the heart, normally supply the myocardium with adequate oxygen and nutrient-rich blood to meet metabolic demands. In the atherosclerotic heart, arteries are chronically dilated beyond narrowed or partially obstructed areas to meet the heart's metabolic demands at rest. Thus when the myocardium requires more oxygen during times of increased work, the coronary arteries cannot increase flow because they are already maximally dilated. An oxygen deficit is created as a result of the oxygen supply being less than the cellular demands.

The oxygen imbalance created with angina can be quite precarious, and many factors can adversely affect this relationship. The demand for oxygen is increased whenever any one of the following is increased: heart rate, afterload (hypertension), wall tension (ventricular volume or pressure), myocardial wall thickness (hypertrophy), or contractility. All of these factors make the heart work harder. Conversely, the oxygen supply is decreased whenever any of the following occur: hypotension (decreased blood volume or hemorrhage), anemia, respiratory insufficiency, or tachycardia, which allows minimal time for diastolic filling.

In the absence of adequate oxygen and glucose, cellular metabolism shifts from the efficient oxidative phosphorylation, which yields a large amount of adenosine triphosphate (ATP) to the inefficient glycolysis; this action not only yields a very small amount of ATP but it also produces lactic acid as a by-product. This acidic environment activates chemical nociceptors, which

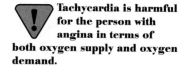 Tachycardia is harmful for the person with angina in terms of both oxygen supply and oxygen demand.

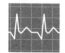 A blood pressure (BP) level that is too high or low is dangerous; therefore monitoring and carefully regulating BP is necessary.

transmit pain impulses to the brain, and the individual experiences chest pain. At this point, the damage is reversible; in other words, if the flow of oxygen and glucose-rich blood is restored, no permanent damage results. However, if the oxygen deficit continues and the lactic acid is allowed to build up, cellular metabolism and function can be altered to the point of irreversible cell death or MI. (Refer to the discussion on MI on page 127 later in this chapter.)

TYPES OF ANGINA

Stable angina is sometimes referred to as *classic* or *exertional* angina. The primary differentiating factor about this type of angina is that it is predictable and occurs intermittently over an extended period. It occurs with the same pattern of onset, duration, and intensity each time. Further, the same precipitating activity (most often physical in nature) usually brings on stable angina. The pain is relieved either when the precipitating event is discontinued or when nitroglycerin is administered in the prescribed fashion. If the pain is unrelieved by either rest or nitroglycerin, the patient may then be at risk for an MI. As previously discussed, stable angina is a result of atherosclerotic plaque that has narrowed the arteries. The chronically dilated vessel is unable to dilate further to meet metabolic demands.

Unstable angina is known by a variety of other names: *progressive*, *crescendo*, and *preinfarction angina* or *acute coronary insufficiency* Unstable angina is potentially life threatening because it signifies advanced ischemic heart disease. This type of angina is most often unpredictable. Moreover, unstable angina attacks tend to occur with increasing frequency, intensity, and duration. No precipitating event is necessary. In fact, these attacks are often brought on at times of complete rest. An individual previously diagnosed with stable angina can progress to unstable angina; alternatively, unstable angina may be the first clinical manifestation in an individual with CAD.

Prinzmetal's angina, the least common type of angina, is also known as *variant angina*. It is unpredictable in onset, duration, and intensity and occurs almost exclusively at rest. Vasospasm of one or more of the major coronary arteries is the underlying cause, which can occur with or without associated atherosclerosis.

CLINICAL MANIFESTATIONS OF ANGINA

The cardinal symptom of angina is chest pain or discomfort. However, many patients describe feeling vague sensations of discomfort, tightness, pressure, heaviness, aching, or squeezing. Others complain of heartburn or indigestion during an attack. The most common location is substernal; however, the pain or discomfort may radiate to the neck, jaw, back, shoulders, left arm, or occasionally the right arm.

When asked to demonstrate or point to the location of the pain, typically patients will clench one or two fists over the substernal region when experiencing myocardial ischemia. This display is known as a positive *Levine's sign*; although not solely diagnostic, this sign can help contribute to the diagnosis. Other associated signs and symptoms include pallor, diaphoresis, cold skin, shortness of breath (SOB), weakness, dizziness, anxiety, and feelings of impending doom.

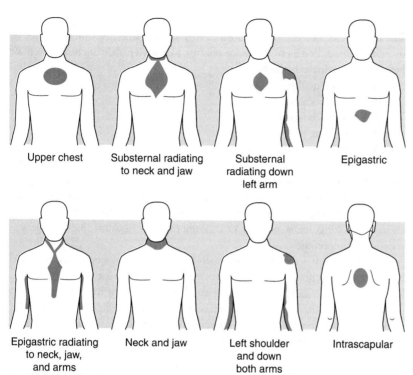

Upper chest   Substernal radiating to neck and jaw   Substernal radiating down left arm   Epigastric

Epigastric radiating to neck, jaw, and arms   Neck and jaw   Left shoulder and down both arms   Intrascapular

> **Many individuals are now recognized as having atypical ischemia, particularly women, but also individuals with diabetes and older adults.**

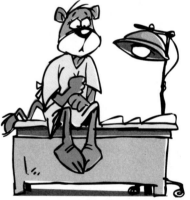

When an individual complains of chest pain, the source of the pain should always be considered cardiac until proven otherwise. However, it is prudent to consider both cardiac and noncardiac causes of chest pain as possible differentials.

Causes of Chest Pain

CARDIAC CAUSES	NONCARDIAC CAUSES
Aortic stenosis	Pneumonia
Mitral valve prolapse	Pulmonary embolism
Dissecting aortic aneurysm	Pneumothorax
Pericarditis	Anxiety or panic disorder
Hypertrophic cardiomyopathy	Pulmonary hypertension
Pericardial tamponade	Lung cancer
	Herpes zoster
	Blunt or penetrating chest trauma
	Gastroesophageal disorders
	Musculoskeletal disorders

DIAGNOSIS OF ANGINA

The importance of a thorough health history and physical assessment cannot be overemphasized. Pertinent questions relating to every episode of chest pain must be asked. They include the following:

- What is the quality of the pain?
- Where is it located?
- What is the duration?
- Does anything relieve the pain?
- Did any precipitating event lead to the onset of the pain?

Any factor that increases the workload of the heart and therefore oxygen consumption of the heart can be a precipitating event that can result in anginal pain. Consequently, questions about specific events such as physical exertion, strong emotions, consumption of a heavy meal, exposure to temperature extremes, cigarette smoking, sexual activity, or consumption of stimulants like caffeine and cocaine are important.

When myocardial ischemia is a possibility, the physical examination should be focused, beginning with the patient's vital signs, pulse oximetry, and general appearance. Is the patient in any apparent distress? Is his or her skin cold, pale, or clammy? Any alteration in orientation or mental status must be assessed. The chest wall should be examined and auscultated for both heart and lung sounds. Extra heart sounds such as an S3 or S4 gallop may be present during an ischemic attack. The carotid arteries must be assessed for bruits and the jugular veins for distention. In addition, the extremities should be assessed for the presence of pulses and edema. An abdominal examination must be performed. Because the clinical presentation of angina can be similar to that attributable to many other causes, much of the physical assessment is designed to exclude other causes of chest pain rather than diagnose the cause as ischemia.

Although many patients with angina have nondiagnostic electrocardiographic (ECG) tracings, this tool remains the "gold standard" for a first-line, noninvasive tool for diagnosing myocardial ischemia. However, because many individuals have a normal ECG in the absence of an angina attack, importantly this tool is only helpful to the diagnostic process during such an attack.

As with any disease process, the clinical presentation is never identical in all patients. Likewise, it must be realized that not all ECG tracings during an anginal attack are identical. However, the most common ECG alterations are those presented in the illustrations on the following page.

Subendocardial ischemia is typically seen as ST segment depressions or T wave inversions, transmural ischemia. Prinzmetal's angina, in contrast, is usually seen as ST segment elevation.

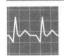
A 12-lead ECG can assist in identifying the area of the heart that is ischemic, injured, or necrotic.

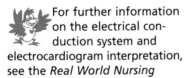
For further information on the electrical conduction system and electrocardiogram interpretation, see the *Real World Nursing Survival Guide: ECGs & the Heart.*

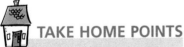
TAKE HOME POINTS

Anginal episodes can occur without any changes in the ECG tracing.

Normal ECG deflections

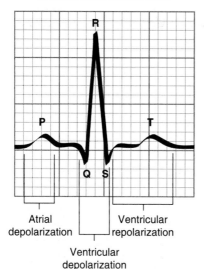

Atrial depolarization

Ventricular repolarization

Ventricular depolarization

ST segment depression

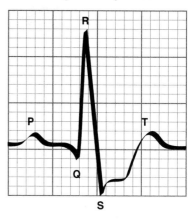

T wave inversion

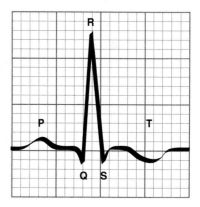

Frequently, a chest x-ray film is reviewed to look for cardiac enlargement, cardiac calcifications, and pulmonary congestion. In addition, serum lipids are drawn to determine a positive coronary risk factor, and cardiac enzyme levels are collected to rule out the possibility of an infarction. Other commonly used but more invasive studies that confirm the diagnosis of angina, especially in the presence of a nondiagnostic ECG or vague clinical picture, include ECG stress tests, nuclear imaging, positron emission tomography (PET), coronary angiography, and stress echocardiograms.

What You DO

With the underlying pathologic imbalance between myocardial oxygen supply and demand in mind, as well as the dangerous potential for thrombus formation, it is easy to not only ascertain the primary goals of anginal treatment but to also understand how the pharmacologic interventions routinely used help achieve these goals. Commonly prescribed antianginal drugs include nitrates, beta-adrenergic blocking agents, and calcium channel blockers. The use of antiplatelet drug therapy is increasingly becoming a standard of care in the pharmacologic management of angina, particularly if unstable. Some of the drugs used in this category are aspirin, dipyridamole (Persantine), sulfinpyrazone (Anturan), or clopidogrel (Plavix). In addition, morphine sulfate is frequently prescribed to not only alleviate chest pain but also to help allay anxiety. Further, morphine has the added benefit of dilating coronary arteries, which improves oxygen delivery to the myocardium.

ST segment elevation

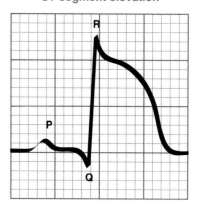

Pharmacologic Interventions to Treat Angina

MEDICATION	ACTION	EFFECT
Nitroglycerin (Tridil)	Predominantly dilates veins	Reduces preload Reduces ventricular wall tension Reduces myocardial oxygen demands
	Dilates peripheral arteries	Reduces afterload Decreases oxygen demand
	Dilates coronary arteries	Increases blood supply to the heart Reduces coronary artery spasm
Beta-adrenergic blocking agent Metoprolol (Lopressor) Atenolol (Tenormin) Propranolol (Inderal) Labetalol (Normodyne)	Blocks sympathetic stimulation of the beta receptors in the heart	Decreases in heart rate Decreases contractility Decreases blood pressure Reduces myocardial oxygen consumption
Calcium channel blockers Nifedipine (Procardia) Verapamil (Calan) Diltiazem (Cardizem)	Decreases the influx of calcium into cardiac cells, causing a decrease in the electrical conduction activity of the heart; smooth muscle relaxation	Reduced myocardial contractility Coronary and systemic vasodilation Reduce myocardial oxygen demands Increases myocardial blood supply Prevents coronary artery vasospasm
Antiplatelet agent Aspirin Ticlopidine (Ticlid) Clopidogrel (Plavix)	Inhibits platelet aggregation	Prevents thrombus development Prevents progression to myocardial infarction

> • **Nitroglycerin loses potency and effectiveness over time and with exposure to both heat and light. Therefore patients should be advised to keep the bottle in a cool, dark place and to replace the supply every 6 to 9 months.**
> • **Beta blockers are contraindicated in patients with atrioventricular (AV) conduction abnormalities, severe left ventricular failure, bradycardia, hypotension, insulin-dependent diabetes, or asthma.**

Nitroglycerin is most often prescribed for use during an attack of chest pain, although it can be taken prophylactically 5 to 100 minutes before an individual with stable angina begins an event that usually precipitates an attack. The standard dosing regimen is one tablet taken sublingually, which should relieve chest pain within 3 to 5 minutes. If unrelieved, the dose may be repeated every 5 minutes for a total of three doses. If the pain remains unrelieved, then the individual is advised to seek emergency medical care.

Nitroglycerin is available in several other forms: ointment, transdermal patches, and sustained-release tablets. All forms are used as maintenance therapies to prevent an attack, and the intravenous (IV) form can be used in emergency situations. The most common side effects of nitroglycerin are hypotension (especially orthostatic) and headaches.

Medical Management of Angina

When any patient complains of chest pain, certain protocols should be instituted while the diagnosis of angina is being included or excluded. Providing supplemental oxygen and IV access are always essential in addition to the ongoing physical assessment that includes frequent vital signs, a 12-lead ECG with subsequent continuous cardiac monitoring, laboratory tests, and prescribed pharmacologic therapies. In the case of new onset chest pain or that which is unrelieved with rest and nitroglycerin, anticipating the need to (1) institute antithrombolytic therapy, (2) admit the patient to the coronary care unit (CCU), and (3) provide advanced cardiac life support (ACLS) if needed are all imperative.

Depending on the extent of the disease process and the degree to which the patient is incapacitated by it, several other treatment modalities for severe atherosclerosis or angina include percutaneous transluminal coronary angioplasty (PTCA), stent placement, arthrectomy, laser angioplasty, or coronary artery bypass grafting (CABG). Although the first four procedures are typically performed in the cardiac catheterization laboratory under local anesthesia, CABG is surgically performed under general anesthesia in the surgical unit.

PTCA involves the passage of an inflatable balloon catheter into the stenotic coronary vessel, which is then dilated, resulting in compression of the atherosclerotic plaque and widening of the vessel. *Stent placement* is usually performed when a vessel that has been previously treated with PTCA is threatening to close. It involves the placement of a meshlike synthetic structure into a narrowed vessel, which then holds the walls of the vessel open. *Arthrectomy* involves the use of a rotational blade, which is guided into the narrowed vessel, and the plaque is then carefully shaved off. *Laser angioplasty* involves the use of a laser guided into the diseased vessel, which then vaporizes the areas of plaque. During a *CABG*, either a saphenous vein from the leg or the left internal mammary artery (LIMA) is harvested and then used to bypass areas of obstruction in the heart.

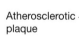

TAKE HOME POINTS

- Nitrates are unable to dilate severely atherosclerotic vessels that are already maximally dilated.
- The administration of nitroglycerin during an unstable angina attack can prevent progression to an MI or death in 51% to 72% of patients.
- For the prevention of an MI, patients are initially given at least 160 mg per day and later maintained on a daily dose of 80 to 325 mg as prescribed by their physicians.

PTCA Balloon Catheter

(compressing atherosclerotic plaque, resulting in widened blood vessel lumen)

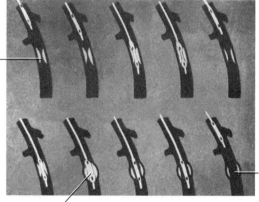

Atherosclerotic plaque

Plaque compressed

Balloon inflated

Nursing Responsibilities

In caring for the patient with angina, the focus of the nurse's role is twofold. The first priority is appropriate management of the acute attack to alleviate discomfort and, if possible, to avert untoward sequelae. The second priority is geared toward extensive education that not only empowers the patient to become an active participant in his or her well being but also imparts practical tools with which the patient can effectively manage the condition at home to achieve the highest level of wellness and independent functioning.

During an acute anginal attack, it is imperative that the nurse perform a rapid and focused physical assessment and health history. Frequent vital signs and continuous cardiac monitoring are essential parts of the ongoing assessment. The most crucial part of the assessment focuses on the current attack; emphasis must be placed on evaluating the pain itself and any precipitating events. The nurse must ask the following questions:

- How severe is the pain? *(scale of 1 to 10)*
- What does the pain feel like?
- Where is the pain? Does it move or radiate? Is it diffused or well localized?
- Did the pain start suddenly or gradually?
- How long does it last?
- How frequently does it occur?
- What makes the pain worse? What brings the pain on?
- What makes the pain better? What resolves the pain?
- Has the pain been increasingly worse with each attack?

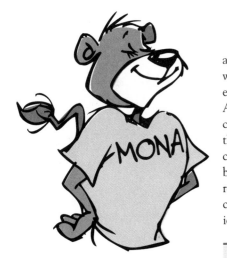

Another critical nursing function is prompt institution of prescribed medical and pharmacologic therapies such as the frequently used acronym **MONA,** which stands for **M**orphine, **O**xygen, **N**itroglycerin, and **A**spirin. Of course, it is equally imperative that the nurse evaluate the effectiveness of all interventions. Any changes in patient condition or ineffective therapies must be immediately communicated to the physician. Other nursing measures that are beneficial to the patient who is suffering an angina attack include helping the patient into a comfortable position, promoting rest and relaxation, and encouraging slow, deep breathing. It is also important for the nurse to offer calming though not false reassuring words, as well as sufficient and appropriate explanations of all medical therapies. All these nursing actions help increase comfort and decrease anxiety, both of which ultimately reduce myocardial oxygen demand.

FIRST-LINE AND INITIAL TREATMENT FOR ANGINA

- Administer pharmacologic therapy such as MONA.
- Obtain a comfortable position.
- Promote rest and relaxation.

Discharge from the hospital, especially after an episode of new-onset or accelerated chest pain, requires the nurse to perform a comprehensive level of patient teaching. Many topics need to be covered in this educational process; they include the following:

- Pathophysiologic explanation of CAD and angina
- Risk factors
- Precipitating factors
- Medicine regimen

A brief and simplistic pathophysiologic explanation is important, but it must be communicated in terms that the patient can understand. Risk factors should be discussed with emphasis on how the patient can reduce the risk of disease process progression. For example, in accordance with the attending physician's recommendations, appropriate information should be provided to encourage the following:

- Complying with blood pressure control regimen
- Ceasing smoking
- Reducing weight
- Increasing physical activity
- Lowering level of low-density lipids (LDL)
- Increasing level of high-density lipids (HDL)
- Reducing alcohol consumption
- Reducing stress
- Tightly controlling blood sugar level, if diabetic
- Adhering to dietary recommendations to decrease fat and sodium intake

The prescribed antianginal medication regimen is a vital topic. The nurse should discuss what each drug does, how it should be taken, its possible side effects, and drug interactions. Special attention must be given to teaching the patient to take nitroglycerin and the importance of seeking emergency medical attention if chest pain is unrelieved after three sublingual tablets, each taken 5 minutes apart. The nurse must also remind the patient to store the nitroglycerin in a cool, dark place, and to replace it every 6 to 9 months, regardless whether the full bottle has been used; the medication may no longer be effective. Above all, the nurse must reassure the patient that if guidelines are closely adhered to, it is possible to continue living a full and productive life.

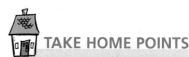

TAKE HOME POINTS

It is important to discuss possible precipitating factors and how the patient can modify his or her lifestyle to minimize the likelihood of future angina attacks.

Conclusion

Angina has a life-threatening potential in the acute scenario and may be life-limiting in the chronic situation. It is imperative to decrease or eliminate risk factors. Nurses armed with a broad knowledge base and excellent clinical skills have the potential to make a crucial difference in the lives of many people. Therefore it is imperative for every nurse to be familiar with the information contained in this chapter to ensure that appropriate and rapid interventions can be made when a patient complains of chest pain.

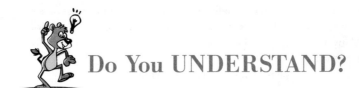

Do You UNDERSTAND?

DIRECTIONS: **Fill in the blanks to complete each of the following statements.**

1. Modifiable risk factors for cardiovascular disease include the following:

   a. _____

   b. _____

   c. _____

   d. _____

   e. _____

   f. _____

   g. _____

   h. _____

2. Unmodifiable risk factors for cardiovascular disease include the following:

   a. _____

   b. _____

   c. _____

   d. _____

Answers: 1. a. elevated serum lipids; b. hypertension; c. smoking; d. sedentary lifestyle; e. diabetes; f. obesity; g. heavy alcohol consumption; h. psychosocial factors; 2. a. age; b. sex; c. heredity; d. race.

3. The myocardial demand for oxygen is increased and the heart is forced to work harder whenever any of the following are increased:

   a. _____

   b. _____

   c. _____

   d. _____

   e. _____

4. Myocardial oxygen supply is decreased whenever any of the following occur:

   a. _____

   b. _____

   c. _____

   d. _____

5. An attack of unstable angina occurs when an unstable plaque ruptures,

   stimulating _____ _____,

   _____ _____ and

   _____ _____, any one of

   which can either partially or completely occlude the lumen of the vessel.

What IS Acute Myocardial Infarction?

As with angina, acute myocardial infarction (AMI) occurs when the heart muscle is deprived of oxygen and nutrient-rich blood. However, in the case of AMI, this deprivation occurs over a sustained period to the point at which irreversible cell

diastolic filling; 5. platelet aggregation, local vasoconstriction, thrombus formation.
or hemorrhage); b. anemia; c. respiratory insufficiency; d. tachycardia, which allows minimal time for
d. myocardial wall thickness (hypertrophy); e. contractility; 4. a. hypotension (decreased blood volume
Answers: 3. a. heart rate; b. afterload (hypertension); c. wall tension (ventricular volume or pressure);

death and necrosis take place. This deprivation leads to structural and functional changes within the affected area of myocardial tissue. As with angina, too, underlying CAD is the most common cause of AMI. With these basic similarities in mind, many components of the AMI disease process and treatment either overlap to some degree or further develop along the continuum of cardiovascular diseases.

With continued advances in medical research and pharmacologic therapies, the nurse has incredible potential for playing a crucial role to not only improve AMI survival rates but to also preserve the highest level of long-term functionality in these patients. Therefore it is absolutely essential that all nurses are able to identify quickly the signs and symptoms of AMI and then execute appropriate life-saving treatments in a rapid and systematic fashion.

What You NEED TO KNOW

Most often, atherosclerosis is the underlying cause of AMI, although in rare cases AMI has been attributed to direct trauma or electrocution. However, it is not clear whether some degree of undiagnosed atherosclerosis actually existed in these cases. Nonetheless, when AMI occurs because of CAD, the offending incident is usually a thromboembolic occlusion of one or more coronary vessels.

In the presence of atherosclerotic plaques, particularly during the more advanced stages, myocardial blood supply is already compromised. In these instances where myocardial reserve is extremely limited, any event that increases the workload of the heart or further impairs the blood supply to the heart places the individual at increased risk for suffering ischemic cardiac changes. The situation is one of simple supply and demand: a demand that outweighs the supply will result in myocardial ischemia and possibly even infarction. Circumstances that cause an imbalance in supply and demand can be called precipitating factors; the following are examples:

- Physical exertion
- Emotional stress
- Weather extremes
- Digestion of a heavy meal
- Valsalva maneuver
- Hot baths or showers
- Sexual excitation
- Pathophysiologic characteristics

As previously discussed, when an individual has CAD, the danger that an area of plaque will rupture at any time is present. This event can lead to two disastrous consequences. A piece of plaque can completely detach and become an embolus that can easily obstruct blood flow in any of the coronary vasculature. Alternatively, even if the plaque does not become an embolus, the irregular surface of this area of damaged endothelium causes platelet aggregation and fibrin deposits, which lead to thrombus formation; partial or total occlusion of the artery will occur—sooner or later. The area of myocardium served by this coronary artery branch is then subjected to a lack of perfusion.

Because insufficient oxygen is available for oxidative phosphorylation to take place, the cells engage in anaerobic metabolism during infarction in an attempt to survive. Lactic acid, a deleterious by-product of anaerobic metabolism, accumulates rapidly within the myocardium and inhibits normal enzyme physiologic activity. Enzymes, which are essential for intracellular function, cease to work in a low pH environment as created by the presence of lactic acid. In addition, the necessary reserves of ATP are exhausted within minutes and the myocardium is unable even to sustain anaerobic respiration. Without ATP, the transmembrane pump fails to work, resulting in free movement of ions across the plasma membrane. The most crucial effect of this ionic movement is the change in membrane potential as sodium moves into the cell and potassium moves out. This change ultimately inhibits the conduction of electrical impulses and thus myocardium contractility. Further, because water follows sodium into the cell, swelling occurs.

Cardiac cells can withstand ischemic conditions for approximately 20 minutes before irreversible cellular death begins. If these ischemic changes are not reversed, then water continues to move into the cytoplasm, eventually causing structural and functional changes, including lysosomal and mitochondrial swelling. Hydrolytic lysosomal enzyme contents spill out when the lysosomal membranes rupture, which causes cellular autodigestion, including the disruption of organelles and genetic material. Eventually, contractile function of the heart stops in the areas of necrosis and the heart is no longer able to pump effectively, which results in a failure to meet adequately the metabolic needs of the body.

Cellular necrosis causes the release of endogenous catecholamines and also activates the body's inflammatory process. The increase in circulating epinephrine and norepinephrine levels stimulates glycogenolysis and lipolysis, which causes a surge in plasma concentrations of glucose and free-fatty acids. In an attempt to heal the injured cells, the inflammatory process initiates the release of leukocytes, which infiltrate the area. These neutrophils and macrophages begin the process of phagocytosis to degrade and remove the necrotic tissue. When this process is completed, a collagen matrix is laid down, which eventually forms scar tissue. Although the scar tissue is strong, it is unable to contract and relax like healthy cardiac muscle, which can lead to ventricular dysfunction or pump failure.

Determining the Severity of Acute Myocardial Infarction

The degree of altered function depends on the specific area of the heart involved, the presence of collateral circulation, and both the size and the duration of the infarction. When describing infarctions in terms of the location of occurrence, the following terms are used: anterior, inferior, lateral, or posterior wall. Common combinations of areas are the anterolateral or anteroseptal MI. The location and area of the infarction correlate with the part of the coronary

TAKE HOME POINTS

- Initially, when blood flow to the myocardium is prevented, ischemia ensues in the area distal to the obstruction. If blood flow is not soon restored, the ischemia progresses to infarction.
- Infarction results from sustained ischemia and is irreversible, causing cellular death and necrosis.

TAKE HOME POINTS

For a period after AMI, a pseudo-diabetic state frequently develops because of glyconeolysis.

The younger person who has a severe MI and has not had sufficient time to develop preestablished collateral circulation is often more likely to have serious impairment than an older person with the same degree of occlusion.

TAKE HOME POINTS

A transmural infarction impairs contractility to a greater extent than does a subendocardial infarction.

Myocardial cell death begins after 20 minutes of ischemia; the damage is not complete and irreversible until after 3 to 4 hours.

TAKE HOME POINTS

Cells in the ischemic area are salvageable if reperfusion therapies and inotropic support is promptly instituted.

circulation involved. For example, inferior wall infarctions are usually the result of right coronary lesions. Left circumflex artery lesions usually cause posterior or inferior AMIs. Lesions in the left anterior descending artery usually cause anterior wall infarctions. (See Color Plate 4 of coronary arteries and localization of AMI.)

The degree of preestablished collateral circulation also determines the severity of infarction. In an individual with a history of heart disease, adequate collateral circulation channels may have been established that provide the area surrounding the infarction site with sufficient blood supply.

Another AMI descriptor refers to the depth or extent of muscle affected. A transmural infarction occurs when the entire thickness of the myocardium in a region is involved, and a subendocardial infarction (nontransmural) exists when the damage has not penetrated through the entire thickness of the ventricular wall, usually only the inner one third to one half.

During the infarction process, so-called *zones* develop. The central core is the *zone of infarction and necrosis*. The tissue immediately beyond the central core is the *zone of hypoxic injury*. The outermost region is the *zone of ischemia*. The amount of tissue included in each area depends on the duration or lack of impaired perfusion. As the area of infarction grows, the degree of resulting functional impairment will also increase.

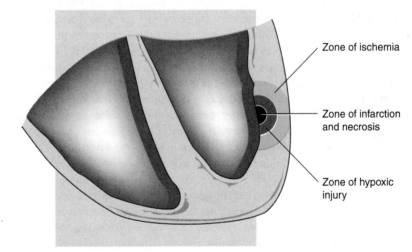

Zone of ischemia

Zone of infarction and necrosis

Zone of hypoxic injury

Clinical Manifestations of Acute Myocardial Infarction

The hallmark of AMI is severe, unrelenting chest pain. As with angina, the pain is typically described as crushing, pressure-filled, tight, constricting, or squeezing. The most common location of the pain is substernal, with radiation to the neck, jaw, or left arm. Less frequently, pain is reported in the shoulders, back, or right arm. In addition, a positive Levine's sign (one or two fists clenched over the chest area when the patient is asked to localize the pain) can contribute to the diagnosis.

The major difference in the clinical presentation of AMI compared with that of angina is the onset, severity, and duration. Chest pain associated with AMI usually has an abrupt onset and can occur during activity, rest, or even sleep. The pain described during AMI is typically more severe than anginal pain, lasting at least 20 to 30 minutes, and it is not relieved with either rest or nitroglycerin. However, not all patients will experience the same clinical presentation.

Some patients who experience cardiac ischemia or infarction can have an atypical clinical presentation, particularly women, individuals with diabetes, and older adults. In these populations, cardiac pain can go unrecognized because of diminished or altered pain perception; in fact, up to 25% of all patients may experience what is known as a *silent infarction*. Usually, individuals experiencing a silent infarction will report one or more of the *associated clinical manifestations*.

During AMI, associated clinical manifestations can range from vague sensations of "just not feeling well" to the loss of consciousness or cardiac arrest. Often the skin is cold and diaphoretic with a pale or ashen appearance, which occurs because of peripheral vasoconstriction as the body shunts blood to the vital core. The initial surge of catecholamines can contribute to a variety of signs and symptoms such as tachycardia, hypertension, anxiety, palpitations, apprehension, and feelings of impending doom. Stimulation of the medulla is mediated via vasovagal reflexes and can result in nausea and vomiting. Fever may be present secondary to the activation of the inflammatory process. As the infarction progresses and the heart's pumping ability becomes impaired, cardiac output drops. Associated with decreased cardiac output is hypotension, restlessness, dyspnea, jugular vein distention, oliguria, and confusion. On auscultation, an S3, S4, or splitting of heart sounds might be heard, which suggests ventricular dysfunction.

Complications of Acute Myocardial Infarction

AMI can result in an array of cardiac functional impairments, which can range from very mild to severe, depending on the factors previously discussed. Physiologic changes can include reduced contractility with abnormal wall motion, decreased stroke volume, altered left ventricular compliance, decreased ejection fraction, increased left ventricular end–diastolic pressure, and sinoatrial node malfunction. These impairments can lead to a variety of clinical complications such as:

- Arrhythmias (affect 90% of patients)
  - First-degree AV block
  - Second-degree AV block
  - Third-degree AV block
  - Atrial fibrillation
  - Ventricular tachycardia
  - Ventricular fibrillation
- Pericarditis
- Cardiac tamponade
- Papillary muscle rupture
- Chordae tendonae cordis rupture
- Myocardial wall rupture
- Pulmonary embolus
- Cerebrovascular accident
- Heart failure
- Pulmonary edema
- Cardiogenic shock
- Cardiac arrest
- Death

TAKE HOME POINTS

Chest pain from an AMI is unrelieved with rest.

Some patients report vague feelings of discomfort or pain that comes and goes, and some will attribute their pain to indigestion.

TAKE HOME POINTS

The conduction disturbances (arrhythmias) may be transient or chronic, and their seriousness depends on the hemodynamic consequences.

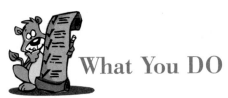

What You DO

A rapid, yet thorough and focused health history and physical assessment are instrumental in the diagnosis of AMI. The goal of the health history is to determine the presence of CAD risk factors, angina, or previous infarctions. As with angina, the physical assessment primarily focuses on the current episode of chest pain, general appearance, determination of frequent vital signs, and continuous monitoring of cardiac and pulse, as well as an ongoing evaluation of mental status, heart, lungs, abdomen, urine output, and extremities. This assessment is helpful in gauging the extent of the infarction and in guiding appropriate therapies.

In addition to the history and physical examination, a 12-lead ECG and serial cardiac enzyme studies are the current gold standard for the diagnosis of AMI. Other clinical findings that are not solely diagnostic but will help contribute to the clinical picture of AMI include fever, hyperglycemia, hyperlipidemia, elevated sedimentation rate, and leukocytosis. Additionally, a chest x-ray film may be examined for cardiac enlargement, cardiac calcifications, and pulmonary congestion. Nuclear imaging is an extremely sensitive, although invasive, diagnostic study that is commonly used to establish a diagnosis of AMI when other data are inconclusive.

Electrocardiographic Tracings

The 12-lead ECG is capable of diagnosing AMI in 80% of patients, making it an indispensable, noninvasive, and cost-effective tool. Because of the pathophysiologic manifestations previously described, the membrane potential is altered in the infarcted area of the myocardium, making it unable to depolarize and repolarize. Thus conduction abnormalities can usually be detected. Whereas routine cardiac monitors look only at the conduction system from one angle, the 12-lead ECG allows the clinician 12 views from many perspectives on the body surface, making it far superior in diagnosing AMI. Because each of the 12 leads correlates with a specific region of the myocardium, the exact location of the infarction can be determined (see Color Plate 4). Conduction abnormalities represented in the leads adjacent to the infarcted area are called *indicative changes*. Conversely, abnormalities seen in the leads opposite the infarcted area are called *reciprocal changes*, and these will be the inverse of those observed in the indicative leads.

Typically, an evolving AMI will show ST segment elevation on an ECG, which indicates acute, evolving myocardial necrosis. To confirm a diagnosis of AMI, these elevations must be greater than 1 ml and be observed in two or more contiguous leads. As AMI evolves, the development of a Q wave may be observed, which signifies further electrical abnormalities. The emergence of Q waves may be an indication of worsening ischemia and necrosis. During the healing process the ST segment gradually returns to normal, however Q waves remain unchanged.

Electrocardiographic Changes Localizing a Myocardial Infarction

LOCATION OF MI	INDICATIVE CHANGES*	RECIPROCAL CHANGES†	AFFECTED CORONARY ARTERY
Lateral	I, aVL, V_5, V_6	V_1-V_3	Left coronary artery—circumflex branch
Inferior	II, III, aVF	I, aVL	Right coronary artery—posterior descending branch
Septum	V_1, V_2	None	Left coronary artery—left anterior descending artery, septal branch
Anterior	V_3, V_4	II, III, aVF	Left coronary artery—left anterior descending artery, diagonal branch
Posterior	Not visualized	V_1, V_2, V_3, V_4	Right coronary artery or left circumflex artery
Right ventricle	V_1R-V_6R		Right coronary artery—proximal branches

*Leads facing affected areas.
†Leads opposite affected areas.

Aehlert B: *ECGs made easy,* ed 2, St Louis, 2002, Mosby.

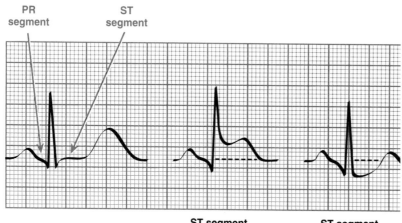

PR segment   ST segment

ST segment elevation   ST segment depression

Anteroseptal Acute Myocardial Infarction

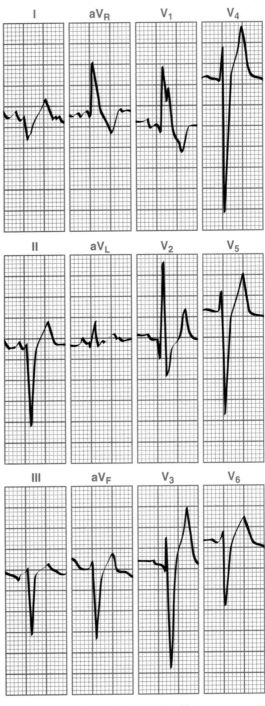

Q wave in leads V_1 to V_3
along with a broad R wave

The diagnosis of AMI solely with the use of ECG is complicated by the fact that not all patients will demonstrate ST elevations. In fact, persistent ST depression and T wave inversion, with or without Q waves, indicate some suben-dothelial infarctions. In addition, left bundle branch block (LBBB), a common arrhythmia seen during AMI, may obscure the detection of ST segment eleva-tions. Further, because the ECG represents the cardiac conduction system, which is a dynamic process that is subject to change over time, one single ECG is not sufficient to confirm or exclude a diagnosis of AMI.

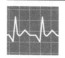 **It is recommended that serial ECGs every 30 minutes for 2 hours be performed for those patients at high risk for AMI.**

Cardiac Enzymes

During the infarction process, cell membranes rupture, allowing intracellular enzymes to spill out into the bloodstream. A blood sample drawn at certain times during or after AMI can be sent to the laboratory where enzymes can be measured and interpreted to determine the presence of an infarction. The prob-lem is that most of these enzymes are not found exclusively in cardiac tissue. Therefore injury to many tissues in the body will cause an elevation in some of the enzymes routinely measured during AMI diagnosis.

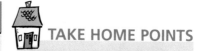 ST segment monitor-ing should be per-formed on all patients at risk for AMI.

Cardiac Enzyme Laboratory Findings

ENZYME	EARLIEST RISE (IN HRS)	PEAK (IN HRS)	RETURN TO BASELINE
CK	2-6	18-36	3-6 days
CK-MB	4-8	15-24	3-4 days
Myoglobin	0.5-1.0	6-9	12 hours
Troponin 1	1-6	7-24	10-14 days

CK, Creatine kinase; *MB,* cardiac muscle marker.

TAKE HOME POINTS

Troponin 1 is the newest cardiac marker and is a protein found only in myocardial cells. It is a quick, rapid test that, if elevated, indicates AMI.

Each of these cardiac markers can be useful in diagnosing AMI. Although some markers are very sensitive for cellular necrosis, others are more specific for cardiac tissue. Some offer the advantage of being able to confirm infarction rapidly, whereas others are useful in diagnosing the presence of AMI when a patient waits a couple of days before requesting medical treatment. Therefore a profile of all these cardiac markers is routinely ordered when AMI is suspected.

Medical Management

When any patient complains of chest pain suggestive of AMI, certain protocols should be instituted while the diagnosis is being made. The physical assessment should be ongoing and must include frequent monitoring of vital signs and pulse oximetry. Serial 12-lead ECGs with subsequent continuous ST segment cardiac monitoring is imperative. Laboratory tests must include a cardiac marker profile and possibly a complete blood count (CBC), basic chemistry, lipid levels, and sedimentation rate. Supplemental oxygen and IV access are essential. In addi-tion to the pharmacologic therapies (fibrinolytics, antiplatelets, anticoagulants, nitrates, morphine, beta blockers, and calcium-channel blockers), it may also be necessary to begin a lidocaine infusion if life-threatening dysrhythmias occur.

FIRST-LINE AND INITIAL TREATMENT FOR AMI

- Provide oxygen.
- Obtain a 12-lead ECG.
- Monitor vital signs and pulse oximetry.
- Order laboratory tests.
- Monitor continuous cardiac rhythm with ST segment monitoring.
- Conduct history and physical examination.
- Administer medications.

The patient will be admitted to the CCU where invasive lines such as an arterial line and a pulmonary artery (PA) catheter may be placed to provide further data to monitor ventricular function and guide the therapeutic regimen. In the event of severe left ventricular dysfunction, an intraaortic balloon pump (IABP) may be used to assist ventricular ejection and promote coronary artery perfusion. Last, reperfusion procedures such as emergency PTCA or CABG should be anticipated if thrombolytics are either contraindicated or unsuccessful.

Pharmacologic Interventions

The American Heart Association (AHA) (2003) reports that more than 85% of all AMIs are due to thrombus formation. Therefore in today's health care arena, thrombolytic and anticoagulant therapies are standards of practice in the treatment of AMI. Other agents frequently used in the management of AMI include nitrates, beta-adrenergic blockers, calcium-channel blockers, morphine sulfate, and antiplatelets such as aspirin (refer to the discussion on angina on page 122).

Thrombolytic Therapy

The survival rate for patients with AMI who receive thrombolytic reperfusion therapy is estimated to be 95%. Prompt and complete restoration of patency reduces infarction size, preserves left ventricular function, reduces morbidity, and prolongs survival. Thus the treatment goals are to institute thrombolytic therapy as quickly as possible to halt the infarction process, salvage the greatest amount of myocardial muscle, and prevent any subsequent infarctions.

Thrombolytics, such as streptokinase, tissue plasminogen activator (t-PA), reteplase (r-PA), and Tenecteplase (TNK-tPA) are administered with the intention of dissolving the clots that occlude coronary arteries, thus promoting vasodilation and restoring myocardial blood flow. However, because thrombolytics produce lysis of the pathologic clot, they may also lyse homeostatic clots such as in those in the cerebrovasculature, gastrointestinal tract, or operative site. Therefore patient selection is important because individuals receiving thrombolytic therapy may have a minor or major bleeding episode as a consequence of the therapy.

An adverse bleeding event is the major complication of thrombolytics, but allergic reaction is also possible because fibrinolytic agents are derived from bacterial proteins.

To be maximally beneficial, thrombolytic treatment should be instituted within 12 hours of symptom onset and ECG changes, although current preference is 6 hours. Beyond 12 hours, few patients will benefit, and no clear evidence exists that confirms whether the benefits outweigh the risk of hemorrhage. All patients with a history and physical examination suggestive of AMI in conjunction with substantiating ECG changes (either ST segment elevation or new LBBB), regardless of age, sex, or race, should be considered for thrombolytic therapy, providing no specific contraindications exist. Successful reperfusion therapy should result in an abrupt cessation of chest pain, a rapid return of the ST elevation to normal, reperfusion arrhythmias or conduction abnormalities, and improved left ventricular function.

Thrombolytic Contraindications

ABSOLUTE	RELATIVE
Aortic dissection	Uncontrolled hypertension
Previous cerebral hemorrhage	(>180/110 mm Hg)
Known history of AVM or cerebral	Current use of anticoagulants
aneurysm	Known bleeding diathesis
Active internal bleeding (excludes	Traumatic head injury (in the past
menstruation)	4 weeks)
Thromboembolic stroke (in past	Major surgery (in past 3 weeks)
6 months)	Internal bleeding (in past 6 months)
Known intracranial neoplasm	Pregnancy
	Active peptic ulcer disease

AVM, Arteriovenous malformation.

Anticoagulant Therapy

Anticoagulant therapy is commonly used in the patient with AMI for three prophylactic reasons. First, after thrombolytic therapy, unfractioned heparin (UFH) or low molecular–weight heparin (LMWH) is frequently administered to prevent reocclusion of the reperfused artery. Second, because pulmonary embolism is a common cause of death as debris or clots break free from the infarcted endocardium, UFH or LMWH is given to prevent this potentially fatal consequence. Third, AMI routinely results in arrhythmias, similar to atrial or ventricular fibrillation, which causes blood to pool in the chambers of the heart; UFH or LMWH can decrease the likelihood for subsequent clot formation. The mechanism by which these drugs work is as follows: UFH or LMWH in low doses prevents the conversion of prothrombin to thrombin; in high doses they neutralize thrombin, which prevents the conversion of fibrin to fibrinogen and, consequently, new clot formation.

TAKE HOME POINTS

Anticoagulants prevent thrombus formation and the extension of existing thrombi; they do not lyse (dissolve) existing thrombi.

Nursing Management

The nurse's primary responsibility during an evolving AMI is to ensure that lifesaving therapies are instituted as quickly and safely as possible to limit the severity of the infarction and thus functional impairment. Long-term nursing responsibilities primarily focus on assisting the patient in returning to a functional, high-quality life with prevention of future AMI being a primary goal.

ACUTE NURSING INTERVENTIONS

During a suspected or evolving AMI, the nurse must perform a rapid and focused physical assessment and health history. Frequent monitoring of vital signs and continuous cardiac monitoring are essential parts of the nurse's ongoing assessment. A critical nursing function is the prompt institution of prescribed medical and pharmacologic therapies, particularly the expeditious administration of thrombolytic agents.

If thrombolytic agents are prescribed, the nurse must frequently assess for signs and symptoms of internal hemorrhage like changes in mental status or level of consciousness, hematuria, hemoptysis, and gastrointestinal pain or bleeding. Although minor bleeding (such as superficial bleeding from IV sites) is to be expected, any sign of major bleeding should be emergently communicated with the physician.

 The administration of thrombolytic agents may cause reperfusion arrhythmias.

During the acute phase, all nursing actions should be aimed at reducing myocardial oxygen demand and increasing supply. Therefore the delivery of oxygen must be ensured via nasal cannula or mask unless otherwise contraindicated, which may be the case in the patient with chronic obstructive respiratory disease (COPD). Continuous monitoring of pulse oximetry is also indicated. The nurse must frequently assess for pain and anxiety and, if present, promptly treat with prescribed agents. A quiet, calm, nonstimulating environment can greatly help reduce stress and anxiety. Bedrest must be enforced, and the nurse should assist with all position changes and personal hygiene to avoid any exertional effort. Accurate measurements of intake and output must be maintained, particularly urine output because this is a reliable indicator of cardiac output and systemic perfusion. A stool softener should be prescribed to prevent straining and possible vasovagal stimulation, which can cause precipitous bradycardia. Emotional support is very important. Therefore the nurse's demeanor should be calming though not false, in the offering of reassurance. In addition, sufficient and appropriate explanations of all medical therapies should be provided.

 TAKE HOME POINTS

As with all nursing interventions, continuous evaluation of effectiveness is essential to modify therapies appropriately.

CHRONIC NURSING MANAGEMENT

The prevention of subsequent coronary events and the maintenance of physical functioning are important aspects of preventative care in patients with AMI. Therefore comprehensive and extensive counseling is essential not only for the patient but also for the family. Of course, education toward preventing a recurrence primarily revolves around risk reduction. However, it is also vital to teach the patient and family the signs and symptoms of myocardial ischemia and the appropriate responsive actions. In addition, the patient must understand the importance of adhering to whichever pharmacologic regimen is prescribed, including specifics of dose, how and when to administer the medication, its side effects, and any drug interactions.

 TAKE HOME POINTS

It is important to determine whether the patient can financially afford his or her prescribed medications.

As addressed earlier, the patient is incapable of altering unmodifiable risk factors. Therefore all efforts must be directed toward identifying and altering modifiable risk factors. Although numerous modifiable risk factors exist for CAD, education should be tailored to each patient's particular risk factors.

Effective management of hypertension requires frequent blood pressure monitoring, adherence to appropriate drug therapy, and nutritional counseling regarding a low sodium diet. In addition, a prescribed exercise program helps control blood pressure levels and promote cardiac rehabilitation in general. Smoking cessation is another focus because cessation has been shown to reduce mortality and reinfarction rates by 50% within 1 year. Interventions in this area include nicotine supplements with subsequent weaning; participation in a support group; relaxation training; instruction on behavioral skills for coping with high-stress situations; and maintenance of long-term, periodic telephone contact. Psychosocial interventions should be directed at identifying and alleviating sources of anxiety and depression, including specific stress management therapies. Patients may need to consider a change in occupation to address this particular risk factor. Overall, MI survivors need to be taught how to individualize the necessary changes in lifestyle and medical treatment to reduce the progression of coronary disease and prevent any recurrence of coronary events.

 TAKE HOME POINTS

- Promotion of cardiac wellness should be a fundamental goal of all nurses.
- Prevention is better than cure, and healthy lifestyle changes that are instituted early in life are not only easier but can also ultimately lead to a longer, more productive and fulfilling life.

 Do You UNDERSTAND?

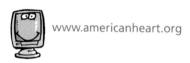 www.americanheart.org

DIRECTIONS: **Fill in the blanks to complete each of the following statements.**

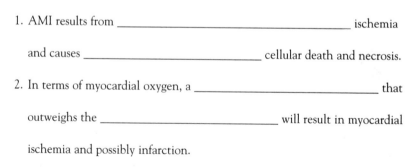

1. AMI results from _____ ischemia and causes _____ cellular death and necrosis.

2. In terms of myocardial oxygen, a _____ that outweighs the _____ will result in myocardial ischemia and possibly infarction.

Answers: 1. sustained, irreversible; 2. demand, supply.

3. Potential precipitating factors of AMI include the following:

   a. ______________________________

   b. ______________________________

   c. ______________________________

   d. ______________________________

   e. ______________________________

   f. ______________________________

   g. ______________________________

4. Cardiac cells can withstand ischemic conditions for approximately

   ____________ minutes before irreversible cellular death begins.

5. After AMI, the degree of altered cardiac function depends on the following:

   a. ______________________________

   b. ______________________________

   c. ______________________________

   d. ______________________________

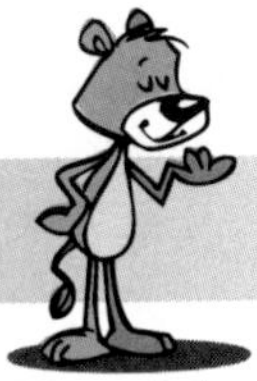

What IS Heart Failure?

Heart failure is a condition in which the ventricles cannot pump forcefully enough to send blood out to meet the metabolic needs of the body. The inadequate tissue perfusion causes fatigue and poor exercise tolerance. Blood backs up from the left ventricle into the veins of the lungs, causing SOB and lung crackles. Blood backs up from the right ventricle into the veins of the systemic circulation, causing edema as a result of fluid retention and volume overload. Not all patients have all of these symptoms. Some patients have no fluid retention but

Answers: 3. a. physical exertion; b. emotional stress; c. weather extremes; d. digestion of a heavy meal; e. Valsalva maneuver; f. hot baths or showers; g. sexual excitation; 4. 20; 5. a. the specific area of the heart involved; b. the presence of collateral circulation; c. the size of the infarct; d. the duration of the infarct.

have exercise intolerance. Some complain of edema but experience few symptoms of dyspnea or fatigue. Because not all patients have volume overload, the term *heart failure* is now preferred over the more common term, "congestive heart failure."

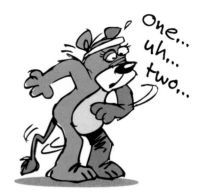

What You NEED TO KNOW

Many causes for heart failure exist. Some of them include the following:
- Injury to the myocardium
- MI
- CAD
- Cardiomyopathy
- Hypertension
- Valvular disease (mitral regurgitation)
- Anemia
- Thyrotoxicosis

Systolic Heart Failure

Systolic heart failure is an impairment in the ability of the heart to contract and empty. It is defined as an *ejection fraction* (EF) of less than 40%. EF is the percentage of blood ejected with each contraction. Normal EF is 65% to 75%. The heart enlarges in systolic heart failure in an attempt to pump more blood, but this is a short-term solution.

Diastolic Heart Failure

Diastolic heart failure is impairment of the heart's ability to relax. The myocardial wall becomes stiff and thickened, impairing the heart's ability to fill. EF is not decreased in diastolic heart failure. Although the ventricle enlarges, it does so concentrically as it thickens more on the inside; consequently, the overall heart size remains normal.

The same symptoms of pulmonary congestion can occur in systolic and diastolic heart failure. Some patients have components of both systolic and diastolic heart failure. Systolic heart failure is seen more commonly than diastolic heart failure; unless otherwise noted, therefore, the focus of this chapter is systolic heart failure. A thorough discussion of diastolic heart failure is beyond the scope of this text.

TAKE HOME POINTS

The term *heart failure* is preferred over the older term, "congestive heart failure," because not all patients have pulmonary or systemic congestion.

For further information on any of these listed disease processes, see the *Real World Nursing Survival Guide: Pathophysiology.*

TAKE HOME POINTS

- Systolic heart failure: An EF less than 40%.
- Diastolic heart failure: When the mitral valve opens, the left ventricle cannot relax to let blood in. Left ventricular (LV) and left atrial (LA) pressures increase, which back up into the pulmonary circulation.

Common Causes of Systolic and Diastolic Heart Failure

SYSTOLIC	DIASTOLIC
Coronary artery disease, MI	Restrictive cardiomyopathy
Idiopathic dilated cardiomyopathy	Hypertrophic cardiomyopathy
Hypertension	Aortic stenosis
Valvular disease (MR)	

MI, Myocardial infarction; *MR,* mitral regurgitation.

Chronic versus Acute Heart Failure

Most heart failure is chronic. *Chronic heart failure* is a gradual, progressive deterioration of left ventricular function. Unless the chronic heart failure is due to a mechanical cause such as coronary artery obstruction or an abnormal heart valve, it cannot be cured but only managed through medications and lifestyle changes. A diagnosis of chronic heart failure is made only after treatable causes have been ruled out. The problem is that once an initial insult has occurred to initiate heart failure, the body's compensatory mechanisms become maladaptive and aggravate the situation. Symptoms of volume overload and decreased cardiac output may be initially mild (decreased exercise tolerance) but gradually progress in severity to symptoms of fatigue and dyspnea, even dyspnea at rest. The immediate goal in treatment is to decrease the workload of the heart by preventing volume overload (preload) and decreasing resistance to pumping (afterload). As heart failure progresses and the heart enlarges, a vicious cycle begins, which can lead to permanent cellular changes and a change in the shape of the heart. This change is called *remodeling.*

Acute heart failure can result from a new onset cardiac event (e.g., MI, dysrhythmias, valve rupture, tamponade). More often, acute heart failure is a complication of chronic heart failure. A patient with chronic heart failure who was previously stable on medications but now comes to the emergency department with extreme SOB (decompensation) is now in acute heart failure. For some reason (see the following box), his or her oral dose of diuretic fails to control congestive symptoms.

REASONS FOR HEART FAILURE EXACERBATIONS

- Noncompliance with drug or diet regimens (increased salt and fluid intake)
- Increased alcohol intake
- Impaired drug absorption
- Underlying disease progression (MI, valvular disease)
- Anemia
- Fever (2° sudden increase in metabolic demand)
- Increased exercise
- Emotion

Left versus Right Heart Failure

Heart failure is a disease of the ventricles of the heart. Although the ventricles may fail independent of one another, left ventricular failure usually occurs first, which causes blood to back up into the pulmonary circulation. This action causes pulmonary hypertension, which leads to right ventricular failure over time. In most chronic advanced heart failure, patients exhibit symptoms of both left and right ventricular failure; consequently, patients with chronic heart failure have combined symptoms of left and right heart failure. (See Color Plate #5 for diagram showing blood flow through the heart.)

Signs and Symptoms of Volume Overload

	LEFT HEART FAILURE (PULMONARY CONGESTION)	RIGHT HEART FAILURE (SYSTEMIC CONGESTION)
Symptoms	Dyspnea* Paroxysmal nocturnal dyspnea* Orthopnea* Fatigue* Dry cough, worse at night Nocturia	Peripheral pitting edema* Weight gain Ascites Liver engorgement or discomfort Anorexia, nausea Abdominal bloating Nocturia
Signs	Cardiomegaly Tachypnea Tachycardia Third heart sound* (listen in left lateral decubitus position) Crackles bilaterally*	Hepatosplenomegaly Jugular venous distention* Positive HJ reflux Elevated CVP

*Classic sign or symptom.
HJ, Hepatojugular; *CVP,* central venous pressure.

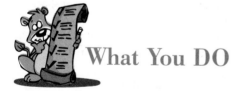

What You DO

Heart failure is largely a clinical diagnosis, which is not based on a single diagnostic or laboratory test but primarily on a careful history and physical examination. Diagnostic tests such as echocardiogram, chest x-ray studies, and radionuclide ventriculography are confirmatory rather than diagnostic in nature.

The signs and symptoms of heart failure (e.g., SOB, fatigue) are often difficult to identify because they are frequently confused with other disorders or attributed to aging, obesity, or lack of conditioning. Exercise intolerance can occur so gradually that patients may adapt their lifestyles to minimize symptoms and thus fail to report them.

Diagnostic tests may include:

- **Echocardiogram.** Two-dimensional echocardiography with Doppler flow is the gold standard of diagnostic tests. It can determine ventricular wall motion and can differentiate systolic from diastolic dysfunction. Periodic echocardiograms may be performed to assess EF; findings in heart failure include dilated left ventricular and decreased EF (<40%). An echocardiogram can evaluate valvular status and assess the pericardium.
- **Chest x-ray studies.** The chest x-ray may be used to rule out other causes of SOB such as COPD or pneumonia. When the patient is first examined, a chest x-ray film will show an enlarged heart and prominent pulmonary vasculature. Early cardiomegaly in symptomatic patients is highly suggestive but not diagnostic of heart failure.
- **ECG.** A 12-lead ECG may show a prior MI, ventricular enlargement, or the presence of dysrhythmias.
- **Radionuclide ventriculography.** Radionuclide ventriculography gives an accurate measurement of global and regional function but is unable to assess directly valvular abnormalities or cardiac hypertrophy.
- **Brain natriuretic peptide (BNP) measurement.** The BNP quickly differentiates symptoms of SOB caused by pulmonary disease as a result of heart failure. BNP is a hormone that is released by the failing ventricle in an attempt to help out by its natural vasodilatory and diuretic responses. A minimal level of BNP supports a lung cause of the SOB. An elevated level is an indication of heart failure.
- **Treadmill stress test and cardiac catheterization.** A treadmill stress test or cardiac catheterization (or both) may be performed to rule out CAD as a treatable cause of heart failure.

Acute Heart Failure

In-Patient Treatment

During acute exacerbations, hospitalization may be necessary. If the clinical signs are mild to moderate, patients may be treated with IV diuretics and sent home. However, if they have symptoms of acute pulmonary edema or shock or both, admission to the coronary care unit is indicated. This situation requires emergency treatment with oxygen and medications. Mechanical ventilation, a PA catheter, or an IABP may be needed, depending on the severity.

FIRST-LINE AND INITIAL TREATMENT FOR ACUTE HEART FAILURE

- Provide oxygen.
- Administer medications.

Medications

Loop diuretics such as furosemide (Lasix), bumetanide (Bumex), ethacrynic acid (Edecrin), or torsemide (Demadex) are intravenously administered to decrease preload. Venous vasodilators such as nitroglycerin may also be given to decrease preload. Morphine sulfate not only decreases anxiety, but it also helps

TAKE HOME POINTS

Acute pulmonary edema occurs when the pressure in the pulmonary vessels becomes so great that fluid floods the alveoli and decreases the availability for air exchange.

decrease preload by venous vasodilation. Nesiritide (Natrecor) is a new class of IV drug that is very effective in acute exacerbations of heart failure; it decreases not only afterload but also preload. Acutely positive inotropic drugs such as milrinone (Primacor) and dobutamine (Dobutrex) or intropin (Dopamine) are used to increase contractility.

Chronic Heart Failure

Outpatient Treatment

Chronic heart failure is usually managed on an outpatient basis. In the past, emphasis was placed on the treatment of symptoms only—digitalis to strengthen the heart and diuretics to unload the extra fluid to decrease SOB. Currently, more emphasis is not only placed on stabilizing the patient but also on stabilizing the disease, breaking the vicious cycle of compensation and preventing the permanent changes of remodeling. This treatment regimen should ultimately lead to an increase in the quality of life and a decrease in hospital readmissions. Treatment of the patient, as well as the disease, is accomplished primarily with medications. Three major classes of drugs are available to treat systolic dysfunction—vasodilators, diuretics, and positive inotropes.

The long-term goal of treatment in chronic heart failure is to break the cycle of hypertrophy and remodeling by suppressing the compensatory mechanisms. How is this done? The harmful effects of the sympathetic nervous system (SNS), renin-angiotensin-aldosterone, and decreased myocardial contractility need to be suppressed by ACE inhibitors, angiotensin II–receptor blockers (ARBs-II), and beta blockers.

The short-term goal of chronic heart failure treatment is to treat the patient's symptoms. Systolic heart failure is treated with vasodilators to decrease afterload, diuretics to decrease preload, and positive inotropes to increase contractility.

Medications

ACE inhibitors help decrease preload by preventing sodium and water reabsorption. They indirectly vasodilate and decrease afterload by interfering with the conversion of angiotensin-1 (AT-1) to angiotensin-2 (AT-2). This interference breaks the cycle and prevents the release of aldosterone. No vasoconstriction and no reabsorption of sodium and water occur.

- An ACE inhibitor is the absolute "number one" drug prescribed for all patients with heart failure.
- Some patients cannot take ACE inhibitors because of cough, renal insufficiency, allergy, or angioneurotic edema. If contraindicated for any reason, an angiotensin-receptor blocker (ARB) should be substituted.
- Side effects of ACE inhibitors may include hypotension and lightheadedness.

Beta blockers are also now considered the standard of care in the treatment of heart failure. Beta blockers block the effects of the SNS so that the compensatory tachycardia, hypertension, and vasoconstriction cannot occur and therefore hypertrophy and remodeling cannot occur.

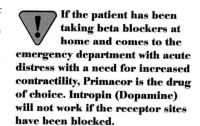 **If the patient has been taking beta blockers at home and comes to the emergency department with acute distress with a need for increased contractility, Primacor is the drug of choice. Intropin (Dopamine) will not work if the receptor sites have been blocked.**

 TAKE HOME POINTS

- A positive inotropic drug increases the force of the heart's contraction, and a negative inotropic drug decreases the force of the heart's contraction.
- IV medications may be switched to those taken orally when the patient transfers out of the coronary care unit, has been hemodynamically stable for 24 hours, and exhibits no remaining symptoms when at rest.
- The patient is still exhibiting chronic heart failure even though the acute episode has been treated.

 Angiotensin-converting enzyme (ACE) inhibitors and beta blockers are not prescribed for acute heart failure.

 TAKE HOME POINTS

An increased heart rate, BP, volume, and vasoconstriction are **BAD** indicators or effects. Any medication that counteracts these effects is **GOOD**.

TAKE HOME POINTS

The *long-term treatment goal* of chronic heart failure is to treat the *disease*. The *short-term treatment goal* of chronic heart failure is to treat the *patient*.

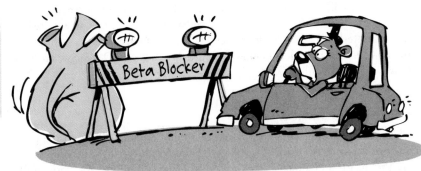

TAKE HOME POINTS

- ACE inhibitors are preventative in nature and therefore not given in acute heart failure.
- An aldosterone blocker such as spironolactone (Aldactone) may also be given along with ACE inhibitors for a more sustained effect in more chronic heart failure.
- Beta blockers are effective at blocking the excessive exercise–induced tachycardia that can limit the patient's activities.
- Beta blockers vasodilate and decrease resistance to flow.
- Beta blockers are not given in acute exacerbations of heart failure.

- At present, **only** carvedilol (Coreg), labetalol (Normodyne, Trandate), metoprolol (Toprol, Lopressor), and bisoprolol (Zebeta) are approved by the Food and Drug Administration (FDA) for the treatment of heart failure.
- Doses of beta blockers must be gradually increased as tolerated. It may take days or weeks before improvement is observed.
- Side effects of beta blockers include fatigue.
- Beta blockers are contraindicated in patients with asthma, COPD, or conduction disorders.

Diuretics are prescribed to prevent and treat the symptoms of fluid overload in patients with chronic heart failure. Loop diuretics are normally used as in acute heart failure, but they are administered by mouth rather than IV routes. Side effects of diuretics include hypotension, dizziness, nocturia, and hypokalemia. If two daily doses are needed, the second dose should be administered no later than 4:00 PM because of the increased potential for nocturia. Potassium supplements are given to prevent hypokalemia.

The major medication prescribed to increase contractility in chronic heart failure is *digoxin* (Lanoxin). Lanoxin is inexpensive and very effective in decreasing symptoms. Signs of toxicity include nausea, blurred vision, and dysrhythmias. A fine line exists between therapeutic digoxin (Lanoxin) doses and toxicity, especially in patients with renal failure.

TAKE HOME POINTS

- Most medications used in acute heart failure are given via IV routes.
- Medications used in patient with chronic heart failure are all administered orally.

Medications Used to Treat Acute and Chronic Heart Failure

DRUG NAME (BRAND)	DRUG NAME (GENERIC)	PURPOSE	USED TO TREAT AHF	USED TO TREAT CHF
Lasix Bumex Demadex Edecrin	furosemide bumetanide torsemide ethacrynic acid	Loop diuretic Decreases preload Is used when symptoms of volume overload appear	Yes	Yes
Nitrobid	nitroglycerin	Decreases preload Dilates venous capacitance beds	Yes	No
Duramorph	morphine sulfate	Decreases preload by dilating venous capacitance vessels	Yes	No
Lanoxin	digoxin	Increases contractility	No	Yes
Primacor	milrinone (phosphodiasterase inhibitor)	Increases contractility	Yes	No
Dobutrex	dobutamine (catecholamine)			
ACE INHIBITORS				
Capoten Vasotec Monopril Zestril Altace Aceon (Use ARBs if ACE inhibitors are contra-indicated)	captopril enalapril fosinopril lisinopril ramipril trandolapril	Prevents conversion of AT-1 to AT-2 Decreases fluid retention Decreases afterload by vasodilation Prevents remodeling	No	Yes
BETA BLOCKERS				
Coreg Normodyne	carvedilol labetalol	Blocks sympathetic response Prevents excessive increases in HR and BP	No	Yes
Trandate, Toprol, Lopressor	metoprolol	Vasodilates to improve symptoms and clinical status		
Zebeta	bisoprolol	Prevents remodeling		
Natrecor	nesiritide	Naturally occurring hormone that counteracts the compensatory responses to heart failure	Yes	No

AHF, Acute heart failure; *CHF,* chronic heart failure; *ACE,* angiotensin-converting enzyme; *AT-1,* angiotensin-1; *AT-2,* angiotensin-2; *ARBs,* angiotensin II–receptor blockers; *HR,* heart rate; *BP,* blood pressure.

TAKE HOME POINTS

- Diastolic heart failure is treated differently than systolic heart failure. Medications such as beta blockers and calcium channel blockers have a negative effect and help relax the work of the left ventricle.
- Vasodilators are used to treat systolic heart failure.

 For further information on any of these listed disease processes, see the *Real World Nursing Survival Guide: Pharmacology*.

TAKE HOME POINTS

Weighing daily is the best indicator for fluid losses or gains in the patient with heart failure; significant weight changes can detect problems before symptoms occur. Approximately 10 pounds of extra fluid must occur before symptoms of increased volume develop.

 A weight change of more than 3 pounds per day is due to fluid, not fat.

TAKE HOME POINTS

What is new in the treatment of heart failure? Scientists have recently begun transplanting skeletal muscle cells (myoblasts) into dead heart muscle or scar tissue in an attempt to regenerate new muscle. Results have been promising.

NONPHARMACOLOGIC TREATMENT

In addition to treating with medication, patients also are advised to do the following:

- Stop smoking.
- Control BP levels.
- Limit sodium and sometimes fluid intake. (Not necessary unless the patient has a problem with fluid overload—usually less than 4 g/day; patients with severe fluid retention may need to limit to 2 g/day.)
- Learn to read medication, food, and herbal labels for sodium content.
- Lose weight, if necessary.
- Limit use of alcohol (can decrease contractility).
- Get plenty of rest.
- Manage stress effectively.
- Weigh daily to maintain fluid volume status; notify physician if weight gain greater than 3 pounds per day or 5 pounds per week occurs.
- Avoid nonsteroidal antiinflammatory drugs (NSAIDs); can increase sodium and water retention.
- Improve physical conditioning with moderate exercise to prevent deconditioning; avoid isometric exercises such as push-ups and weightlifting.
- Report worsening of symptoms or new symptoms such as hypotension or dizziness that might be drug-related developments.

Other treatment options include the following:

Cardiac resynchronization therapy. This type of biventricular pacemaker leads are inserted into the left and right ventricles and the coronary sinus to *resynchronize* the contractility of the ventricles. This treatment is indicated for severe heart failure and useful only in patients with asynchrony of the ventricles (i.e., bundle branch block). Indications include a QRS greater than or equal to 130 msec. Cardiac resynchronization therapy allows the ventricles to regain synchrony in pumping, which is lost in bundle branch block. The use of a regular pacemaker is not an appropriate treatment for heart failure because the problem lies with the mechanical system (contractility), not the electrical system.

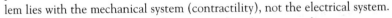

Heart transplantation. Several centers perform heart transplants on appropriate patients. Obviously, heart transplantation is a drastic step, and the entire patient profile must be carefully considered. Heart failure must be end stage, and the other organs must be healthy. Other considerations include the stress of surgery, side effects of antirejection immunosuppressive drugs, and the cost and need for frequent follow-up maintenance.

Left Ventricular Assist Device (LVAD) or mechanical heart pump. An LVAD may help a failing heart until a donor heart becomes available. Age considerations and co-morbidity do not restrict its use as significantly as that for heart transplantation. The costs are approximately the same.

COMPLICATIONS

Heart failure can result in an array of cardiac impairments that include the following:

- Mitral regurgitation may result from the dilated ventricle stretching the mitral valve leaflets.
- Atrial fibrillation may result from increased LA pressures and stretching caused from the backflow of blood.
- Thrombi may result from stagnant blood flow as a result of incomplete emptying in a dilated inefficient heart or because of atrial fibrillation.
- Ventricular dysrhythmias may result from ischemia or electrolyte imbalances.

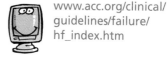

www.acc.org/clinical/
guidelines/failure/
hf_index.htm

Do You UNDERSTAND?

DIRECTIONS: Select the best answer to complete the following statements. Place the corresponding letters in the spaces provided.

_____ 1. Which condition best describes heart failure?
   a. The heart stops beating.
   b. The heart cannot beat enough to meet the needs of the body.

_____ 2. Which of the following is considered the patient's responsibilities?
   a. Compliance with prescribed medications
   b. Monthly weighings and reporting any sudden headache
   c. Compliance with weekly uses of cathartics
   d. Performing aerobic and strength exercises within 1 week of AMI.

_____ 3. Heart failure is one of the most common causes of recurrent readmissions to hospitals, some of which may be avoided. What affect does the nurse have to help decrease the readmission rate?
   a. Allow the patient to stay an extra 2 days in the hospital before discharging.
   b. Double the diuretic dose on discharge.
   c. Ask the patient to move physically closer to his or her primary care provider.
   d. Provide adequate patient education information on discharge and follow up on the patient within 7 days of discharge from the hospital.

_____ 4. A patient can have chronic and acute heart failure at the same time.
   a. True
   b. False

Answers: 1. b; 2. a; 3. d; 4. a.

DIRECTIONS: **Provide a short answer to the following question.**

5. Which diagnostic test is the gold standard for diagnosing systolic heart failure?

_____

_____

DIRECTIONS: **Circle the correct word in each group that accurately describes the goals in the treatment of systolic heart failure.**

6. Preload: *increase* or *decrease*

7. Afterload: *increase* or *decrease*

8. Contractility: *increase* or *decrease*

9. Heart rate and BP: *increase* or *decrease*

10. *Vasodilation* or *vasoconstriction*

DIRECTIONS: **Match the following drug names in Column A with the actions used to treat heart failure in Column B.**

Column A

_____ 11. Increases the pumping ability of the heart (contractility)

_____ 12. Prevents the conversion of AT-1 to AT-2, thereby reducing afterload by dilating peripheral arterioles

_____ 13. Decreases heart rate and BP (oxygen demand to the heart)

_____ 14. Decreases preload by its diuretic action

_____ 15. May be substituted for ACE inhibitors if they are contraindicated

_____ 16. Natural-occurring hormone that counteracts the body's compensatory responses to heart failure

_____ 17. Dilates venous capacitance beds to decrease preload

Column B

a. Nesiritide
b. Furosemide
c. Lanoxin
d. ACE inhibitors
e. Beta blocker
f. Morphine
g. ARB

DIRECTIONS: **With the clues given, find the answers in the "Word Search" puzzle below.**

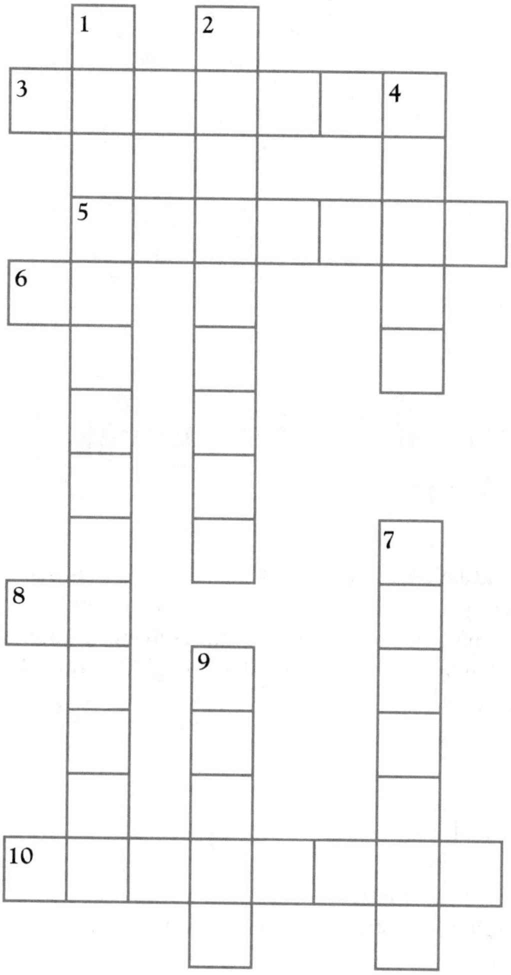

(crossword puzzle grid with numbered cells 1–10)

Down

1. Generalized cardiomegaly—ischemic or nonischemic—that causes heart failure
2. Type of heart failure with stiff, noncompliant LV
4. When chronic heart failure symptoms become uncontrolled
7. Neck vein distention and peripheral _____ that occur in right-sided heart failure
9. When permanent degenerative changes occur in heart failure

Across

3. Symptom of left-sided heart failure—tiredness
5. Symptom of left sided heart failure—shortness of breath
6. Necrosis of heart tissue—can cause heart failure (abbreviation)
8. When chronically elevated, _____ can cause heart failure (abbreviation)
10. Type of heart failure—LV ejection fraction less than 40%

Answers: **Down:** 1. cardiomyopathy; 2. diastolic; 4. edema; 7. chronic; 9. acute. **Across:** 3. fatigue; 5. dyspnea; 6. MI; 8. BP; 10. systolic.

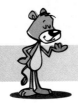

What IS Mechanical Ventilation?

Mechanical ventilation is a form of artificial ventilation that takes over all or part of the work performed by the respiratory muscles and organs. It is initiated when the patient's ability to oxygenate and exchange carbon dioxide (CO_2) is impaired. Mechanical ventilation may be indicated for the following reasons:

- Hypoxemia
- Respiratory distress
- Atelectasis
- Aspiration
- Pulmonary edema
- Pulmonary embolism (PE)
- Respiratory muscle fatigue
- Acute respiratory distress syndrome (ARDS)
- Over sedation
- To reduce intracranial pressure
- To stabilize the chest wall

The main goal of mechanical ventilation is to support gas exchange until the disease process or condition is resolved.

TAKE HOME POINTS

Before mechanically ventilating a patient, other oxygen delivery devices such as nasal cannulas and face masks may be used. A nasal cannula delivers low-flow oxygen (1 to 6 L/min) through prongs inserted into the nose; a face mask, which covers the nose and mouth, delivers higher concentrations of oxygen (40% to 60%).

What You NEED TO KNOW

Positive-Pressure Ventilation

Positive-pressure ventilation is the most common form of mechanical ventilation used in the acute care setting. This form of ventilation forces oxygen into the lungs, either through an endotracheal tube or a tracheostomy tube, mimicking respiration. Four types of positive-pressure ventilators are available. *Volume-cycled ventilators* deliver a breath until a preset volume is reached. *Pressure-cycled ventilators* deliver a breath until a preset pressure is achieved within the airway. *Flow-cycled ventilators* deliver a breath until a preset flow rate is reached. *Time-cycled ventilators* deliver a breath over a preset period. Newer ventilators are capable of providing some or all of these types of ventilation.

Modes of Ventilation

There are various modes of ventilation that may be used to ventilate and oxygenate the patient. Essentially, these modes are ways in which ventilation is triggered; they allow the patient some or all control over his or her breathing.

Controlled ventilation (CV) delivers a preset volume or pressure at a preset rate. This mode takes away all control of breathing from the patient; it is primarily used for patients who have no respiratory effort at all. Sedation must be used for any patient who has spontaneous breathing.

Assist-control ventilation (ACV) delivers a preset volume or pressure whenever the patient initiates a breath. If the patient does not initiate a breath by a preset time, the ventilator will give one. This mode is used primarily for the patient with normal breathing but who has weak respiratory muscles or who cannot achieve an adequate volume on his or her own. Sedation may be used if the patient has excess spontaneous breathing.

Synchronized intermittent mandatory ventilation (SIMV) delivers a preset volume at a preset rate and is synchronized with the patient's effort. This mode allows for spontaneous breathing between ventilated breaths and prevents competition between the patient and the ventilator. When a spontaneous breath occurs, it is at the patient's own rate and tidal volume. SIMV is the most common mode used and allows for weaning from the ventilator. Respiratory muscle fatigue may develop from the increased work of breathing.

Pressure-controlled ventilation (PCV) delivers a positive-pressure breath until a maximum amount of pressure is reached; then the breath stops. The maximum pressure limit is preset and helps prevent barotrauma (i.e., damage from the pressure) to the lungs. The amount of volume that is delivered varies, based on airway resistance and lung compliance. Usually the maximal pressure limit is set to achieve a goal tidal volume that is designated by the physician. This mode improves gas exchange and compliance of the lungs.

For patients with chronic lung disease (i.e., chronic obstructive pulmonary disease [COPD]), high levels of oxygen must be cautiously delivered because too much oxygen can cause them to lose their drive to breathe. Therefore low-flow oxygen devices are usually tried first.

TAKE HOME POINTS

- The most common type of mechanical ventilation is positive pressure.
- CV takes control of breathing from the patient.

TAKE HOME POINTS

- ACV delivers the preset tidal volume each time the ventilator breathes or the patient takes a spontaneous breath.
- SIMV delivers the preset tidal volume with each set breath, and the patient receives his or her own initiated tidal volume for each spontaneous breath taken.

⚠ To ensure adequate volume and pressure delivery with PCV, sedation and muscle paralysis may be required.

⚠ Sedation and neuro-muscular blockade (chemical-induced muscle paralysis) is usually required for IRV to work effectively.

⚠ A CPAP of >10 cm H_2O pressure may increase intrathoracic pressure to the point that it affects the patient's venous return, decreasing cardiac output and blood pressure. CPAP at this level may also cause a pneumothorax to occur.

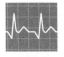 CPAP of >10 cm H_2O pressure may cause a pneumothorax to occur.

Inverse-ratio ventilation (IRV) is used when the inspiratory time is increased and the expiratory time is decreased. With IRV the inspiration-expiration (I/E) ratios used most are 1:1 and 2:1. This mode of ventilation allows for a longer period for gas exchange to improve oxygenation. This mode is generally used in patients with ARDS and in conjunction with PCV or SIMV. This type of ventilatory mode creates an abnormal breathing pattern for the patient; consequently, the patient may become uncomfortable and anxious.

Constant positive airway pressure (CPAP) provides positive pressure during spontaneous breaths; the ventilator will not initiate any breaths. This mode increases oxygenation by opening any closed alveoli that may occur at end-expiration, thereby increasing the functional residual capacity (FRC). CPAP can be used as a method to wean patients from the ventilator and generally ranges from 5 to 10 cm water (H_2O) pressure.

Pressure support ventilation (PSV) allows for a preset positive pressure to assist during inspiration of the patient's spontaneous breaths. This mode can be used with full spontaneous breathing, with SIMV, or to wean the patient from the ventilator. When used for full spontaneous breathing, the patient maintains full control over the rate and volume of each breath. When used in conjunction with SIMV, this mode allows for a larger tidal volume to be obtained. PSV increases patient comfort and decreases the amount of work needed by the patient for spontaneous breathing through an endotracheal tube or tracheostomy tube.

High-frequency ventilation (HFV) or jet ventilation is a mode that delivers a small amount of tidal volume at a very increased rate. Tidal volumes can range from 50 to 400 ml per breath with rates from 60 to >200 breaths per minute. The small amount of tidal volume decreases airway and intrathoracic pressures; therefore a decreased risk of barotrauma and hemodynamic changes occur. This mode is generally used on patients who cannot tolerate the normal tidal volumes or airway pressures of the other modes such as CV or ACV. Sedation and muscle paralysis are usually required.

Positive end-expiratory pressure (PEEP) adds positive pressure during expiration of each ventilated breath. PEEP can be used as a supplement to most modes of ventilation. PEEP can range from 5 to 20 cm H_2O pressure, prevent alveoli from collapsing at end-expiration, improve oxygenation, and increase FRC. The use of PEEP increases intrathoracic pressure and decreases venous return and cardiac output; therefore it may cause hypotension. PEEP >20 cm H_2O pressure can cause overdistention of the alveoli leading to barotrauma, pneumothorax, hypotension, increased intracranial pressure, and alveolar ventilation–perfusion mismatch.

**Effect of Application of PEEP
on the Alveoli**

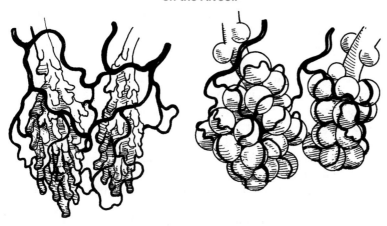

Ventilator Settings

Ventilator settings must be individualized to each patient to allow for optimal gas exchange. Settings are generally based on arterial blood gas (ABG) measurements. Most acute care institutions have respiratory therapists who set up and manage the ventilator. All nurses should be familiar with the control panels of ventilators to verify at least once every shift the ventilator modes, settings, and alarms.

Ventilator Settings, Descriptions, and Ranges

VENTILATOR SETTING	DESCRIPTION	RANGES
VT	Amount of oxygen delivered to patient with each preset ventilated breath	5-15 ml/kg (average 10 ml/kg)
Respiratory rate	Number of breaths/min that ventilator is set to deliver	4-20 breaths/min
FiO$_2$	Percentage of oxygen delivered by ventilator with each breath	21%-100%
I/E Ratio	Duration of I/E time	1:2 (unless IRV is used)
Sensitivity	Determines amount of effort patient must generate before ventilator will give a breath	Too low—patient will have to work harder to obtain a breath Too high—patient may fight ventilator
Flow rate	Determines how fast VT will be delivered during inspiration	High—increase airway pressure Low—decrease airway pressure
Pressure limits	Regulates maximum amount of pressure the ventilator will generate to deliver preset VT	Ventilated breath is stopped when pressure limit is reached

VT, Tidal volume; *FiO$_2$,* fraction of inspired oxygen; *I/E,* inspiratory to expiratory; *IRV,* inverse-ratio ventilation.

TAKE HOME POINTS

Ventilator setting adjustments are based on arterial oxygen saturation (SaO_2) level and ABG results.

TAKE HOME POINTS

A patient needing long-term ventilatory management will need a tracheostomy placed at some point. Endotracheal tubes (oral or nasal) are not intended for long-term management and may lead to other problems such as mucosal breakdown, skin ulcerations (lips), sinusitis, and vocal cord paralysis or damage (or both).

TAKE HOME POINTS

Successful weaning is a team effort among physicians, nurses, respiratory therapy personnel, and patient.

Mechanical Ventilation Complications

Barotrauma occurs when high airway pressures cause over-distention of the alveoli, rupture, and leakage of air. Barotrauma can cause a pneumothorax, subcutaneous emphysema, or crepitus. Air can leak under the mediastinum or into the pericardium or peritoneum, causing problems with organs located in these areas.

Hypotension associated with mechanical ventilation occurs because positive-pressure ventilation and PEEP cause an increase in intrathoracic pressure. The increased intrathoracic pressure decreases venous return to the right side of the heart, creating a decrease in preload, which in turn decreases cardiac output.

Stress ulcers, gastrointestinal (GI) bleeding, inadequate nutrition, and paralytic ileus are some of the more common GI problems associated with mechanical ventilation. Providing adequate nutrition and the administration of histamine H_2-receptor antagonists such as ranitidine or cimetidine help reduce the incidence of these occurrences.

When an artificial airway is placed in a patient, it bypasses many of the body's normal defense mechanisms in the upper respiratory system, such as the cough reflex and ciliary clearance of mucus. Secretions can pool above the cuffs of artificial airways and leak into the lower respiratory tract, making suctioning a needed intervention. Within 24 hours the secretions can become contaminated with bacteria. Positioning, nasogastric tubes, and gastric reflux can all lead to bacterial contamination of respiratory secretions.

Weaning from Ventilation

Weaning from mechanical ventilation is the gradual withdrawal of ventilatory support, allowing the patient to breathe more on his or her own. The length of the weaning process can vary according to the length of time on the ventilator and the patient's condition. Patients who need short-term ventilator support generally wean more quickly than those who need long-term support. Factors related to whether the patient is ready to wean include status of the underlying disease process that required the mechanical ventilation, nutritional status, cardiovascular status, respiratory status, and whether the patient will be able to participate in the weaning process. The different weaning methods that are most commonly used include T-tube and T-piece, SIMV, CPAP, and PSV.

Use of the T-tube and T-piece for weaning requires that the patient be removed from the ventilator for short periods, as if on a trial basis, and then placed back on ventilatory support. Supplemental oxygen is placed through the T-tube and T-piece while the patient spontaneously breathes. Gradually the length of time off the ventilator is extended until ventilatory support is no longer needed. This method allows the patient to build respiratory muscle strength and endurance.

When SIMV is used for weaning, the respiratory rate is gradually decreased at regular intervals until the patient is able to breathe completely on his or her own. This decrease in rate is generally two breaths per minute, and ABGs are assessed 30 to 45 minutes after each change. This method can take a few hours or a few days, depending on how long ventilatory support was required.

CPAP is commonly used in conjunction with T-tube and T-piece or SIMV modes to help facilitate the weaning process. The use of CPAP during the weaning process helps prevent atelectasis during shallow breathing and improves oxygenation by increasing the FRC.

PSV weaning is commonly used with SIMV to assist in the weaning process. Once a rate of two to four breaths per minute are achieved during weaning in SIMV, the mode is changed to PSV and the pressure is set to facilitate a spontaneous tidal volume of 10 to 12 ml/kg. Once 5 cm H_2O pressure is reached and tolerated by the patient, extubation can be considered.

Noninvasive Mechanical Ventilation

Noninvasive mechanical ventilation is positive-pressure ventilation implemented through a facemask instead of an endotracheal or tracheostomy tube. The ventilating unit provides either PSV or inspiratory positive airway pressure (IPAP) to increase tidal volume and PEEP or expiratory positive airway pressure (EPAP) to facilitate spontaneous breathing. This type of ventilation is used when invasive mechanical ventilation is contraindicated. It is also used to support patients after extubation and provide comfort to the patient with end-stage respiratory disease.

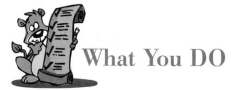

What You DO

The following are practices performed for patients receiving mechanical ventilation.

- The respiratory status is assessed every 4 hours and more frequently when a change in condition occurs. Close attention is paid to breathing sounds and the amount of patient effort.
- Signs of hypoxia are assessed. These signs include restlessness, anxiety, increased heart rate and blood pressure, increased respiratory rate, and oxygen saturation via pulse oximetry (SpO_2) less than 90%.
- Endotracheal or tracheostomy tube placement is maintained by properly securing the tube and preventing inadvertent extubation by staff or patient. Placement is maintained until extubation.
- The endotracheal tube is repositioned per institutional policy to prevent pressure sores.
- Secretions are suctioned to maintain an open airway. Amount, color, and consistency of the secretions are noted, as well as how well the patient tolerated the procedure.
- Ventilator settings and alarms are verified once a shift or when any changes occur.
- Continuous pulse oximetry and ABGs are monitored for assessing the oxygenation status; the physician is notified of any changes in parameters.
- The patient is frequently positioned to allow for optimal ventilation, to prevent complications, to mobilize secretions, and to promote comfort.

- Ventilator circuit is monitored for moisture or water trapping in tubing and emptied when necessary. Moisture may impede the flow of oxygen and may provide a medium for bacterial growth.
- A functioning manual resuscitation bag is maintained at bedside at all times in case of malfunctioning equipment.
- The patient is medicated as needed to decrease anxiety and facilitate oxygenation.
- Alternative methods of communication are provided for patients to decrease anxiety and maintain some control over their environment.
- Mouth and lip care is provided at least once every shift to keep mucous membranes moist.

Do You UNDERSTAND?

DIRECTIONS: **Match the mode of ventilation in Column A with the corresponding descriptions in Column B.**

Column A	Column B
_____ 1. SIMV	a. Preset volume or pressure given when patient breathes
_____ 2. PSV	b. Ventilated breath ends when pressure limit is met
_____ 3. AC	c. Prevents competition between patient and ventilator
_____ 4. PCV	d. Preset positive pressure given during inspiration
_____ 4. PCV	

DIRECTIONS: **Match the following descriptions of ventilator settings in Column A with the types of ventilators in Column B.**

Column A	Column B
_____ 5. Determines how fast the tidal volume will be delivered	a. I/E ratio
_____ 6. Number of breaths per minute	b. Respiratory rate
_____ 7. Duration of inspiratory time to expiratory time for each breath	c. Flow rate
_____ 8. Percentage of oxygen set to be delivered with each breath	d. FiO_2

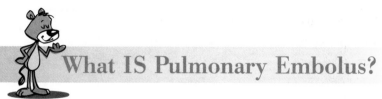

What IS Pulmonary Embolus?

PE is a thrombotic (blood clot) or nonthrombotic (fat) emboli that lodges in the pulmonary artery (PA) system. This blockage obstructs blood flow to the lung tissue supplied by the affected vessel. Thrombotic emboli mainly originate from the deep veins of the legs, right ventricle (RV) of the heart, or pelvis. Nonthrombotic emboli mainly originate from fat release after skeletal injuries, amniotic fluid, air, and foreign bodies.

What You NEED TO KNOW

Causes

A decrease in blood flow (venous stasis), a problem with blood clotting, and some form of injury to the vessel wall are three factors that can lead to the development of venous thrombi. These three factors together are called *Virchow's triad*. The box that follows shows conditions and risk factors that can predispose a patient or that can precipitate the formation of venous thrombi.

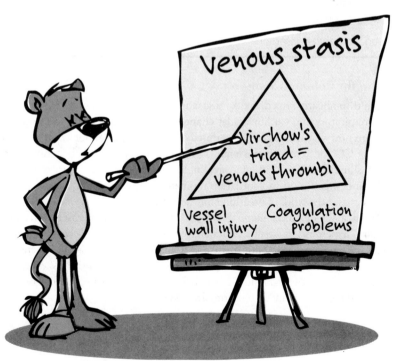

VENOUS THROMBI: CONDITIONS AND RISK FACTORS

Predisposing Factors to the Development of Venous Thrombi

Atrial fibrillation

Immobility

Infection

Atherosclerosis

Polycythemia

Conditions that Can Precipitate the Formation of Venous Thrombi

Heart failure

RV heart failure

Cardiomyopathy

Surgery (orthopedic, vascular, abdominal)

Trauma

Pregnancy

OTHER RISK FACTORS FOR PULMONARY EMBOLISM

Immobilization

Obesity

Varicose veins

Long bone fractures

Atrial fibrillation

Venous catheter insertion

TAKE HOME POINTS

Virchow's triad consists of decrease blood flow (venous stasis), blood-clotting problem, and vessel wall injury.

TAKE HOME POINTS

Some patients with hypercoagulable states are prone to the development of thrombi, which can ultimately result in a PE.

Pathophysiologic Changes

When thrombi are formed, break loose, and lodge in the pulmonary vasculature, both respiratory and cardiovascular changes occur. Alveoli distal to the occlusion are now ventilated but not perfused. Gas exchange cannot occur, and the level of CO_2 decreases in this area. This decrease causes bronchoconstriction, which shunts blood to ventilated areas of lungs, increases pulmonary resistance, and causes a perfusion-to-ventilation mismatch. This mismatch causes hypoxia and increases the work of breathing for the patient.

When a PE obstructs more than 50% of the pulmonary vasculature, pulmonary hypertension results. Pulmonary vasoconstriction occurs from the release of mediators at the injury site and from hypoxia. As resistance increases, the workload of the RV of the heart also increased. Failure of the RV eventually occurs, which leads to failure of the left ventricle, decreased cardiac output, decreased blood pressure, and eventually shock.

Clinical Manifestations of Pulmonary Embolism

Clinical manifestations of PE are often nonspecific, and a thorough history and physical are usually required to help with the diagnosis. The duration and the extent of the embolism often influence the clinical manifestations.

Shortness of breath (SOB) is one of the most common clinical manifestations patients present with of a PE, although up to 20% of patients have no SOB. SOB can have a sudden onset or occur on exertion. Cough and hemoptysis can be observed in up to one half of patients diagnosed with PE. Hemoptysis occurs when an area of infarction at or near the periphery of the lung begins to hemorrhage. Tachypnea (a respiratory rate >24 breaths per minute) is a response to the hypoxia that develops from impaired gas exchange.

Chest pain occurs in over one half of patients diagnosed with PE. The pain generally comes from an infarction of the pulmonary vessel near the area in which the pleural nerves innervate. The pain is usually worse when taking a deep breath. Tachycardia (a heart rate >100 beats per minute) is a response to the decrease in oxygenation and impaired gas exchange. Jugular vein distention (JVD) occurs as a result of pulmonary hypertension and the decreased effectiveness of the RV. Hypotension can be observed in patients with a large PE and is related to the decrease in cardiac output after ventricular dysfunction.

Other clinical manifestations that may occur but are not specific to PE include apprehension, palpitations, syncope, rales and crackles, fever, diaphoresis, murmur or gallop, and cyanosis.

Diagnosis

A thorough history and physical examination must be obtained and must include risk factors (see boxes titled, "Venous Thrombi: Conditions and Risk Factors" and "Other Risk Factors for Pulmonary Embolism"), recent medical and surgical history, and any physical findings. SOB and chest pain should be described and include time of onset, when it occurs (rest or exertion), how long it lasts, location, duration, and position.

Common initial diagnostic tools include chest radiograph (CXR), ABG analysis, D-dimer testing, and electrocardiogram (ECG) findings. The CXR cannot diagnose the presence of a PE, but it can exclude other reasons that may cause the same clinical manifestations. Patients with a PE may show PA distention, an elevation of the diaphragm, and small infiltrates or pleural effusions. ABG analysis can reveal respiratory alkalosis, low partial pressure of oxygen (pO_2), and low partial pressure of CO_2 (pCO_2). A D-dimer blood test will detect clot fragments that have been produced from clot lysis. Abnormal ECG findings usually involve transient nonspecific ST segment and T wave changes.

Differential diagnostic studies include a ventilation-perfusion (V/Q) scan, an echocardiogram, the spiral computed tomographic (CT) scan, and pulmonary angiography. When compared with other diagnostic studies, V/Q scans can sometimes be inconclusive and other diagnostic studies need to be performed. An echocardiographic study is quick, readily available, and can be very helpful in the differential diagnosis of PE. It can determine the presence of RV overload,

PA dilation, tricuspid regurgitation, pericardial fluid, hypovolemia, ventricular dysfunction, and valvular disease. A spiral CT scan is the newest approach to diagnosing PE. It is quick, readily available, and noninvasive. When intravenous contrast is given, vessels and thrombotic emboli can be visualized. Pulmonary angiography is the most definitive test for diagnosing a PE, but it is expensive, invasive, and not available in all settings.

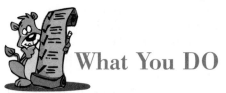

What You DO

The best treatment for PE is prevention. When patients are at risk for developing PE, prophylactic measures should be instituted such as intravenous or subcutaneous heparin, low molecular–weight heparin (Lovenox), or oral anticoagulants such as warfarin (Coumadin). The goal of therapy is to prevent thrombi formation, limit thrombi growth, and encourage breakdown of existing thrombi. Management of hypoxia may require supplemental oxygen, intubation, and mechanical ventilation.

FIRST-LINE AND INITIAL TREATMENT FOR HYPOXIA

- Administer oxygen.
- Provide intubation.
- Provide mechanical ventilation.

**Greenfield
Stainless Steel Filter**

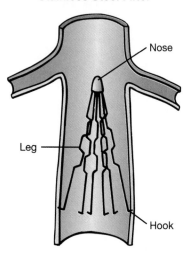

Nose

Leg

Hook

Heparin therapy is started with a bolus (usually based on the patient's weight) and a continuous infusion adjusted every 4 to 6 hours, depending on the institution's protocol. Activated partial thromboplastin time (aPTT) should be maintained at 1.5 to 2.0 times the normal value. Heparin therapy is generally continued for 7 to 14 days while the patient is on bedrest. If oral anticoagulant therapy is used, it is generally started 2 to 3 days after heparin therapy has begun, once the aPTT levels have stabilized and infusion is at a maintenance level. Oral anticoagulant doses are adjusted until the international normalized ratio (INR) is 2 to 3 times the normal value; then therapy is maintained for 3 to 6 months. Once discharged from the hospital, the patient requires that the INR be checked every 2 weeks for any adjustment in dose.

The placement of an umbrella-type filter (i.e., Greenfield) is used whenever a patient cannot, for some reason, receive anticoagulant therapy. The filter is placed in the inferior vena cava to prevent any potential thrombi from reaching the lungs.

Thrombolytic therapy may be used for patients who have had a major PE and those who present in shock or who are hemodynamically unstable. Drugs in this category include streptokinase, urokinase, and tissue plasminogen activator (t-PA). Thrombolytic therapy is used to break down the clots that have formed and are generally given within the first 24 to 48 hours of onset. If any of these medications are used, heparin therapy is to be started within 24 hours after the initial dose is given. Hemorrhage is a major concern with this type of therapy.

Surgical intervention is rarely used and is considered a last resort. Pulmonary embolectomy is the removal of a clot from the larger vessels of the pulmonary vasculature. This surgery carries a high risk of death and is only used in those patients who do not respond or have contraindications to the other interventions.

Hemodynamic changes associated with PE stem from the development of pulmonary hypertension. Pulmonary hypertension causes increased PA pressures and a dilated RV. Measures that can be taken include the use of fluid to increase RV preload and improve contractility and the use of inotropic agents to improve contractility and cardiac output. (For more information on heart failure, refer to the discussion in Chapter 4).

Nursing Responsibilities

The main nursing goal is to prevent the development of deep venous thrombosis (DVT) that may lead to a thrombotic PE. Interventions should include early ambulation, use of pneumatic stockings or boots, support hose, and passive range-of-motion (ROM) exercises. All of these improve venous blood flow and increase circulation.

Other nursing interventions include the following:

- Signs and symptoms of DVT are monitored in the lower extremities (calf pain or tenderness, redness, swelling, warmth, pain on dorsiflexion of foot [Homan's sign]).
- Prescribed oxygen therapy is maintained, and the patient is asked to cough and deep breathe every 2 hours.
- Signs and symptoms of respiratory distress or a worsening of pulmonary status (heart failure, pulmonary edema) are monitored, and the physician is notified of any developments.
- ABG analysis is monitored, and pulse oximetry is continuously taken. The physician is notified of any changes in parameters (SpO_2 <90, oxygen tension in the arterial blood [PaO_2] <80, SaO_2 <90).
- Patient is positioned for comfort and optimal oxygenation, as well as to promote the expulsion of secretions. When PE has occurred, patient should be turned to his or her unaffected side to improve perfusion and to ventilate these areas.
- Pillows are placed under the patient's knees in an attempt to improve venous return. When knees are bent, venous blood flow can be impeded.
- Signs and symptoms of bleeding are monitored when anticoagulant or thrombolytic therapy is in progress (i.e., blood in stool or urine, pale mucous membranes, petechia, ecchymosis, complaints of back or flank pain).
- Anticoagulant laboratory values (complete blood count [CBC], aPTT, INR, fibrinogen) are monitored for any abnormal or out of therapeutic range levels.
- Signs of cardiac arrhythmias such as atrial fibrillation and flutter are monitored; these may predispose the patient to thrombi formation.

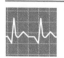
The therapeutic range for a patient taking heparin is based on the aPTT, which should be 1.5 to 2.0 times the normal value.

The reversal agent for heparin is protamine sulfate; the reversal agent for warfarin (Coumadin) is vitamin K or fresh-frozen plasma (FFP).

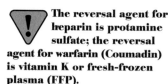 **TAKE HOME POINTS**

An inferior vena cava filter is not a treatment for PE; rather, it is a device used in an attempt to prevent a PE from occurring in patients with a known venous thrombus or at high risk for developing thrombi.

 TAKE HOME POINTS

Administration of thrombolytics will break down the clots.

Hemorrhage is a major concern with the administration of thrombolytic therapy.

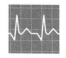
A PE will result in an increase in PA pressures.

If Homan's sign is positive, then do NOT retest it; doing so may dislodge the clot.

- Medication is administered to decrease anxiety and pain.
- Areas of skin puncture sites (venipuncture, lumbar puncture, bone marrow aspiration) are assessed for leakage, hemorrhage, and hematoma.
- Distraction is provided during the periods of bedrest. Patients are on bedrest to prevent mobilization of any other thrombi and to preserve oxygen demands during activity.

Patient Education

Topics to be covered in educating the patient and family include the following:

- An explanation of the definition of PE is given to the patient and family. This explanation includes how it develops, its signs and symptoms, and the interventions involved in the treatment and prevention of occurrences.
- If the patient is receiving anticoagulant or thrombolytic therapy, then an explanation of the signs and symptoms of bleeding is provided to the patient and family.
- If the patient is discharged while still receiving oral anticoagulant therapy, discussions about the drug, doses, side effects, food and drug interactions, importance of follow-up laboratory work, and physician visits are conducted.
- The patient receives instruction on the application of antiembolic leg hose, as well as the importance of not crossing the legs, of avoiding prolonged sitting, and of wearing constrictive clothing.
- The patient is taught the importance of adequate hydration.

Do You UNDERSTAND?

DIRECTIONS: **Choose the correct answer to each of the following questions, and write the corresponding letter in the space provided.**

_____ 1. Which of the following is a risk factor for the development of a PE?
     a. Anticoagulated blood
     b. Early ambulation
     c. Use of pneumatic stockings
     d. Injury to vessel wall

_____ 2. Which of the following is caused by the decrease in CO_2 related to ventilation-perfusion mismatch?
     a. Bronchoconstriction
     b. Decrease in pulmonary resistance
     c. Increase in oxygenation
     d. Shunting of blood to affected areas of lung

Answers: 1. b; 2. a.

_____ 3. A clinical manifestation of PE includes which of the following?
   a. Chest pain on expiration
   b. Hypertension
   c. Wheezing
   d. Dyspnea
_____ 4. Heparin therapy is maintained at a therapeutic level that is _____ times normal.
   a. 1.0 to 1.5
   b. 2.0 to 2.5
   c. 1.5 to 2.0
   d. 0.5 to 1.5

What IS Acute Respiratory Distress Syndrome?

Acute respiratory distress syndrome (ARDS) is a syndrome with inflammation and increased permeability of the alveolocapillary membrane that occurs as a result of an injury to the lungs. This inflammation causes noncardiogenic pulmonary edema with severely impaired gas exchange. The mortality rate can be as high as 60%, mostly from multisystem organ failure. Of those who survive, many have long-term impairment of lung function.

What You NEED TO KNOW

Causes

A multitude of possible causes for ARDS result from direct and indirect injury to the lungs themselves. Some of the more common conditions that can precipitate ARDS are the following:

- Sepsis
- Aspiration of gastric contents
- Near drowning
- Trauma
- Severe burns
- Multiple blood transfusions

Pathophysiologic Changes

When an injury occurs to the lungs, an inflammatory response is initiated by the immune system. This response stimulates the activation of neutrophils, macrophages, and endotoxins into the lungs and the release of mediators. Permeability of the alveolocapillary membrane is increased, allowing large molecules, such as protein-rich fluid, to enter into the lung tissue; this action causes the alveoli to collapse. Severe hypoxia develops, leading to respiratory acidosis, narrowing of small airways, and pulmonary vasoconstriction. As hypoxia increases, the patient begins to hyperventilate, which creates fatigue and eventually respiratory failure. Pulmonary vasoconstriction can lead to pulmonary hypertension with RV dysfunction and decreased cardiac output.

Stages of Edema Formation

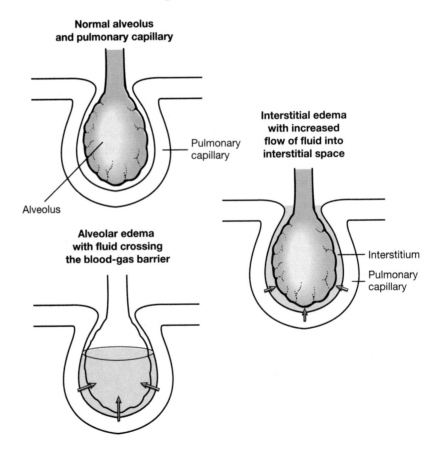

Clinical Manifestations

A review of the patient's history and the potential risk factors related to ARDS development is needed for early assessment, diagnosis, and intervention. Most patients exhibit symptoms 24 to 48 hours after the initial insult to the lungs. Apprehension and restlessness, hyperventilation and SOB with the use of accessory muscle are some of the first signs leading to respiratory failure. Auscultation of lungs may reveal clear lung fields and crackles or rales. Other signs and symptoms of ARDS include tachycardia, hyperthermia, cyanosis, and cough.

Diagnosis

ABG analysis reveals a low PaO_2, despite the increase of supplemental oxygen concentration. This increase is known as refractory hypoxemia and is an important factor in diagnosis. $PaCO_2$ will decrease, initially related to the patient's hyperventilating, but the $PaCO_2$ will eventually increase as the patient becomes fatigued, which leads to respiratory acidosis. CXR findings may reveal bilateral infiltrates as a result of the increased alveoli permeability. Terms such as "patchy" infiltrates or "white out" may be associated with these CXR results. Hemodynamic monitoring with a PA catheter reveals a pulmonary capillary wedge pressure (PCWP) of less than 18.

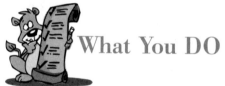

What You DO

Treatment

The main goals in the treatment of ARDS include improving and maintaining oxygenation, maintaining fluid and electrolyte imbalances, providing adequate nutrition, and preventing respiratory and metabolic complications.

Supplemental oxygen is the first step in the treatment of ARDS. These patients generally require intubation and mechanical ventilation to maintain adequate gas exchange. FiO_2 as high as 100% and intubation may be needed to help with tissue oxygenation. Maintaining a PaO_2 of >60 mm Hg and an SaO_2 of 90 mm Hg using the lowest amount of FiO_2 possible is the main goal of oxygen therapy. If greater than 60%, then FiO_2 is used for longer than 24 to 48 hours and oxygen toxicity may develop. Oxygen toxicity can increase damage to lung tissue by increasing membrane permeability and alveolar damage.

Mechanical ventilation after intubation is often needed in response to fatigue and respiratory failure, and it allows for the underlying problem to be treated. The goal of mechanical ventilation is to improve ventilation function while decreasing the work of breathing and the oxygen concentration. PEEP is often added to the mode of ventilation to assist in improving oxygenation by opening alveoli that have closed. The use of PEEP generally leads to improved gas exchange and allows for lower concentrations of oxygen to be used.

TAKE HOME POINTS

Most often patients who develop ARDS exhibit symptoms within 24 to 48 hours after the initial insult to the lungs.

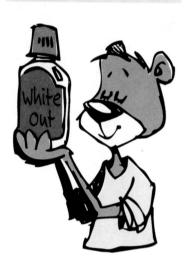

In patients with ARDS, PaO_2 will be low, despite oxygen administration; pCO_2 will decrease as a result of hyperventilation.

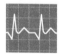 The PCWP reading from a PA catheter is normal (<18 mm Hg), which means that the pulmonary edema is not cardiogenic in nature.

Oxygen toxicity may develop if high concentrations of oxygen are used for longer than 24 to 48 hours.

TAKE HOME POINTS

PEEP may need to be at high levels (>7.5); the astute nurse watches for possible complications such as a pneumothorax.

TAKE HOME POINTS

IRV ventilation improves oxygenation through increasing the inspiratory time.

Patients in respiratory failure from ARDS have a tendency to continue to hyperventilate and breathe against the ventilator once they are placed on it. The use of sedation allows for the ventilator to take over the work of breathing; decreasing anxiety helps the patient rest. Neuromuscular-blocking agents may be used in conjunction with sedatives, enabling the patient to be adequately sedated.

IRV is a mode of ventilation that has been used in patients with ARDS to improve oxygenation. Normally, expiratory time is longer than inspiratory time. With IRV, inspiratory time is longer than expiratory time. This characteristic allows for alveoli that have been closed to reopen and lowers airway pressures. The change in I/E time often makes patients uncomfortable and increasingly anxiousness; therefore sedation is frequently required with this mode of ventilation.

The use of mechanical ventilation can have complications such as increased airway pressures, increased inflammation, and hemorrhaging in the alveoli by over distending the lung tissue. These complications can increase the injury to the lungs and increase the rates of mortality. Ventilatory support with small tidal volumes (6 ml/kg) has been used to decrease airway resistance, decrease the stretch on lung tissue, and possibly reduce mortality.

HFV is a new therapy that is being investigated for the treatment of ARDS. HFV delivers a small amount of tidal volume at a rapid respiratory rate. The use of HFV helps prevent overdistention of alveoli, decreases airway pressures, and maintains $PaCO_2$ and PaO_2 levels.

The use of extracorporeal membrane oxygenation (ECMO) is another new treatment that is being investigated for use on patients with ARDS who experience refractory hypoxemia and do not improve with maximal supportive care. ECMO, like cardiopulmonary bypass, can be used for long-term support of a patient. It is used to improve oxygenation and to allow the lungs to rest and recover. To date, the use of ECMO has not yet been shown to reduce mortality in patients with ARDS, and its use in research is limited to the major institutions.

Liquid ventilation is a promising new treatment for patients with ARDS. Liquid fluorocarbon has low-surface tension (allowing alveoli to open), dissolves a high amount of oxygen (improving oxygenation), and spreads evenly throughout lung tissue (improving oxygen distribution). It is poorly absorbed by the body and evaporates through the lungs. Fluorocarbon is dense; therefore gravity pulls it toward the dependent lung regions. The weight and pressure of the fluid pushes blood from the damaged areas to areas that receive more ventilation, thereby improving oxygenation.

Partial liquid ventilation (PLV) is a type of ventilation in which liquid fluorocarbons are instilled into the lungs through the endotracheal tube until the FRC is reached. A normal ventilator is then used to deliver oxygen and a tidal volume and to remove CO_2. PLV is still in clinical trials and is generally used on patients when all other measures have been exhausted.

Hemodynamic Monitoring

The use of an arterial pressure line and a PA catheter are often seen in patients with ARDS. Together, they are used for monitoring blood pressure, collecting ABGs, measuring cardiac output, and monitoring fluid management. The use of PEEP can cause a decrease in venous return (low central venous pressure [CVP]), cardiac output, and blood pressure. Pulmonary vasoconstriction that can occur with ARDS may lead to pulmonary hypertension and RV dysfunction. The use of hemodynamic monitoring is essential in early recognition and intervention of these possible complications.

Mixed Venous Oxygen Saturation

Monitoring mixed venous oxygen saturation (SVO_2) indicates the amount of oxygen available after the tissues have been perfused. A fiberoptic network located in specialized PA catheters is how it is measured. Four components are used to measure SVO_2: (1) SaO_2, (2) hemoglobin, (3) cardiac output, and (4) oxygen consumption (VO_2). Normal values of SVO_2 range from 60% to 80%. Values less than 50% are an indication of increased tissue oxygen demand.

Fluid Management

The goal of fluid therapy is to maintain tissue perfusion. Fluid restriction is generally observed in these patients to prevent further leakage of fluid into the alveoli and to decrease pulmonary edema, but fluid restriction can also cause a decrease in cardiac output and blood pressure. Studies have shown that intravascular volume should be given to keep the CVP between 4 and 12 mm Hg or the PCWP between 6 and 14 mm Hg. When a decrease in blood pressure occurs, vasopressors such as dobutamine may be used to keep mean arterial pressure (MAP) above 65 mm Hg. This level maintains tissue perfusion to the extremities and major organs.

Positioning

Prone positioning is an intervention that may improve oxygenation by decreasing edema and atelectasis, thereby providing an improved distribution of oxygen throughout the lungs. Prone positioning requires several nursing professionals to implement safely; airway protection is of utmost concern. More studies are needed to develop guidelines on the use of prone positioning to obtain maximal benefits for these patients. Hemodynamic instability and activity intolerance with increased oxygen consumption are contraindications to prone positioning.

Nutrition

Energy expenditure during respiratory failure is high and is caused by the increased work of breathing. The goal of nutritional support is to provide the needed nutrients to maintain the patient's current level of metabolism, energize the immune system, and maintain end-organ function. Enteral GI feeding is the route of choice to provide the calories and nutrients needed and to assist in maintaining normal GI function. If the patient is unable to tolerate enteral feedings, then a parenteral (intravenous) route is necessary until the patient can tolerate enteral feedings.

For further information on hemodynamics, refer to Chapter 1 in the *Real World Nursing Survival Guide, Hemodynamic Monitoring*.

For further information on the electrical conduction system and ECG interpretation, see the *Real World Nursing Survival Guide, Hemodynamic Monitoring*.

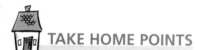

TAKE HOME POINTS

Fluid restriction is necessary; however, tissue perfusion and cardiac output should not be compromised.

Increased oxygen consumption and hemodynamic instability (unstable blood pressure) are contraindications for prone positioning.

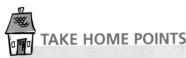

Corticosteroid Therapy

Corticosteroids may be prescribed as antiinflammatory agents to decrease the permeability of the alveolocapillary membrane and to prevent further leakage of fluid into the alveoli. Corticosteroid therapy may increase the risk of nosocomial infections related to immune suppression.

Nursing Responsibilities

The main nursing goals are to optimize oxygenation, maintain tissue perfusion, provide adequate nutrition, and provide emotional support to the patient and family and include the following:

- Respiratory status is assessed every 1 to 2 hours, documenting rate, rhythm, breathing pattern, and use of accessory muscles.
- Breath sounds are assessed at least every 4 hours for abnormal findings such as crackles or rales.
- The patient is assessed for restlessness, anxiety, change in level of consciousness, and tachypnea; any one of these symptoms may indicate a progression of respiratory distress.
- The patient is positioned for optimal gas exchange and comfort (prone position is recommended if not contraindicated).
- ABGs are monitored, and the physician is notified of any significant changes related to oxygenation status (e.g., PaO_2 <80, SaO_2 <90%, acidosis).
- Supplemental oxygen is administered at the lowest flow to provide adequate oxygen saturation.
- Mechanical ventilation is maintained and monitored (see discussion on mechanical ventilation earlier in this chapter).
- The patient is provided with adequate periods of rest by grouping nursing activities.
- Good pulmonary hygiene such as cough, deep breathing, and suctioning the endotracheal tube is provided when needed.
- Hemodynamics are monitored when a PA catheter is in use, observing for trends and notifying the physician if significant increases in CVP or PCWP readings occur and if cardiac output or blood pressure levels decrease.
- Adequate nutrition is provided. If receiving enteral feedings, residual amounts are measured every 4 hours. The physician is notified if the residual amount is $1^1/2$ to 2 times the infusion rate (indicating that the patient is not tolerating feedings).
- Changes in skin integrity related to bedrest, compromised immune system, and poor nutritional state are monitored.

Patient and Family Education

Topics to be covered in educating the patient and family include the following:

- An explanation is given to the patient and family about ARDS.
- An explanation is given to the patient and family about the signs and symptoms of respiratory distress.
- The patient and family are taught the treatments and interventions designed to decrease levels of anxiety.

- An explanation is given to the patient and family about the reason for frequent laboratory testing and ABG monitoring.
- An explanation is given to the patient and family about monitors and what is being monitored.
- An explanation is given to the family about the role of sedation during ventilatory support.

Do You UNDERSTAND?

DIRECTIONS: Choose the correct answer to each of the following questions, and write the corresponding letter in the space provided.

_____ 1. The increased permeability that is seen in ARDS increases fluid accumulation in which of the following areas?
   a. RV
   b. Brain tissue
   c. Pericardial sac
   d. Alveoli

_____ 2. Symptoms of respiratory distress associated with ARDS begins within _____ hours of insult to lungs?
   a. 6 to 12
   b. 12 to 24
   c. 24 to 48
   d. 48 to 72

_____ 3. The addition of PEEP to the mode of ventilation may cause which of the following to occur in the patient with ARDS?
   a. Increased venous return
   b. Decreased cardiac output
   c. Decreased oxygen saturation
   d. Increased work of breathing

_____ 4. Which of the following medications may be used to maintain tissue perfusion during periods of low cardiac output?
   a. Dobutamine (Dobutrex)
   b. Neosynephrine
   c. Nitroglycerin
   d. Sodium nitroprusside (Nipride)

6 Nervous System

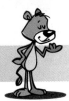

What IS a Seizure?

A seizure is a sudden, abnormal, excessive discharge of electrical activity within the brain that disrupts the brain's usual system for nerve conduction. A seizure is a nonchronic disorder. Epilepsy is a chronic disorder, characterized by recurrent seizure activity.

What You NEED TO KNOW

Three phases of seizure activity exist. The first phase is the *prodromal phase*. It consists of mood or behavior changes that may precede the seizure by hours or days. An aura occurs in some individuals before the seizure. It is a sensory warning such as an unusual taste or smell, metallic taste, or flash of lights. The second phase is the *ictal phase*, which is the seizure activity itself. The third phase is the *postictal phase* that follows the seizure. There may be behavior changes, lethargy, or confusion.

Classification of Seizures

The International Classification of Epileptic Seizures recognizes three broad categories of seizure disorders. Seizures are classified as (1) *partial (focal) seizures*, (2) *generalized seizures*, or (3) *unclassified seizures*. Simple partial seizures occur in about 15% of patients with seizures. Symptoms may be motor, cognitive, sensory, autonomic, or affective, depending on the area of cerebral cortex involved. Consciousness is not impaired with this type of seizure. Complex partial seizures occur in approximately 35% of patients with seizures. Consciousness is partially or completely impaired, but no initial generalized tonic-clonic activity occurs.

TAKE HOME POINTS

- A seizure is an outward sign of the disruption of the brain's electrical activity.
- A seizure is a symptom, not a disease.
- A seizure will frequently result in changes in behavior, movements, sensation, perception, or consciousness.

A patient may experience an aura before seizing.

Clinical presentation does vary, but patients usually experience an aura, automatism, postictal confusion, or tiredness. They will have no memory of the events during the seizure.

Generalized seizures account for 40% of patients with epilepsy. The manifestations of generalized seizures indicate involvement of both hemispheres, most commonly impairment of consciousness with bilateral motor involvement. Patients usually have amnesia of the event.

- Absence or petit-mal seizures are most common in children.
- Head trauma and injury is a common cause of seizures in young adults.

Types of Generalized Seizures and Signs and Symptoms

TYPE OF SEIZURE	SIGNS AND SYMPTOMS
Absence (petit-mal)	Occurs in 5% of patients with seizures Occurs primarily in children Vacant, blinking stare Some body movements may occur No convulsions or postictal signs or symptoms
Atonic (drop attacks)	Sudden loss of postural muscle tone
Myoclonic	Brief symmetric jerking of the extremities that usually involve the upper extremities
Clonic	Repetitive, rapid motor activity
Tonic	Rigidity
Tonic-clonic (grand-mal)	Occurs in 25% of patients with seizures Most common type of generalized seizures in adults Tonic stiffening (extension) followed by jerking movements (clonic phase) May produce cyanosis, labored respirations, bowel or bladder incontinence (or both), involuntary tongue biting, and postictal fatigue, confusion, or stupor

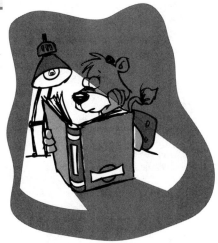

TAKE HOME POINTS

- Unclassified seizures are idiopathic; they occur for an unknown reason and do not fit into the partial or generalized classifications.
- Seventy-five percent of seizures are idiopathic in nature.
- A seizure may occur in isolation or with an acute problem within the CNS (low blood sugar, drug or alcohol withdrawal, head injury).
- Brain tumors are the most common cause of seizures. Seizures are often the first manifestation of an intracranial mass.

Cause of Seizures

Seizures may be triggered by toxic states, electrolyte imbalances, anoxia, cerebral tumors, inflammation of the central nervous system (CNS) tissue, cerebrovascular disease, hyperpyrexia, increased intracranial pressure (ICP), trauma, Huntington's disease, multiple sclerosis, Alzheimer's disease, or idiopathic causes.

Myths and Stigmas Associated with Seizures

Many myths and stigmas are associated with seizures, all of them untrue:
- Epilepsy is synonymous with stupid.
- Epilepsy is contagious.
- Seizures are an act of the supernatural.
- Epileptics have psychiatric problems.
- Epileptics cannot participate in sports or other normal activities of daily living.
- Epileptic employees have a higher rate of on-the-job injuries and absenteeism.

- Adults are usually instructed to stay up late the night before the EEG and to awaken early.
- For a sleep-deprived EEG, children and infants should not be allowed to nap before the scheduled test.

Diagnostic Tests

Blood tests should include a sodium, potassium, calcium, phosphorus, magnesium, blood urea nitrogen (BUN), glucose level, and a toxicology screen. Other laboratory tests that may be used to look for abnormalities that may result in seizures include oxygen tension in the arterial blood (PaO_2) (hypoxemia), low anticonvulsant medication therapeutic levels, and associated blood identifying disorders (lead poisoning, leukemia, sickle cell anemia). An electroencephalogram (EEG) is the most definite test to diagnose seizure activity. An EEG may determine the presence of a seizure focus, it measures electrical activity of the brain through electrodes that are placed on the scalp. The standard 21-lead, 30-minute EEG may be falsely negative; it has a sensitivity of only 50% to 60%. A 24-hour EEG may be necessary to establish a definitive diagnosis.

Sleep-deprived EEG may be ordered because sleep deprivation may evoke abnormal brain patterns, and most EEGs require the patient to sleep the last part of the EEG test.

A computed tomography (CT) scan of the head with contrast is particularly useful in the setting of a focal seizure, neurologic deficit, absence of a history of alcohol abuse, or possible trauma. Magnetic resonance imaging (MRI) of the head is indicated after a tonic-clonic seizure. MRI will show an abnormality in 10% to 20% of patients with a generalized tonic-clonic seizure and a normal CT scan. Single photon emission computed tomography (SPECT) scans are also done to help diagnose seizure disorders. This scan uses several of the common radionuclides that are commercially prepared. A SPECT scan is the scan of choice for a diagnostic evaluation of certain types of CNS disorders; it is used to provide information about the metabolism of and the blood flow through the brain tissue. A cerebral arteriogram may be prescribed to visualize vascular abnormalities not seen on the CT scan. Skull radiographs may be done if head trauma is involved. Finally, a lumbar puncture (LP) is indicated if infection or hemorrhage is suspected as the cause of the seizure activity, and a bone marrow aspiration is conducted if leukemia is suspected.

Treatment

Medication therapy is the hallmark of seizure management. However, less than 75% of seizures are fully controlled by anticonvulsant drug therapy. Seizure type and the patient's tolerance for side effects determine drug choices. Combination therapy results in total control of seizures in 10% of patients not controlled with monotherapy, and an additional 40% have a reduction in seizure frequency. The doses of the anticonvulsant medication are determined by clinical response, not serum drug level. If the patient is seizure free, increasing the dose will not reduce the risk of future seizures but will increase toxicity, even if the drug level is subtherapeutic. Finally, the usual effective plasma concentration may be exceeded to achieve seizure control if the patient is not having significant drug toxic effects.

Antiepileptic Drugs

DRUG	THERAPEUTIC SERUM DRUG LEVEL (mg/ml)	INDICATION FOR USE	COMMON SIDE EFFECTS
Acetazolamide (Diamox)	Not established	Second choice for myoclonic seizures	Lethargy, paresthesias, appetite suppression, renal calculi, metabolic acidosis
Carbamazepine (Tegretol)	6-12 Toxic is >14	First choice for partial simple and complex and tonic-clonic	Dizziness, diplopia, leukopenia
Clonazepam (Klonopin)	0.02-0.08	Second choice for myoclonic seizures	Sedation, confusion, ataxia, depression
Ethosuximide (Zarontin)	40-100	First choice for typical absence seizures Second choice for atypical absence seizures	Gastrointestinal (GI) side effects: nausea/vomiting; lethargy, anorexia, skin rash
Gabapentin (Neurontin)	Not established	Second choice for partial simple and complex seizures	Somnolence, ataxia, dizziness, fatigue, weight gain
Lamotrigine (Lamictal)	Not established	Second choice for partial simple and complex seizures, typical and atypical absence seizures, and tonic-clonic seizures	Weight gain, somnolence, rash, ataxia, dizziness, diplopia, headache, nausea/vomiting
Levetiracetam (Keppra)	Not established	Second choice for partial complex seizures	Psychiatric symptoms, somnolence, asthenia
Oxcarbazepine (Trileptal)	Not established	First choice for partial complex seizures and tonic-clonic seizures	Diplopia, ataxia, dizziness, somnolence
Phenobarbital	10-40 Toxic level >60	Second choice for tonic-clonic seizures	Dizziness, ataxia, rash, sedation, cognitive impairment, drowsiness
Phenytoin sodium (Dilantin)	10-20 Toxic level >40	First choice for partial simple and complex seizures and tonic-clonic seizures	Gingival hyperplasia, gastric distress, rash, ataxia, nystagmus, osteomalacia, lymphadenopathy, macrocytosis, hypertrichosis
Primidone (Mysoline)	5-12	Second choice for tonic-clonic seizures	Nystagmus, ataxia, nausea, dizziness, sedation, vertigo
Topiramate (Topamax)	Not established	Second choice for tonic-clonic seizures	Weight loss, nervousness, somnolence, ataxia, confusion, dizziness
Valproic acid (Depakene)	50-100 Toxic level >150	First choice for partial simple and complex seizures and for typical and atypical absence seizures and tonic-clonic and myoclonic seizures	Somnolence, nausea/vomiting, anorexia, hair loss, increased liver enzymes, bruising
Zonisamide (Zonegran)	Not established	Second choice for partial complex seizures and for myoclonic seizures	Headache, dizziness, ataxia, somnolence, renal calculi

TAKE HOME POINTS

- Monotherapy (or the use of one anticonvulsant) is preferred; however in some cases combination therapy is needed.
- Clinical response to the medication is the key for dosing and managing the seizure patient, not serum drug levels.
- Most seizures decrease in frequency but are not totally eliminated when a corpus callosotomy is done.

Surgical management is another consideration for some patients experiencing seizures. Resective procedures to remove the brain tissue that is the focus of the seizure activity is one type of surgical treatment. With resective procedures the goal is to remove the maximal amount of seizure producing tissue without causing any sort of neurologic deficit. Another type of surgical treatment is a palliative corpus callosotomy. The corpus callosum is a fibrous network of nerves that join the brain hemispheres; therefore this procedure stops the spread of seizures and thus prevents loss of consciousness.

The use of vagus nerve stimulation (VNS) is achieving more attention in the treatment of seizures. The VNS is a pacemaker-like device connected to a programmable generator. It stimulates the left vagus nerve (the nerve that affects parts of the brain that propagate seizures) in the neck and can modestly reduce seizure frequency. The patient can also trigger it with a hand held device (magnet) if he or she experiences an aura, and often the seizure is prevented or the severity of the seizure is lessened.

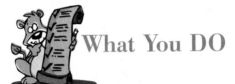

What You DO

Seizure Precautions

Seizure precautions vary from institution to institution and are performed to prevent the patient from injury if a seizure does occur. In most institutions it is recommended that oxygen (O_2) and suction equipment with an airway be readily available in the patient's room. It is also appropriate to have intravenous (IV) access at all times for a patient with a history of seizures, this allows IV medication to be given if needed. The use of padded side rails is controversial; side rails are rarely a source of significant injury for the patient with seizures. However, they should always be left up to prevent a fall from the bed. Because of the social stigma that is attached to seizures, the padded side rails may be a source of embarrassment for the patient and the family. The bed must be in the lowest position at all times in case the patient falls out of bed.

FIRST-LINE AND INITIAL TREATMENTS FOR SEIZURES

- Have O_2 and suction equipment ready for use if a patient is placed on seizure precautions.

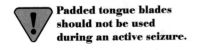

Padded tongue blades should not be used during an active seizure.

Padded tongue blades are rarely kept at the bedside, and they should not be inserted into the patient's mouth after the seizure begins. After the seizure begins, the jaw may clench down; forcing a tongue blade or airway into the mouth is more likely to chip the teeth and cause aspiration of tooth fragments rather than to prevent the patient from biting the tongue. In addition, improper placement of a padded tongue blade can cause obstruction of the airway.

The actions taken by the nurse should be appropriate for the type of seizure. A complete description of the type of seizure activity that occurs, along with the presence or absence of an aura, and the events surrounding the seizure assists in determining the best plan of care. The following nursing interventions should be completed when a patient has a seizure:

- The patient should be protected from injury, and his or her movements should be guided if necessary.
- Objects that are in the patient's way should be removed to prevent injury.
- The patient should never be restrained.
- Any restrictive clothing worn by the patient should be loosened.
- A tongue blade or airway should not be forced into the patient's mouth.
- The patient should be turned onto his or her right side.
- The patient should be suctioned as needed to maintain the airway.
  At the end of the seizure the medical team should:
- Assess the patient's vital signs.
- Perform neurologic checks.
- Keep the patient on his or her side.
- Allow the patient to rest.
- Document the seizure.
  When documenting a seizure the following should be included:
- Onset: Was it sudden or preceded by an aura (if an aura was present, describe the aura)?
- Duration: What time did the seizure start and end?
- Frequency and number: Did the patient have one seizure or several seizures?
- State of consciousness: Was the patient unconscious? If so, for how long? Could he or she be aroused? (Any changes in consciousness should be noted.)
- Eyes and tongue: Did the pupils change in shape, size, equality, or in their reaction to light? Did they deviate to one side?
- Teeth: Were they opened or clenched?
- Motor activity: Where did the motor activity begin? What parts of the body were involved? Was there a pattern of progression of the activity? Describe his or her movements.
- Body activities: Did the patient become incontinent of urine or stool? Did he or she have any oral bleeding, or vomit, or salivate?
- Respirations: What was the respiratory rate and quality? Was there any cyanosis?
- Drug response: If any drugs were given during the seizure, how did the patient respond? Did the seizures stop or worsen?
- Seizure awareness: Is the patient aware of what happened? Did he or she immediately go into a deep sleep after the seizure? Was he or she upset or seem ashamed? How long did it take for the patient to return to preseizure status?

The nursing interventions outlined in the Status Epilepticus section that follows will need to be performed if the patient develops status epilepticus.

TAKE HOME POINTS

An airway is inserted into the patient's mouth wrong side up and then turned onto the correct side once it is in the middle of the mouth. This prevents the tongue from being pushed back and occluding the airway.

What IS Status Epilepticus?

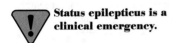

Status epilepticus is a clinical emergency.

Status epilepticus is defined as continually recurring seizures that occur in rapid succession and do not allow for recovery at the end of the postictal phase. It is a potential complication of all seizure types. Principal concerns with convulsive status epilepticus are anoxia, arrhythmias, and acidosis. The usual causes of status epilepticus are as follows:

- Withdrawal from anticonvulsant medication
- Acute alcohol withdrawal
- CNS infections
- Metabolic disturbances
- Head injuries
- Brain tumors
- Cerebral edema
- Cerebrovascular disease

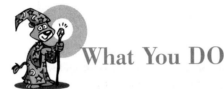

What You DO

If status epilepticus does occur, the nurse must notify the physician immediately and support the airway, breathing, and circulation of the patient. Immediate interventions include providing O_2 via nasal cannula or face mask, preparing for intubation, protecting the patient from injury, establishing IV access, and infusing an IV of normal saline (NS) solution. In addition, inserting a nasogastric (NG) tube and connecting it to gastric suction will assist in preventing the patient from vomiting and possible aspiration. Cardiac rate and rhythm, along with continuous blood pressure (BP), should also be monitored.

FIRST-LINE AND INITIAL TREATMENTS FOR STATUS EPILEPTICUS

- Monitor ABCs (airway, breathing, circulation).
- Notify the physician.
- Establish IV access.
- Prevent injury.
- Monitor heart rate, ECG rhythm, and BP.
- Prepare to administer medications.

Medications should be administered as prescribed, usually IV diazepam (Valium) 10 to 20 mg at 5 mg/min (adult patient). Onset of action is almost immediate; duration of action is 30 to 60 minutes. Lorazepam (Ativan) may also be prescribed at 4 mg IV over 2 to 5 minutes every 10 to 15 minutes if seizures persist. Onset of action of Lorazepam is approximately 15 minutes. These medications induce respiratory depression; therefore the patient's vital signs must be monitored closely. Flumazenil (Romazicon) may be administered if the patient's respiratory status becomes compromised. Flumazenil is a benzodiazepine receptor antagonist that helps decrease the respiratory depression of the patient. It is administered IV to adults in doses as follows: 0.2 mg given over 30 seconds; wait 30 seconds, then give 0.3 mg over 30 seconds; further doses of 0.5 mg can be given over 30 seconds at intervals of 1 minute up to a cumulative dose of 3 mg. Phenytoin (Dilantin) may also be prescribed, total dose of 15 to 18 mg/kg slow IV push (no more than 50 mg/min). The onset of action is 10 to 20 minutes; the duration of action is 24 hours.

Phenytoin can infiltrate easily and is very caustic to tissues. Treatment of infiltrated tissue with phenytoin varies; the literature states to elevate the extremity and apply dry heat and cool compresses. The use of topical nitroglycerine is also suggested to increase intravascular absorption and relieve vasospasms. Because of the possible infiltration and hemodynamic side effects (hypotension, bradycardia) of phenytoin, sometimes Fosphenytoin will be administered. Fosphenytoin's action is like phenytoin without the potentially detrimental side effects. Fosphenytoin is administered IV at 15 to 20 mg/kg or up to 150 mg/min. Phenobarbital may also be given IV at a dose of 5 to 8 mg/kg at 60 mg/min. The onset of action is 5 to 20 minutes; the duration of action is about 24 hours.

If seizure activity is not stopped with the previously mentioned medications, high-dose pentobarbital therapy may be used. Loading dose is 5 to 10 mg/kg over 1 hour and then 5 mg/kg per hour three times. Maintenance dose is 1 to 3 mg/kg per hour. Continuous EEG monitoring is required, along with monitoring serum levels (therapeutic level is 25 to 40 mg/dl).

For status epilepticus, the nurse or other members of the medical team should do the following:

- Maintain the patient's airway. A nasal airway lubricated with water-soluble lubricant can be inserted while someone else is notifying the physician.
- Administer O_2 via nasal cannula or face mask; prepare for intubation.
- Turn the patient on his or her side to allow for secretions to drain from the oral cavity.
- Suction the airway as needed.
- Start an IV of NS solution to keep the vein open. The IV insertion site should not be in the wrist or antecubital area, because the catheter could become dislodged.
- Remove any objects that can harm the patient.
- Connect the patient to a cardiac and O_2 saturation via pulse oximetry (SpO_2) monitor and automatic BP device.
  - Administer medications as ordered.
  - Insert an NG tube and connect to suction.
  - Plan for transfer to the intensive care unit (ICU), if not already there.
  - Remember that patient education is vital for any patient diagnosed with a seizure disorder.

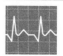 When administering phenytoin, one must assess for hypotension, bradycardia, or the development of heart blocks.

- Phenytoin should not be mixed with any dextrose solution because it will form precipitation or crystallization of the solution.
- Because of the adverse side effects of phenytoin, Fosphenytoin is an alternative medication that may be administered.

Respiratory depression, hypotension, and depression of consciousness may occur with phenobarbital; therefore one must also monitor vital signs and neurologic status.

The patient should be told to do the following:

DOs	DON'Ts
• Stay well hydrated. • Follow proper nutrition, and eat a balanced diet. • Learn to identify an aura and assume a safe position. • Tell the important people in his or her life so that they may react calmly and safely when a seizure occurs. • Take anticonvulsant medications as prescribed and on time, never missing a dose. • Wear a medical alert necklace or bracelet. • Contact the Epilepsy Foundation of America (www.epilepsyfoundation.org) or other organized epilepsy groups. • Join a seizure support group. • Investigate local and state laws covering driving as an epileptic.	• Ingest too much caffeine. • Use illegal drugs or alcohol. • Get excessively fatigued. • Tackle too many stressful activities at once. • Take any medications that the physician is unaware of, including over-the-counter and herbal medications.

Do You UNDERSTAND?

DIRECTIONS: Unscramble the letters in italics to form types of seizures or seizure management, treatment, or terminology.

1. _____
   (cocinymlo)

2. _____
   (ttssua iispptcelue)

3. _____
   (tinobbaehlpar)

4. _____
   (cneehoraltocgerlaemp)

5. _____
   (raua)

Answers: 1. myoclonic; 2. status epilepticus; 3. phenobarbital; 4. electroencephalogram; 5. aura.

What IS Meningitis?

Meningitis is an inflammation of the membranes covering the brain and spinal cord (arachnoid and pia mater). Viruses, bacteria, fungi, chemicals, trauma, or tumors can cause it. The infective agent can be introduced by way of the sinuses, or ear canal, which may be caused by a basilar skull fracture resulting in dural tears with cerebrospinal fluid (CSF) leak or otitis media or sinusitis, bloodstream at the blood-brain barrier, or through a penetrating head wound, gunshot wounds, depressed skull fracture, ICP monitoring device, dental abscess or recent dental therapy, septicemia or septic emboli, ruptured cerebral abscess, or surgical procedure. The organism can then migrate throughout the CNS via the subarachnoid space, producing an inflammatory response in the arachnoid, pia mater, CSF, and ventricles. The exudates, which are formed during the inflammatory response, may spread to both the cranial and spinal nerves, thus causing further neurologic deterioration.

What You NEED TO KNOW

Bacterial Meningitis

Bacterial meningitis, in 80% to 90% of cases, is caused by streptococcal pneumonia, *Haemophilus influenzae*, or *Neisseria meningitides*. Bacterial meningitis is seen most frequently in the fall and winter when upper respiratory tract infections are more common.

Bacterial meningitis largely occurs in areas of high population density, such as refugee groups, college dormitories, military barracks, prisons, and crowded living areas. Transmission occurs through direct contact with infectious respiratory secretions. More often the patient who develops bacterial meningitis has a predisposing condition, such as otitis media, pneumonia, acute sinusitis, or sickle cell anemia. A fractured skull or spinal or brain surgery may also contribute to the development of meningitis. Treatment is focused on antimicrobial therapy. Patients with meningococcal meningitis must be kept in isolation to prevent the spread of the disease. Ten to 15% of patients with meningococcal meningitis will die, and of those who recover, as many as 10% will have long-term effects such as arthritis, myocarditis, and hearing loss.

Viral or Aseptic Meningitis

Viral or aseptic meningitis often occurs as a sequela to a variety of viral illnesses. For example, respiratory or gastrointestinal (GI) illnesses that are common with enteroviruses can cause viral meningitis. Enteroviruses, which include echoviruses and coxsackieviruses, account for most cases of viral meningitis in

TAKE HOME POINTS

- Meningitis is an inflammation of the brain's membranes and involves the subarachnoid space and CSF.
- Meningococcal meningitis is the only type of bacterial meningitis that occurs in outbreaks.

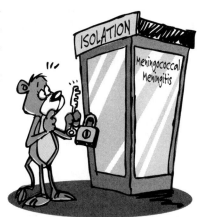

Vulnerable populations include patients with infections elsewhere in the body, those who are immunosuppressed, have immunocompromised disorders, and older adults, especially those with chronic debilitating diseases.

TAKE HOME POINTS

- The causative virus is unidentified in approximately 50% of cases.
- Prevention of some types of viral meningitis is accomplished by vaccines for polio, varicella, and measles-mumps-rubella.

The majority of patients with viral meningitis (70%) are children younger than 5 years old.

Typically, Haemophilus meningitis is seen in patients 1 month to 6 years of age.

The incidence rate of Haemophilus meningitis is three times higher in Native Americans and Eskimos than in the general population.

Pneumococcal meningitis is the most common meningitis in adults.

the United States. Other viral causes include measles, mumps, herpes simplex, and herpes zoster. Transmission of viral meningitis most often occurs through contact with respiratory secretions, but mode of transmission, communicability, and incubation times vary with the infecting virus.

Symptoms of viral meningitis are usually milder than bacterial meningitis, including headache, muscle aches and pains, and abdominal and chest pain, but most patients recover without permanent neurologic deficits.

Fungal Meningitis

Cryptococcus neoformans is the most common cause of fungal meningitis in patients with immune deficiency disorders (such as acquired immunodeficiency syndrome [AIDS]), reticuloendothelial system disorders (such as sarcoidosis), and those who are on corticosteroid therapy. Fulminant invasive fungal sinusitis is also a cause of fungal meningitis. Clinical manifestations vary among patients because of their compromised immune system, which affects the inflammatory response. Some patients may have a fever while others do not. Almost all patients have nausea, vomiting, headache, and a decline in mental status. Transmission is suspected to occur by inhalation. The fungus can be isolated from the bark and foliage of some eucalyptus trees, pigeon nests, and soil. The patients may have symptoms of kidney, lung, prostate, and bone infections. Untreated patients will die within weeks to months.

Haemophilus Meningitis

Haemophilus meningitis is caused by *Haemophilus influenzae*. Transmission occurs through droplets and contact with nasal and throat secretions during the communicable period of the disease (until the patient has 24 to 48 hours of effective antibiotic therapy). Infection may follow otitis media or an upper respiratory tract infection. Treatment is centered on antimicrobial therapy, but the use of corticosteroids may reduce the risk of hearing loss. The disease has a 5% mortality rate, even for those patients who are treated. Fifty percent of patients have neurologic defects, including learning disorders and abnormal speech and language development.

Pneumococcal Meningitis

Pneumococcal meningitis is caused by streptococcus pneumoniae. Transmission and incubation are linked to the underlying disease or condition, which typically is otitis media, bacteremia, mastoiditis, pneumonia, infective endocarditis, or basilar skull fracture. The mortality rate for this type of meningitis is approximately 25%.

Neonatal Meningitis

Neonatal meningitis is often caused by group B streptococcus, as well as mono-cytogenes and *Escherichia coli.* Infants are thought to become infected when passing through the birth canal or nosocomially. If the infant is infected within the first week of life, it is usually due to transmission via the birth canal. Incubation of disease acquired nosocomially usually takes 2 weeks to 2 months. Neonatal meningitis is not usually transmitted through normal social contact between people. The mortality rate for this type of meningitis is high at 50%.

Syphilitic Meningitis

Treponema pallidum causes syphilitic meningitis, and the risk factor for develop-ing this disease is having a previous infection with syphilis. It is a potential con-sequence of untreated secondary or early latent syphilis. Clinical manifestations may include psychologic changes, altered vision or sensation, cerebrovascular accident, tremors, ataxia, or seizures.

Tuberculous Meningitis

Tuberculous meningitis is caused by mycobacterium tuberculosis, and the risk factor for developing this disease is a history of tuberculosis. Clinical manifesta-tions include a loss of appetite and weight loss.

Regardless of the cause of meningitis, the signs and symptoms are usually sim-ilar. For adults they are severe headache, fever, nausea, vomiting, nuchal rigidi-ty, positive Kernig's sign, positive Brudzinski's sign, photophobia, seizures, men-tal status changes, skin rash, and petechiae or purpura. Neurologic abnormalities will reflect which cranial nerve (CN) is involved. Potential complications of meningitis include Waterhouse-Friderichsen syndrome (adrenal hemorrhage) with resulting hemorrhage and shock, encephalitis, hydrocephalus, cerebral edema, hearing or vision loss, brain damage, muscle paralysis, and disseminated intravascular coagulation (DIC).

Neonatal meningitis is an infection that develops at 2 weeks to 2 months of life and could be related to birth or nosocomially.

TAKE HOME POINTS

Syphilitic meningitis cannot be trans-mitted from person to person.

TAKE HOME POINTS

Transmission occurs from the spread of tuberculosis infection from another site of the patient's body and cannot be transmitted from person to person.

If tuberculous meningi-tis is not treated, it is usually fatal in 18 weeks to 5 years.

Brudzinski's Sign

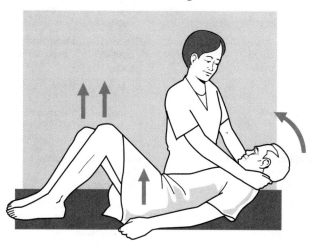

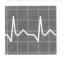 Petechiae or purpura is most common in meningococcal meningitis.

 Signs and symptoms of young children with meningitis include, fever, behavioral changes, lethargy, refusal of feeding, vomiting, arching of the back or neck retraction, blank-stare facial expression, bulging fontanels, seizures, and pale or blotchy skin.

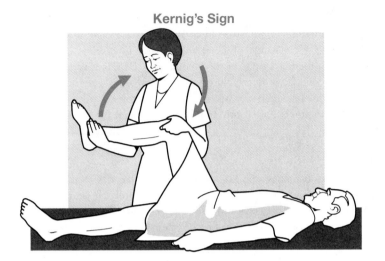

Kernig's Sign

Diagnostic Tests

LP for a specimen of CSF is used to diagnose most cases of meningitis. The result will depend on the type of organism causing the meningitis. An LP is not usually done if increased ICP is suspected.

Cerebrospinal Fluid (CSF) Findings in Meningitis

CSF FINDING	WBCs (CELLS/mm³)	PROTEIN (mg/dl)	GLUCOSE (mg/dl)	DIFFERENTIAL CELL COUNT	GRAM STAIN	CULTURE
Viral meningitis	Increased (6-1000)	Elevated (40-150)	Normal (50-75)	Mostly lymphocytes	Negative	Viruses may be isolated
Meningococcal meningitis	Increased (>100)	Elevated	<40% of simultaneous blood glucose level	Mostly polymorphonuclear cells	Gram-negative diplococci	*Neisseria meningitidis*
Haemophilus meningitis	Increased (>100)	Elevated (50-1000)	<40% of simultaneous blood glucose level	Mostly polymorphonuclear cells	Gram-negative bacilli	*Haemophilus influenzae*
Pneumococcal meningitis	Increased (>100)	Elevated (50-1000)	<40% of simultaneous blood glucose level	Mostly polymorphonuclear cells	Gram-positive cocci	*Streptococcus pneumoniae*
Neonatal meningitis	Increased or decreased	Elevated (50-1000)	<40% of simultaneous blood glucose level	Mostly polymorphonuclear cells	Gram-negative bacilli	Usually group B streptococcus, may be *Listeria monocytgenes* or *Escherichia coli*
Cryptococcal meningitis	Increased (10-500)	Elevated (50-1000)	<40% of simultaneous blood glucose level	Mostly lymphocytes	May resemble leukocytes	Negative
Tuberculosis meningitis	Increased (25-500)	Elevated (50-1000)	Normal (50-75)	Mostly lymphocytes	Negative	*Mycobacterium tuberculosis*

CSF, Cerebrospinal fluid.

Blood tests also help diagnose meningitis. A complete blood count (CBC) may be prescribed with the white blood cell (WBC) count being elevated well above normal. Serum electrolytes may also be obtained with the focus on the sodium level.

CT scan may be normal in acute uncomplicated meningitis, but it may show hydrocephalus and diffuse enhancement in severe cases. Radiographic films of the air sinuses, mastoids, and chest are taken to determine the presence of infection or a basilar skull fracture. MRI may be prescribed to identify the presence of a brain abscess, or increased ICP. An EEG may show generalized slow wave activity.

Medical Management

The physician will prescribe antibiotics specific to the bacterial or fungal causative agent. The medication of choice for household contacts; nursery, preschool, and school contacts; and health care providers who have been exposed to bacterial meningitis is rifampin (Rifadin).

• Performing an LP on a patient with increased ICP could be detrimental and cause herniation of the brainstem as a result of the sudden release of ICP.
• Dilutional hyponatremia may be present due to syndrome of inappropriate antidiuretic hormone (SIADH), which is a common complication of bacterial meningitis.

Empiric Therapy for Meningitis

ORGANISM	ANTIBIOTIC/AGENT
Virus	Acyclovir (Zovirax)
Neisseria meningitidis	Penicillin
	Cephalosporins
Haemophilus influenzae	Ceftriaxone (Rocephin)
	Cefotaxime (Claforan)
Streptococcus pneumoniae	Penicillin
	Cefotaxime (Claforan)
	Ceftriaxone (Rocephin)
	Rifampin (Rifadin)
	Vancomycin (Vancocin)
Treponema pallidum (causing syphilitic meningitis)	Penicillin G
	Procaine penicillin plus probenecid
Fungus (*Cryptococcus neoformans*)	Amphotericin B with 5-fluorocytosine
	Fluconazole (Diflucan)
Mycobacterium tuberculosis	Four-drug therapy with isoniazid (INH), rifampin (Rifadin), ethambutol (Myanbutol), and pyrazinamide (Tebrazid)
Staphylococcus	Vancomycin
	Ceftazidime (Fortaz)

FIRST-LINE AND INITIAL TREATMENTS FOR BACTERIAL MENINGITIS

- Remember that for individuals exposed to someone with bacterial meningitis, rifampin (Rifadin) is the drug that will be prescribed.

Treatment of viral or aseptic meningitis is mainly supportive, however acyclovir may be used to treat herpes virus and varicella-zoster virus, along with IV hydration.

FIRST-LINE AND INITIAL TREATMENTS FOR HAEMOPHILUS MENINGITIS

- Remember that for individuals exposed to someone with Haemophilus meningitis, rifampin is the drug that will be prescribed.

Treatment for pneumococcal meningitis is based on antimicrobial therapy, and prevention of this type of meningitis is achieved through vaccination with the pneumococcal vaccine to prevent pneumonia. Treatment for neonatal meningitis is also based on antimicrobial therapy, and prevention is aimed at screening pregnant women for group B streptococcus and then initiating group B streptococcus prophylaxis by administering antibiotics before delivery of the infant. If indicated, the mother should also be prepared for cesarean section.

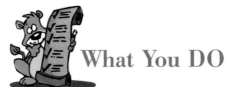 What You DO

To help decrease morbidity and mortality, it is vital that an accurate and immediate assessment be made of a patient with suspected meningitis. This can be accomplished by gathering a good nursing history. Subjective and objective findings may include the following:
- Headache that has grown progressively worse
- Nausea and vomiting
- Photophobia
- Neck or back pain upon flexion
- Seizures
- Irritability, confusion
- Medications, such as immunosuppressant drugs
- Presence of causative or precipitating factors: a highly suspect injury, procedure, or pathologic condition
- Social history, such as IV drug abuse
  The nurse must then examine the patient for the following:
- Signs of infection: Chills, fever, tachycardia, skin rash (petechiae or purpura most common in meningococcal meningitis)
- Meningeal irritation: Headache, nuchal rigidity, Brudzinski's reflex, Kernig's sign

- Neurologic abnormalities: Decreased level of consciousness (LOC), seizures, focal neurologic signs (hemiplegia, hemiparesis)
- CN involvement:
  - Optic (CN II): Papilledema may be present; blindness can occur
  - Oculomotor, trochlear, abducens (CN III, CN IV, CN VI): Impairment of ocular movement, ptosis and unequal pupils, and diplopia commonly found
  - Trigeminal (CN V): Photophobia
  - Facial (CN VII): Facial paresis
  - Acoustic (CN VIII): Tinnitus, vertigo, deafness
  - Complications: Waterhouse-Friderichsen syndrome (adrenal hemorrhage) with resulting hemorrhage and shock (may be seen in fulminating meningococcal meningitis), DIC, hydrocephalus, cerebral edema, brain abscess, subdural effusions, encephalitis

The nurse must then examine the laboratory and radiologic findings of the patient:

- CSF: Results depend on type of organism
- Protein levels: Higher level in bacterial than in viral meningitis
- Glucose levels: Low glucose levels in most cases of bacterial meningitis; may be normal in viral meningitis
- Purulent and turbid in most cases of meningitis; may be clear with some viruses
- Cells: Mostly lymphocytes in viral form, and polymorphonuclear leukocytes in bacterial form
- Cultures: Specimens from CSF, blood, drainage from sinuses or wounds to help identify the organism; nurse should make sure that specimens are transported to laboratory expeditiously (prompt culturing necessary for certain organisms)
- EEG: May show generalized slow wave activity
- Electrolytes: Hyponatremia may be present
- Nasopharyngeal smear: Causative bacteria may be present
- Radiologic findings: CT scan may be normal in acute uncomplicated meningitis but show diffuse enhancement in some types or reveal hydrocephalus; skull radiographs may reveal infected sinuses or basilar skull fracture

Nursing interventions are focused on the accurate monitoring and recording of the patient's neurologic status, vital signs, and vascular assessment. The nurse should do the following:

- Assess vital signs and perform gross neurologic examinations every 2 to 4 hours, or as prescribed.
- Do CN assessments with particular attention to CN numbers II, III, IV, V, VI, VII, VIII.
- Provide interventions to treat or prevent increased ICP (see Increased Intracranial Pressure).
- Protect the patient from injury from potential seizures (see previous section on seizures).

- Manage pain through nursing interventions such as assessment of symptoms of pain and administration of pain medications as prescribed. Monitor and record side effects and effectiveness of pain medications. Perform comfort measures to promote restfulness. Plan activities with patient to provide distraction such as radio, television, visitors, or reading if the patient is able. Manipulate the environment to promote periods of uninterrupted rest, such as turning down lights (this would assist in decreasing irritability [photophobia]). Help place the patient in a comfortable position.

- Nursing interventions to help with hyperthermia are also vital in the care of the patient with meningitis. These include administering antibiotic therapy as prescribed and at the first suspicion of infection, even before CSF results are obtained from the cultures. Monitor temperature every 2 to 4 hours, or as ordered. Administer antipyretic medications, such as Tylenol. Use cooling measures as indicated; remove blankets; use a hypothermia blanket; or use tepid water, alcohol sponges, or a fan (ambient cooling). Monitor systemic response to infection or fever such as vital signs, respiratory rate, LOC.

- Perform vascular assessment and monitor for vascular changes that may be caused by septic emboli. The patient's temperature, color, pulses, and capillary refill of all extremities should be assessed.

- Maintain isolation precautions as per the health care institution's policy.

- Make sure that those individuals exposed to the patient with bacterial meningitis are treated prophylactically with rifampin.

Do You UNDERSTAND?

DIRECTIONS: **Fill in the blanks to complete the sentences using the words listed on the following page. Words are used only once, and not all words are used.**

1. To help prevent _____, one can

   position the patient with the head of the bed elevated 15 to 30 degrees.

2. Nursing interventions to help with hyperthermia include the use of

   _____ water and alcohol sponges.

3. Individuals exposed to a patient with bacterial meningitis are treated

   prophylactically with _____.

4. Manipulating the environment of a patient with meningitis, such as turn-

   ing down lights, would help to decrease _____.

5. Meningeal irritation is caused by meningitis and is indicated by a positive

   Brudzinski's reflex, nuchal rigidity, and a positive _____

   sign.

vancomycin	rifampin	acyclovir
decreased	increased	intraabdominal
cold	Kernig's	Waterhouse-Friderichsen
tepid	photophobia	ICP

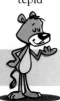

What IS Spinal Cord Injury?

Spinal cord injury occurs when a force is exerted on the vertebral column, resulting in damage to the spinal cord.

Injuries to the spinal cord are classified by the area and mechanism of injury. The area of injury refers to the level of the spine where the injury occurred (cervical, thoracic, lumbar, or sacral). The higher the spinal level, the greater the degree of injury. The mechanism of injury includes hyperflexion, hyperextension, axial loading and vertical compression, or penetrating injury. The spinal cord may remain intact or undergo a destructive process.

Spinal Segments and Nerve Supply

SPINAL SEGMENTS/ROOTS	NERVE SUPPLY
Cervical	C4—diaphragm
	C5—deltoid and biceps
	C6—wrist extensors
	C7—triceps
	C8—hand
Thoracic	T2-T7—chest muscles
	T9-T12—abdominal muscles
Lumbar	L1-5—leg muscles
Sacral	S2-5—bladder, bowel, and sexual functioning

MECHANISMS OF INJURY

Hyperflexion/Flexion Injury

Cervical flexion injury: Head is suddenly and forcefully accelerated forward

Lower thoracic/lumbar: Flexion injury when trunk is suddenly flexed on itself, as with a fall on the buttocks

- Posterior ligaments are stretched or torn
- Vertebrae may fracture or dislocate
- Causes hemorrhage, edema, necrosis

Hyperextension Injury

- Occurs most often with auto accidents (hit from behind) or falls where chin is struck
- Head is suddenly accelerated and then decelerated
- Anterior longitudinal ligaments are stretched or torn
- Vertebrae may fracture or subluxate
- Intervertebral disks may possibly rupture

Axial Loading/Vertical Compression Injury

- Most often caused by diving or fall from a ladder
- Vertebrae shatter with the blow
- Pieces of bone enter spinal canal and damage the spinal cord

Penetrating Injury

- Low velocity (knife): Causes damage directly at the site; localized damage to cord or spinal nerves
- High velocity (gunshot wound): Causes direct and indirect damage; spinal cord edema develops; necrosis of cord from compromised capillary circulation and venous return

**Destructive
Spinal Cord Process**

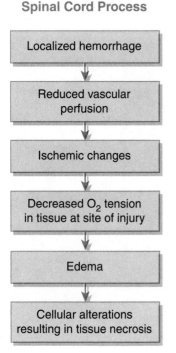

The *anatomic level of injury* refers to damage of the upper and lower motor neurons. The upper motor neurons descend from the brain to the spinal cord and begin and end with the CNS. The lower motor neurons originate in the anterior horns of the spinal cord and end in the muscles and tissues. If damage to an upper motor neuron occurs above the level of decussation (crossing) at the medulla, ipsilateral (same side) dysfunction is seen; if damage occurs below the level of decussation for upper or lower motor neurons, contralateral (opposite side) dysfunction occurs.

Spinal Card Injury Functional Activity Chart

Functional Activities

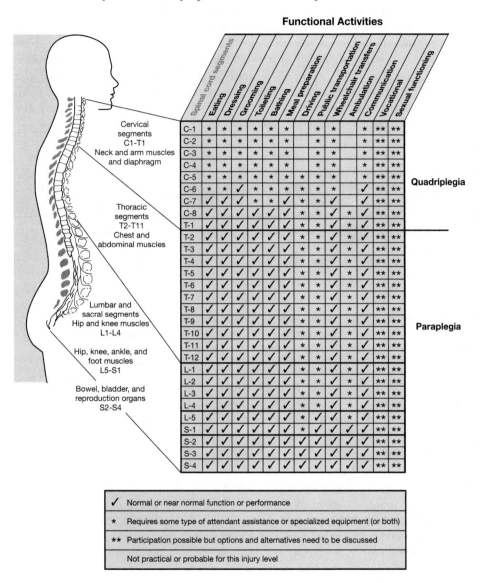

Spinal cord segments	Eating	Dressing	Grooming	Toileting	Bathing	Meal preparation	Driving	Public transportation	Wheelchair transfers	Ambulation	Communication	Vocational	Sexual functioning	
C-1	★	★	★	★	★	★		★	★		★	★★	★★	Quadriplegia
C-2	★	★	★	★	★	★		★	★		★	★★	★★	
C-3	★	★	★	★	★	★		★	★		★	★★	★★	
C-4	★	★	★	★	★	★		★	★		★	★★	★★	
C-5	★	★	★	★	★	★	★	★	★		★	★★	★★	
C-6	★	★	✓	★	★	★	★	★	★		✓	★★	★★	
C-7	✓	✓	✓	★	★	✓	★	★	✓		✓	★★	★★	
C-8	✓	✓	✓	✓	✓	✓	★	★	✓	★	✓	★★	★★	
T-1	✓	✓	✓	✓	✓	✓	★	★	✓	★	✓	★★	★★	
T-2	✓	✓	✓	✓	✓	✓	★	★	✓	★	✓	★★	★★	
T-3	✓	✓	✓	✓	✓	✓	★	★	✓	★	✓	★★	★★	
T-4	✓	✓	✓	✓	✓	✓	★	★	✓	★	✓	★★	★★	
T-5	✓	✓	✓	✓	✓	✓	★	★	✓	★	✓	★★	★★	
T-6	✓	✓	✓	✓	✓	✓	★	★	✓	★	✓	★★	★★	
T-7	✓	✓	✓	✓	✓	✓	★	★	✓	★	✓	★★	★★	
T-8	✓	✓	✓	✓	✓	✓	★	★	✓	★	✓	★★	★★	
T-9	✓	✓	✓	✓	✓	✓	★	★	✓	★	✓	★★	★★	Paraplegia
T-10	✓	✓	✓	✓	✓	✓	★	★	✓	★	✓	★★	★★	
T-11	✓	✓	✓	✓	✓	✓	★	★	✓	★	✓	★★	★★	
T-12	✓	✓	✓	✓	✓	✓	★	★	✓	★	✓	★★	★★	
L-1	✓	✓	✓	✓	✓	✓	★	★	✓	★	✓	★★	★★	
L-2	✓	✓	✓	✓	✓	✓	★	★	✓	★	✓	★★	★★	
L-3	✓	✓	✓	✓	✓	✓	★	★	✓	★	✓	★★	★★	
L-4	✓	✓	✓	✓	✓	✓	★	★	✓	★	✓	★★	★★	
L-5	✓	✓	✓	✓	✓	✓	★	✓	✓	★	✓	★★	★★	
S-1	✓	✓	✓	✓	✓	✓	★	✓	✓	✓	✓	★★	★★	
S-2	✓	✓	✓	✓	✓	✓	✓	✓	✓	✓	✓	★★	★★	
S-3	✓	✓	✓	✓	✓	✓	✓	✓	✓	✓	✓	★★	★★	
S-4	✓	✓	✓	✓	✓	✓	✓	✓	✓	✓	✓	★★	★★	

Cervical segments C1-T1 — Neck and arm muscles and diaphragm

Thoracic segments T2-T11 — Chest and abdominal muscles

Lumbar and sacral segments — Hip and knee muscles L1-L4

Hip, knee, ankle, and foot muscles L5-S1

Bowel, bladder, and reproduction organs S2-S4

✓	Normal or near normal function or performance
★	Requires some type of attendant assistance or specialized equipment (or both)
★★	Participation possible but options and alternatives need to be discussed
	Not practical or probable for this injury level

The functional level of injury refers to the extent of disruption of normal spinal cord function; they are classified as *complete* or *incomplete* injuries. Complete injuries generally result in total loss of motor, sensory, and reflex activity below the level of injury; the cord is completely transected; it occurs infrequently. Complete injuries can result in spinal or neurogenic shock, which lasts between 1 to 6 weeks, at which point 50% of patients regain some degree of spinal cord function. Incomplete lesions have preservation of a mixed pattern of motor, sensory, and reflex function. Five syndromes exist that are secondary to incomplete spinal cord lesions.

Syndromes Secondary to Incomplete Spinal Cord Injuries

INCOMPLETE LESION	ASSOCIATED WITH	LOSS OF FUNCTION	INTACT FUNCTION
Anterior cord syndrome	Flexion and dislocation injuries of the cervical cord	Pain and temperature sensations and motor function Babinski reflex pathologically positive and spastic paralysis seen	Touch, proprioception, pressure, and vibration senses
Posterior cord syndrome	Hyperextension of the cervical spine	Proprioception and sensation of light touch	Pain and temperature sensations and motor function
Central cord syndrome	Hyperextension of the cervical spine and in older patients in whom degenerative changes of the vertebrae and disks allow central cord compression to occur	Upper extremity motor function with an accompanying but less significant loss of lower extremity motor function	Some patients do not experience loss of lower extremity motor function Sensory function, varying degrees remain intact
Brown-Sequard's syndrome	Penetrating wounds, such as knife or bullet wounds, that cause hemisection of the cord; also seen in surfers who suffer traumatic injury caused by the surfboard hitting them in the neck	Ipsilateral (same side of the lesion) motor, proprioception, vibration, and deep touch Contralateral (opposite side of the lesion) pain, temperature, and light touch	Contralateral motor, proprioception, vibration, and deep touch Ipsilateral pain, temperature, and light touch
Cauda equina or conus medullaris	Damage to spinal nerve roots in the sacral area from trauma-induced fracture dislocation	Variable pattern of motor or sensory loss results in neurogenic bowel and bladder	Neurologic deficits specific to the nerve roots involved

Anterior Cord Syndrome

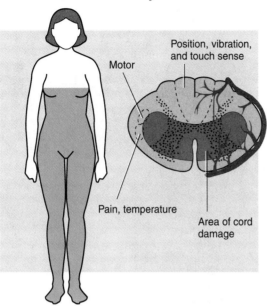

Motor

Position, vibration, and touch sense

Pain, temperature

Area of cord damage

Central Cord Syndrome

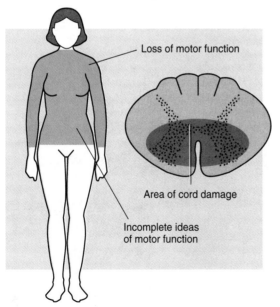

Loss of motor function

Area of cord damage

Incomplete ideas of motor function

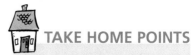

TAKE HOME POINTS

- Total loss of all reflex activity occurs below the level of injury in complete spinal cord injuries.
- A mixed loss of reflex activity or a preservation of some reflexes is found with incomplete lesion.

Brown-Séquard Syndrome

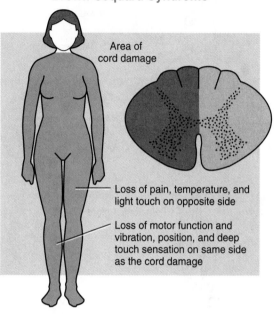

Area of
cord damage

Loss of pain, temperature, and
light touch on opposite side

Loss of motor function and
vibration, position, and deep
touch sensation on same side
as the cord damage

Conus Medullaris and
Cauda Equina Syndromes

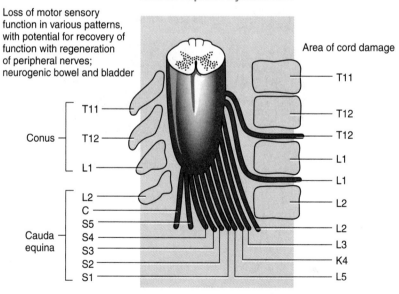

Loss of motor sensory
function in various patterns,
with potential for recovery of
function with regeneration
of peripheral nerves;
neurogenic bowel and bladder

Area of cord damage

Conus
- T11
- T12
- L1

Cauda
equina
- L2
- C
- S5
- S4
- S3
- S2
- S1

- T11
- T12
- T12
- L1
- L1
- L2
- L2
- L3
- K4
- L5

What You NEED TO KNOW

Diagnostic Tests

A variety of diagnostic tests are used with spinal cord injuries. Spinal radiographs assess for fractures, dislocations, and degenerative changes of the vertebral column. A CT scan may demonstrate bony pathology, myelography may show cord compression, and MRI may show soft tissue injury. In addition, in patients with gunshot or stab wounds, an angiography may be prescribed to assess vascular injuries.

Medical Management

Immobilization or stabilization of the spinal injury is the priority of initial care along with treatment of acute symptoms. Emergency surgery may be necessary to repair fractures, remove bone fragments, evacuate hematomas, remove penetrating objects (bullet), or decrease pressure on the spinal cord. For cervical spine injuries, Gardner-Wells tongs or a halo fixation device with jacket may be applied to the patient's head to help immobilize the cervical spinal column. Spinal fusion with bone plugs or wires and rods may be required to stabilize spinal injuries.

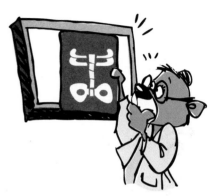

FIRST-LINE AND INITIAL TREATMENTS FOR SPINAL CORD INJURY

- Immobilize the patient.
- Monitor ABCs (airway, breathing, circulation).

Medication therapy is also used after a spinal cord injury. Atropine is used to treat bradycardia; dopamine (Intropin) is used to treat hypotension; and methylprednisolone (Solumedrol), a steroid, will be started within 8 hours of injury, with an IV loading dose initially. Treatment with methylprednisolone is started within the first 3 hours and is continued with an IV drip for 24 hours; treatment initiated between 3 hours and 8 hours is continued for 48 hours. This is used to decrease cord swelling, inflammation, glutamate release, and free-radical accumulation; therefore limiting spinal cord injury.

TAKE HOME POINTS

In an attempt to preserve any possible function, the stabilization of the spinal cord is important

---

FIRST-LINE AND INITIAL TREATMENTS FOR SPINAL CORD INJURY

- Remember that methylprednisolone may be started within hours after the injury in an attempt to decrease the edema associated with the destructive process that occurs in a spinal cord injury.

Crystalloid and colloid fluid replacement is used to maintain normal BP, along with vasopressors. Plasma expanders, such as Dextran, are used to increase capillary blood flow within the spinal cord.

Hyperbaric oxygenation is used in some facilities after 12 to 24 hours of injury. It supplies 100% O_2 in a pressurized chamber, which allows the blood to carry more O_2 and is thought to improve O_2 perfusion to the spinal cord, thus decreasing ischemic injury.

Autonomic Dysreflexia

Damage to the spinal cord at T6 or above can lead to autonomic dysreflexia, an emergency clinical condition that can occur after the period of spinal shock is completed. It results in uninhibited sympathetic discharge to a noxious stimulus below the level of the spinal cord injury. The spinal cord injury prevents the message from reaching the brain, so the sympathetic nervous system's (SNS's) response is unopposed, resulting in life-threatening hypertension. Symptoms of this sympathetic discharge include diaphoresis and flushing above the level of injury, with chills and severe vasoconstriction below the level of injury, the dramatic increase in BP produces a pounding headache. Other signs and symptoms include nasal congestion, nausea, bradycardia, and unusually frequent spasms of the lower extremities or abdomen.

The noxious stimulus that most frequently triggers this response is a distended bladder or bowel. Other triggers are a hot or cold stimulus (sitting in a drafty hall), skin pressure (such as tight clothing or staying in one position too long), pressure ulcers, ingrown toenail, or bowel and bladder stimulation during bowel and bladder training regimens. Autonomic dysreflexia usually occurs suddenly.

Physicians treat autonomic dysreflexia by removing the noxious stimulus and administering antihypertensive medications to avoid a stroke from the hypertension. If the noxious stimulus is relieved immediately, the dysreflexia may resolve on its own. If the physician is unable to relieve the noxious stimulus, he or she may order topical nitroglycerine ointment, oral or sublingual (SL) nifedipine, or IV hydralazine hydrochloride to reduce the BP.

TAKE HOME POINTS

Autonomic dysreflexia is a clinical emergency that can happen at any time after injury.

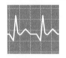

Patients with autonomic dysreflexia have severe, life-threatening hypertension.

TAKE HOME POINTS

A noxious stimuli is the triggering event for autonomic dysreflexia.

A stroke may occur from the hypertension.

FIRST-LINE AND INITIAL TREATMENTS FOR AUTONOMIC DYSREFLEXIA

- Remove the noxious stimulus (i.e., urinary catheterization, manual rectal decompaction).
- Administer antihypertensive medications.

What You DO

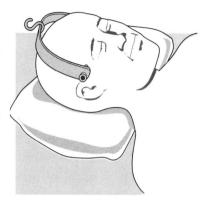

Gardner-Wells tongs

If the patient's spinal cord has been immobilized by Gardner-Wells tongs, which consist of two tongs inserted in the outer aspect of the skull with traction added, nursing care is focused on the traction of this device and on infection control. To accomplish this, the nurse should do the following:

- Ensure that the prescribed weights are on the device and are hanging freely at all times.
- Make sure the patient is in proper alignment, and that the ropes remain in the pulley device.
- Assess neurologic signs at least every 4 hours or more frequently as prescribed.
- Inspect pins for signs and symptoms of infection, and administer pin care with $1/2$ hydrogen peroxide and $1/2$ NS solution every shift (or as the hospital policy and procedure manual dictates).

If the patient is in a halo fixation device with jacket, four pins are inserted into the skull with the fixation device and then the jacket is applied, which stabilizes the halo from the chest. To maintain cervical stability and patient safety, the nurse must do the following:

Halo Fixation Device with Jacket

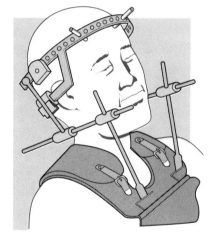

- Assess the skin and jacket to make sure no pressure areas are present. One should be able to insert one finger easily under the jacket.
- Assess pins for a secure tight fit, administer pin care, check for signs and symptoms of pin infection, and perform neurologic checks as previously discussed.
- Ensure that a "key" or Allen wrench is taped to the outer chest of the jacket for easy removal in the event of a cardiac arrest.

The nurse should remember that immobilization places the patient at increased risk for hypoventilation, pneumonia, and pulmonary embolism. To avoid these complications the nurse should do the following:

- Perform respiratory assessment and breath sounds assessment every 2 hours or as prescribed.
- Suction as necessary to keep airway clear using aseptic technique,
- Provide chest physical therapy as per unit protocol.
- Monitor sputum cultures.
- Ensure adequate hydration to help liquefy secretions.
- Use antiembolic stockings, pneumatic compression devices, or both.
- Get the patient out of bed three to four times a day when the spinal cord is stabilized.
- Encourage deep breathing and use of incentive spirometry every hour while the patient is awake (coughing may increase spinal cord pressure).
- Measure vital capacity and tidal volumes, and monitor pulse oximetry and ABGs.

If the patient had a surgical intervention to immobilize a portion of the spinal cord with bone plugs or wires and rods, the nurse should initiate the following postoperative measures:

- Empty Jackson Pratt (JP) drains and record drainage at least every shift.
- Assess neurologic signs (motor and sensory) based on the level of the spinal cord injury to detect changes from baseline values.
- Change spinal cord dressing as ordered, usually after a few days it is left open to air.
- Prevent further damage by immobilizing the area, using special beds and equipment. Logroll the patient from side to side, and use additional help as needed.
- Assess for hypotension, bradycardia, and vasovagal reflex, which may result in cardiac arrest; be prepared to institute advanced cardiovascular life support (ACLS).
- Hyperoxygenate before and after suctioning to prevent hypoxia and vasovagal reactions.
- Avoid placing IV lines in paralytic limbs.
- Prevent deep vein thrombosis (DVT) and skin breakdown with proper positioning, frequent turning, therapeutic range-of-motion exercises, antiembolism stockings, and prophylactic anticoagulant therapy as ordered.
- Apply splints or high-top tennis shoes to feet on a 2-hours-on and 2-hours-off schedule to maintain normal alignment and prevent foot drop.

Fluid volume deficit may result from hemorrhage, gastric dilation (vomiting), or gastric ulceration. Urine retention may occur due to anatomic bladder or areflexia and can result in urinary tract infections (UTIs), stone formation, or renal deterioration. The nurse will need to consider the following interventions when addressing these issues:

- Administer histamine-2 antagonists, antacids, gastric lavage, and fluids as ordered.
- Inspect the abdomen for distension.
- Indwelling urinary catheters are necessary during hemodynamic instability.
- Monitoring urine cultures are necessary.
- When the patient's condition stabilizes, intermittent catheterization or self-catheterization programs may be initiated.
- Begin patient teaching regarding self-catheterization as soon as feasible.
- Provide supportive care and treatment of complications resulting from the injury, such as arrhythmias, especially tachycardia and bradycardia, which are common in patients with spinal cord injuries. Respiratory disturbances are also common and associated with the level of injury. High cervical neck injuries result in respiratory nerve paralysis; therefore the patient is ventilator dependent.

For those patients with T6 or above lesions who are susceptible to autonomic dysreflexia, one must be aware of the algorithm (www.pva.org) to follow:

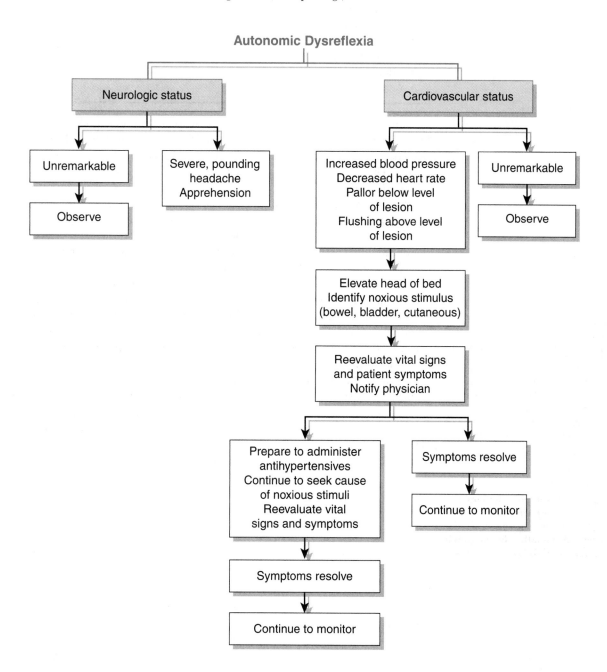

FIRST-LINE AND INITIAL TREATMENTS FOR AUTONOMIC DYSREFLEXIA

- Elevate HOB.
- Identify and remove noxious stimulus.
- Administer antihypertensives.
- Administer nitroglycerine ointment.
- Administer nifedipine SL.
- Administer hydralazine IV.

Patient and family education regarding how to prevent an episode of autonomic dysreflexia is essential. The patient and family should be educated on the elimination of drafts, good skin and nail care, and regular bowel and bladder regimens. They should also be given written material on how to identify and remove noxious stimuli.

The patient and family members will need assistance coping with the emotional repercussions of these devastating injuries. Patient issues involve impaired adjustment related to depression, change in body image, or role performance. Disrupted self-concept, related to sexuality issues and feeling of powerlessness, are also common patient findings. Fertility is an especially important component of postinjury care. In men, erectile and ejaculatory dysfunction is present. Semen quality and motility is reduced secondary to recurrent UTIs, scrotal hyperthermia, drugs, prostatic fluid stasis, spermatazoan contact with urine through retrograde ejaculation, testicular denervation, and changes in seminal fluid. Patient education can be conducted by educating the patient that treatment of erectile dysfunction includes mechanical interventions and pharmacological interventions, and that ejaculatory dysfunction can be treated pharmacologically. Assisted reproductive methods include intrauterine insemination, intracytoplasmic sperm injection, and in-vitro fertilization. Family coping may be ineffective, given the situational crisis and long-term burden of care. Professional consultative support is often needed from a psychologist, psychiatrist, or clinical nurse specialist in psychiatric mental health.

TAKE HOME POINTS

Education for females who experience a spinal cord injury is that they remain fertile and can conceive and deliver. They should use a method of birth control that does not increase the risk of clot formation, such as a diaphragm, foam, or condom.

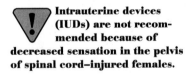

Intrauterine devices (IUDs) are not recommended because of decreased sensation in the pelvis of spinal cord–injured females.

Do You UNDERSTAND?

DIRECTIONS: **Write the letter that matches the items in column A with the correct items in column B. (Not all items in column B will be used.)**

Column A

1. _____ A lesion that would result in quadriplegia
2. _____ Damage to spinal cord at this level or above can result in autonomic dysreflexia
3. _____ A classic symptom of autonomic dysreflexia
4. _____ Results in loss of upper extremity motor function with an accompanying but less significant loss of lower extremity motor function
5. _____ Occurs most often with auto accidents

Column B

a. Hypertension
b. Central cord syndrome
c. Tachycardia
d. A complete C7 injury
e. Hyperextension injury
f. Hyperflexion or flexion injury
g. T6
h. Anterior cord syndrome
i. T7

7 Gastrointestinal System

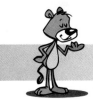

What IS Gastrointestinal Bleeding?

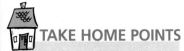
Gastrointestinal (GI) bleeding is a symptom of an underlying disease. Bleeding can result from a variety of diseases that occur in the esophagus, stomach, small intestine, large intestine, or rectum, such as peptic ulcer disease, Mallory-Weiss syndrome, esophageal or rectal varices, neoplasms, esophagitis, stress ulcers, or inflammatory bowel disease. GI bleeding can also result from underlying clotting disorders, such as those with liver disease.

Bleeding can be chronic or acute. Symptoms of GI bleeding can occur without warning and be sudden and severe or have a slow onset. Acute GI bleeding can be a life-threatening condition if the cause of bleeding cannot be treated or controlled. Assessment of the patient for the underlying cause of the bleeding and his or her hemodynamic stability are key factors in the initial care of the patient.

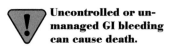

Uncontrolled or unmanaged GI bleeding can cause death.

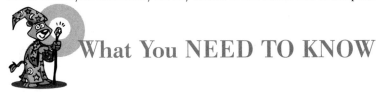

What You NEED TO KNOW

Clinical Manifestations

Clinical manifestations such as anorexia, nausea, vomiting, constipation, diarrhea, weakness, fatigue, weight loss, abdominal pain, and discomfort may precede GI bleeding and be indicative of the underlying disease.

The feces and vomitus often are the first clues that reveal evidence of GI bleeding. The presence of blood in the stomach is an irritant and a stimulus for vomiting. Hematemesis is bright-red, bloody vomitus or vomitus with a coffee ground appearance. Bright-red vomitus is associated with fresh bleeding. Coffee ground vomitus is blood that has been exposed to the acid and pepsin action of the stomach for a period of time.

Examination of the stool in a patient with GI bleeding can reveal hematochezia, a bright, red or maroon blood passed via the rectum. Black, tarry stool is called *melena*. The black appearance of melena is caused by the breakdown of blood by intestinal bacteria and digestive enzymes. Occult blood is another clinical manifestation of GI bleeding. It cannot be identified on visual examination and is detected by guaiac testing.

Hematemesis and melena are associated with upper GI diseases that cause bleeding. Hematochezia is generally associated with diseases of the lower GI tract. If hematochezia is caused by an upper GI bleed, the loss of blood is usually significant. The amount of blood found in the vomitus or stool will depend on the volume and rate of blood loss, the cardiovascular status of the patient, and the underlying disease state causing the bleeding.

Causes

Peptic ulcer disease is caused by an imbalance of defensive and aggressive factors found in the stomach. The mucosal lining of the stomach forms a protective barrier against the acid-pepsin action of the stomach contents. This lining has the ability to renew and regenerate. Adequate blood flow is necessary for the mucosal layer to regenerate. Any alteration in mucosal blood flow can cause decreased cellular renewal and weaken the defensive barrier. Chronic ingestion of aspirin, alcohol, and nonsteroidal antiinflammatory drugs (NSAIDs) weaken the gastric mucosal barrier against the acid and pepsin action of the stomach. Aspirin and NSAIDs cause gastric mucosal irritation and inhibit prostaglandin synthesis that increases gastric secretion. Other defensive factors include the secretion of bicarbonate and the production of prostaglandins. Bicarbonate balances the acid secretion of the stomach. Prostaglandins protect the stomach by suppressing gastric acid secretion, promoting the secretion of bicarbonate and mucus and maintaining submucosal blood flow.

Aggressive factors include the presence of *Helicobacter pylori*. *H. pylori* are bacteria found in the majority of patients with gastric and duodenal ulcerations. The bacteria thrive in an acidic environment and may result in injury to the mucosal barrier of the stomach. This disruption causes the underlying layers of the stomach to be more susceptible to the acid and pepsin action of the stomach. Acid, pepsin, stress, and smoking are also thought to be aggressive factors that can lead to peptic ulcer disease. The three stimuli that promote the secretion of gastric acid by the parietal cells of the stomach are (1) acetylcholine, (2) histamine, and (3) gastrin. Vagal stimulation causes the release of acetylcholine for which a parietal cell muscarinic receptor exists that promotes hydrochloric acid release. Mast cells release histamine. Histamine 2 (H_2) receptors are found on the parietal cell and respond with the release of hydrochloric acid. G cells release gastrin, which is received by parietal cell G-cell receptors and results in hydrochloric acid release. Pepsin is an enzyme responsible for the breakdown of proteins. Chief cells in the stomach release pepsinogen and, in the presence of the acidic stomach environment, form pepsin. Without an adequate mucosal protective barrier, pepsin will break down proteins found in the underlying layers of the stomach wall.

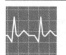

Bright-red blood indicates fresh bleeding; whereas secretions appearing like coffee grounds indicate old bleeding.

TAKE HOME POINTS

- The appearance of melena in the stool means that the blood has gone through the digestive tract.
- Signs of shock include hypotension; tachycardia; decreased capillary refill; cool, clammy skin; shortness of breath; changes in level of consciousness; anxiety; and decreased urine output.
- Clinical manifestations of chronic blood loss include weakness, fatigue, shortness of breath, lethargy, and faintness.

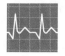

Patients who have acute blood loss will exhibit progressive signs of hemorrhagic shock.

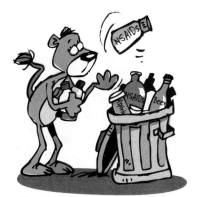

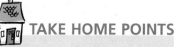

TAKE HOME POINTS

Anything that destroys or weakens the mucosal stomach lining can contribute to GI bleeding.

Persons who are immunosuppressed have an increased risk of developing ulcers and treatment needs to be proactive.

TAKE HOME POINTS

- Smoking is thought to promote a decrease in mucosal blood flow and slow the mucosal renewal process.
- Peptic ulcer disease must be managed in an attempt to prevent GI bleeding.

A Mallory-Weiss tear is an arterial bleed.

Mallory-Weiss syndrome is most commonly seen in men.

TAKE HOME POINTS

- Bleeding from a Mallory-Weiss tear is treated through surgery.
- Because of the stress of illness and hospitalization, stress ulcers can readily form in the critically ill patient.

An imbalance in the defensive or aggressive factors in the stomach can create conditions that promote cellular damage and cause erosion and ulceration. Progressive erosion into the underlying vascular layers of the stomach can result in GI bleeding. The treatment of peptic ulcer disease consists of pharmacologic and nonpharmacologic management. If this treatment is not effective and GI bleeding results, surgical intervention may be needed. Surgical intervention for peptic ulcer disease can include procedures such as total or partial gastrectomy, Bilroth I or Bilroth II procedures, antrectomy, vagotomy, or pyloroplasty.

Mallory-Weiss syndrome is characterized by a linear tear of the gastric mucosa found at the stomach and esophageal junction, which is caused by retching during vomiting. Mild-to-massive GI bleeding is a result. Associated findings that can contribute to the development of Mallory-Weiss syndrome include aspirin or NSAID use, alcohol abuse, bulimia, hiatal hernia, gastritis, or esophagitis. Surgical intervention is used to repair the tear. Angiography may be useful in identifying the site of bleeding and in control of hemorrhage through the infusion of pharmacologic vasoconstrictors.

A superficial erosion of the gastric mucosa usually characterizes stress ulcers, which are often seen in the critically ill population. Patients who are diagnosed with immunosuppression, acute respiratory distress syndrome, sepsis, shock, burns, trauma, acute head injury, or multisystem organ failure are at risk for the development of stress ulcerations. Stress ulceration is caused by mucosal ischemia that results in the loss of the defensive, mucosal barrier. A situation is created where the stomach lining is susceptible to acid and pepsin action of the stomach contents. The treatment of stress ulceration focuses on the underlying cause of the mucosal ischemia.

Neoplasms, both benign and malignant, of the esophagus, stomach, and small and large intestine can lead to GI bleeding. Tumors that are not caught in their early stages can spread and erode into the vascular layers of the GI tract, resulting in GI bleeding. Treatment of GI neoplasms includes surgical removal, chemotherapy, or radiation (or both). The type of treatment depends on the location, type, and progression of the cancer.

Gastritis is a diffuse inflammation of the gastric mucosa and is diagnosed as acute or chronic. Factors that can cause acute gastritis include the ingestion of alcohol, aspirin, and bacterial endotoxins. Chronic gastritis is thought to be caused by inflammation associated with *Helicobacter pylori*. Acute or chronic gastritis can result in GI bleeding. Treatment of gastritis consists of removal of the irritant causing the inflammatory process such as cessation of alcohol consumption and treatment of positive *H. pylori* with appropriate antibiotics.

Esophageal Varices

Varices are engorged, distended veins that are susceptible to hemorrhage. They result from portal hypertension, an increase in pressure within the liver's portal circulation, usually related to chronic alcoholism. These distended esophageal veins result in esophageal varices. Rupture of the friable veins can result in life-threatening GI bleeding. Treatment of varices focuses on the reduction of portal pressures through the use of pharmacological therapy and changes in behavior such as no ingestion of alcohol. Pharmacological agents such as vasopressin

(Pitressin), octreotide acetate (Sandostatin), beta blockers, and nitrates are used to reduce portal pressures. Endoscopy is used as a diagnostic tool to identify the site of bleeding and is also used as a form of interventional treatment. Treatment of varices is accomplished via endoscopic sclerosis or ligation (banding) of the fragile, distended veins. Endoscopic ligation (banding) involves the suctioning of the vein into a chamber in the endoscope. The vein is ligated with a small band. A loss of blood flow occurs through the banded vein and, over time, thrombosis and fibrosis occur and the banded vein sloughs off. Sclerosis involves the injection of an agent that causes initial thrombosis and hemostasis. Repeated injections of a sclerosing agent result in mucosal fibrosis and less venous bleeding.

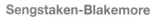

FIRST-LINE AND INITIAL TREATMENTS FOR ESOPHAGEAL VARICES

- Administer vasopressin (Pitressin), octreotide acetate (Sandostatin), beta blockers, and nitrates.
- Treat with endoscopy, sclerosis, ligation (banding), and balloon tamponade.
- Use Sengstaken-Blakemore, Minnesota, or Linton-Nachias tubes.

Another esophageal varices treatment involves the use of balloon tamponade. Several types of tubes are used for the procedure: Sengstaken-Blakemore, Minnesota, and Linton-Nachias. In general, the tubes have three ports: (1) a gastric balloon port, (2) gastric aspiration port, and (3) an esophageal balloon port. The tube is anchored in the stomach via a gastric balloon. The stomach balloon exerts pressure on the fundus of the stomach and causes compression of esophageal blood flow. The esophageal balloon is then inflated, and this places direct pressure on the varices. The balloon pressures are monitored and maximum inflation time identified. Once placed, it is essential to prevent upward tube migration. The migration could lead to airway occlusion. Oropharyngeal and gastric secretions must also be managed.

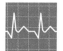 Because of the pressures exerted from the tubes for balloon tamponade, it is crucial that airway patency be continually assessed.

Sengstaken-Blakemore

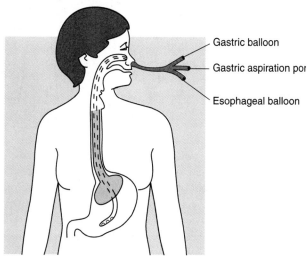

Gastric balloon

Gastric aspiration port

Esophageal balloon

Minnesota Tube

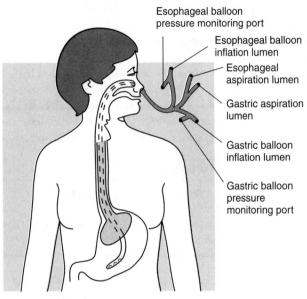

Esophageal balloon
pressure monitoring port

Esophageal balloon
inflation lumen

Esophageal
aspiration lumen

Gastric aspiration
lumen

Gastric balloon
inflation lumen

Gastric balloon
pressure
monitoring port

Linton-Nachias Tube

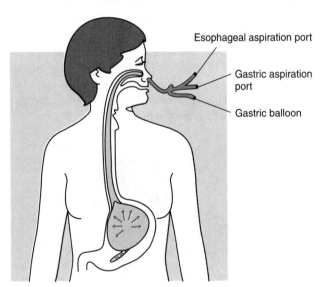

Esophageal aspiration port

Gastric aspiration
port

Gastric balloon

If these treatment modalities do not effectively manage esophageal varices, radiographic or surgical intervention is considered. The radiographic procedure involves the placement of a stent that creates a portosystemic shunt and reduces portal pressures. Surgical techniques to reduce portal hypertension include the placement of portacaval, mesocaval, or splenorenal shunts. The surgical shunts divert blood flow and result in a reduction of portal pressures.

Inflammatory Conditions of the Gastrointestinal Tract

Esophagitis is an inflammation of the esophagus often seen in association with gastroesophageal reflux disease (GERD). The acidic contents of the stomach flow back into the esophagus through the lower esophageal sphincter. Severe forms of GERD can result in esophageal tissue erosion and ulceration, which can lead to GI bleeding. The treatment of esophagitis focuses on suppressing gastric acidity, improving gastric emptying, and decreasing pressure on the lower esophageal sphincter. In some cases, surgical intervention to strengthen the lower esophageal sphincter may be needed.

Ulcerative colitis and Crohn's disease are two types of inflammatory bowel disease that can result in GI hemorrhage. Ulcerative colitis is commonly found in the colon and rectum and is characterized by abdominal pain, diarrhea, and rectal bleeding. Crohn's disease is an inflammatory process that affects the proximal colon and the terminal ileum. Ulcers form that extend into all the layers of the GI wall. Clinical manifestations of Crohn's disease include abdominal pain, diarrhea, and GI bleeding. Treatment of both inflammatory bowel processes focuses on reduction of the inflammatory process by pharmacological intervention, diet, and in some cases surgical intervention. In patients with GI bleeding from inflammatory bowel disease, the diseased portion of the colon or small intestine is removed.

Diagnostics

Endoscopy is a diagnostic tool that provides direct visualization of the GI tract and the bleeding site. Esophagogastroduodenoscopy (EGD) is visualization of the esophagus, stomach, and duodenum. Colonoscopy provides for visualization of the colon, and sigmoidoscopy allows for rectal visualization. Enteroscopy is used for visualization of the small bowel. Endoscopy can also be used to treat and control bleeding by obtaining biopsies and for electrocoagulation, ligation, sclerosis, or laser therapy.

Radiographic procedures, such as an upper GI series and barium enema, can be used to diagnose GI bleeding. An upper GI series can be used to detect varices, ulcers, neoplasms, and inflammation of the upper GI tract. A barium enema can assist with the identification of underlying disease processes such as neoplasms and inflammatory bowel disease, all of which can be a bleeding source.

Dye can be injected via angiography to identify the site of a bleeding vessel when the source of bleeding is not accessible to an endoscope. Medications, such as vasoconstrictors, can also be administered directly via angiographic means and assist in controlling hemorrhage.

Radionuclide scanning is a noninvasive diagnostic tool. A small amount of a radioactive substance is injected into the patient. Scans are then completed that locate the site of bleeding.

Complete blood counts (CBC), basic and complete metabolic profiles, coagulation profiles, liver function tests, arterial blood gases (ABGs), and gastric or stool aspirate for guaiac are diagnostic tests used for patients with GI bleeding. Hemoglobin and hematocrit laboratory values may not be helpful when obtained immediately after blood loss. An elevation in blood urea nitrogen (BUN) may

TAKE HOME POINTS

All treatment modalities for varices are not without side effects and potential complications such as variceal hemorrhage, hypovolemic shock, rebleeding after treatment, and airway occlusion from migration of a balloon tamponade tube.

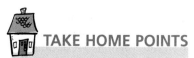

TAKE HOME POINTS

Endoscopy is considered the gold standard for diagnosis of GI bleeding.

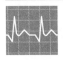

The patient's creatinine should be monitored for any signs of inadequate renal perfusion associated with hypovolemia and hemorrhagic shock—a complication associated with massive GI bleeding. An elevated creatinine indicates a slowing of the glomerular filtration rate (GFR) and a decrease in the functioning of the renal nephrons.

For patients with massive hemorrhage, the lactic acid will elevate, indicating the body's conversion from aerobic to anaerobic metabolism and inability to meet cellular needs.

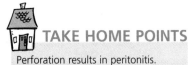

be seen up to 24 hours after a GI bleed that results in hematemesis or melena. Coagulation studies should be assessed for any abnormalities. Platelets and white blood cells (WBC) may initially be elevated after a GI bleed. An initial elevation in blood glucose may be seen. The glucose elevation is seen because of the stress response. Because the liver plays a role in the metabolism of clotting factors, liver function tests should be obtained to rule out any underlying liver abnormality, which could be contributing to the GI bleeding. If the patient is vomiting, hypokalemia and a metabolic alkalosis may result from the loss of hydrogen ions with vomiting. Patients who are suspected of having chronic GI bleeding should have guaiac testing for occult blood in the feces and vomitus.

Patients with peptic ulcer disease and chronic gastritis should be tested for the presence of the *Helicobacter pylori* bacteria. Invasive and noninvasive tests are available for determining the presence of the bacteria. Blood and breath tests are available as noninvasive means, and tissue samples can be taken via invasive endoscopy as an invasive means.

Complications

To care for the patient with GI bleeding, it is important to understand the potential complications including hemorrhagic shock, perforation, and obstruction.

If GI bleeding is massive, hemorrhagic shock can occur. Hemorrhagic shock is characterized by a decrease in preload (venous return) to the heart, caused by the loss of blood volume. Losses of at least 15% of blood volume occur before the clinical manifestations of hemorrhagic shock are apparent.

Peptic ulcer disease, neoplasms, varices, and inflammatory bowel disease may cause perforation. Perforation occurs when an erosion of all the layers of the GI wall occurs and the contents of the GI tract spill into the peritoneum, resulting in peritonitis. Clinical manifestations of perforation include abdominal sudden onset of severe pain, tenderness, and distention. The abdomen often becomes rigid and boardlike. Other results include nausea, vomiting, fever, tachycardia, hypotension, paralytic ileus, and fluid and electrolyte imbalances. If perforation occurs, the area is surgically closed or patched; otherwise the peritonitis can progress to sepsis, septic shock, and death. GI obstruction can also be an associated complication of GI bleeding.

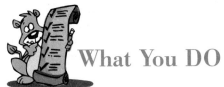

What You DO

In addition to the traditional patient history, particular questions should be directed to the patient with GI bleeding. Questions should include:

- *Are you taking any medications that could be compounding the bleeding problem?* The patient should be assessed for use of anticoagulants (Warfarin), NSAIDs, antiplatelets (aspirin), or recent use of thrombolytic medications.
- *Do you have any previous history of GI disease or surgery?* Bleeding from an operative site can be a postoperative complication.

Plate 1: Anaphylactic Shock Mediator Response and Clinical Manifestations

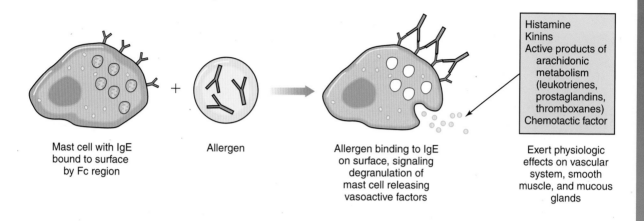

Mast cell with IgE bound to surface by Fc region

Allergen

Allergen binding to IgE on surface, signaling degranulation of mast cell releasing vasoactive factors

Histamine
Kinins
Active products of arachidonic metabolism (leukotrienes, prostaglandins, thromboxanes)
Chemotactic factor

Exert physiologic effects on vascular system, smooth muscle, and mucous glands

Clinical Manifestations of Type 1 Hypersensitivity Reactions

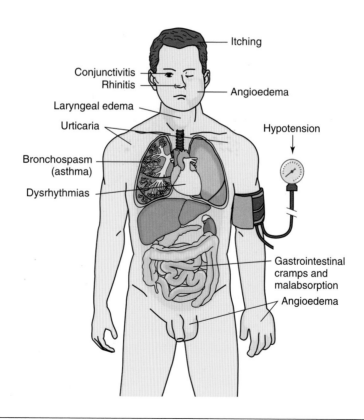

Itching

Conjunctivitis
Rhinitis

Angioedema

Laryngeal edema

Urticaria

Hypotension

Bronchospasm (asthma)

Dysrhythmias

Gastrointestinal cramps and malabsorption

Angioedema

Reprinted with permission from Phipps W et al: *Medical-surgical nursing: health and illness perspective*, ed 7, St Louis, 2003, Mosby (page 1635).

Plate 2: Intraaortic Balloon Pump

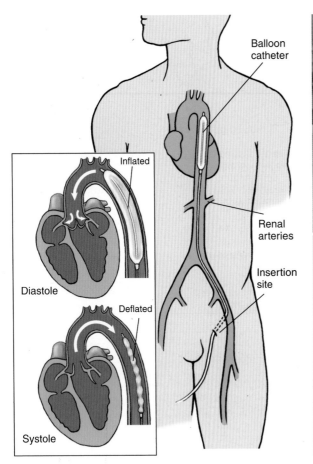

Balloon catheter

Renal arteries

Insertion site

Inflated

Diastole

Deflated

Systole

Plate 3: Application of Cricoid Pressure

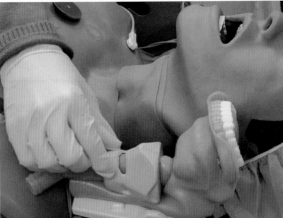

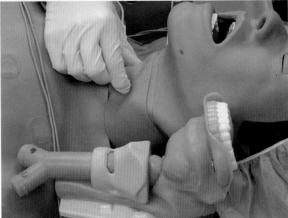

Plate 2: Reprinted with permission from Phipps W et al: *Medical-surgical nursing: health and illness perspective*, ed 7, St Louis, 2003, Mosby (page 296).
Plate 3: Courtesy of Matthew W. Kervin, MN, CRNA.

Plate 4: Coronary Arteries and Myocardial Infarction Localization

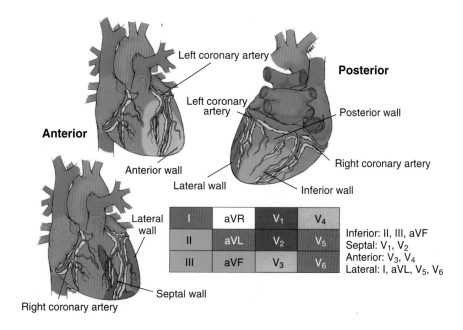

Anterior

Left coronary artery

Left coronary artery

Anterior wall

Lateral wall

Posterior

Posterior wall

Right coronary artery

Inferior wall

Lateral wall

Right coronary artery

Septal wall

I	aVR	V$_1$	V$_4$
II	aVL	V$_2$	V$_5$
III	aVF	V$_3$	V$_6$

Inferior: II, III, aVF
Septal: V$_1$, V$_2$
Anterior: V$_3$, V$_4$
Lateral: I, aVL, V$_5$, V$_6$

Plate 5: Blood Flow through the Heart

Plate 6: Osmosis and Diffusion

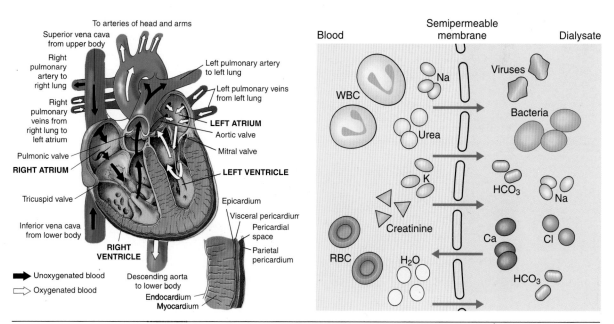

To arteries of head and arms

Superior vena cava from upper body

Right pulmonary artery to right lung

Right pulmonary veins from right lung to left atrium

Pulmonic valve

RIGHT ATRIUM

Tricuspid valve

Inferior vena cava from lower body

RIGHT VENTRICLE

Left pulmonary artery to left lung

Left pulmonary veins from left lung

LEFT ATRIUM
Aortic valve

Mitral valve

LEFT VENTRICLE

Epicardium

Visceral pericardium
Pericardial space
Parietal pericardium

Descending aorta to lower body

Endocardium
Myocardium

➡ Unoxygenated blood
⇨ Oxygenated blood

Blood — Semipermeable membrane — Dialysate

WBC

Na

Urea

K

Creatinine

RBC

H$_2$O

Viruses

Bacteria

HCO$_3$

Na

Ca

Cl

HCO$_3$

Plate 4: Reprinted with permission from Achlert B: *ECGs made easy*, ed 2, St Louis, 2002, Mosby (page 209). **Plate 5:** Reprinted with permission from Ignatavicus, Workman: *Medical-surgical nursing: critical thinking for collaborative care*, ed 4, Philadelphia, 2002, WB Saunders (page 620). **Plate 6:** Reprinted with permission from Lewis, Heitkemper, Dirksen: *Medical-surgical nursing: assessment and management of clinical problems*, ed 5, St Louis, 2000, Mosby (page 1321).

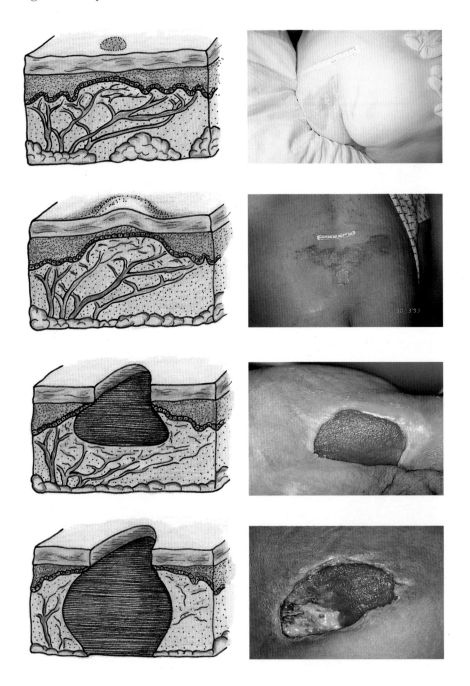

- *Do you have any known liver disease?* One of the functions of the liver is to metabolize clotting factors. In the presence of liver disease, these factors are not metabolized and can result in coagulopathies.
- *Do you have any known bleeding or coagulation problems?* Other associated diseases such as thrombocytopenia, leukemias, and lymphomas can result in bleeding and coagulation defects. An assessment for the presence of these disorders assists in ruling out the underlying cause of the bleed.
- *What types of medications (prescribed, over the counter, and herbal) are you currently taking?* Of particular interest would be the use of NSAIDs. The nurse should remember to ask about herbal supplements when taking a medication history. Garlic, feverfew, and *Ginkgo biloba* can suppress platelet aggregation and increase the risk of bleeding when taken in association with anticoagulant or antiplatelet drugs.
- *Do you drink alcohol and if so, how often?* Alcohol is a known irritant to the defensive mucosal barrier and an associated cause for bleeding.

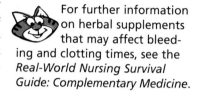

For further information on herbal supplements that may affect bleeding and clotting times, see the *Real-World Nursing Survival Guide: Complementary Medicine.*

The nurse should also perform a physical exam in addition to the history. A complete abdominal assessment should be performed, including inspection, percussion, auscultation, and palpation. Clues may be found on the physical exam that may identify the underlying cause of GI bleeding. For example, the presence of spider nevi, petechiae, and bruising in the presence of a palpable nodular liver may indicate liver cirrhosis. A rigid, boardlike, tender abdomen can indicate perforation. The presence of blood in the gut often stimulates peristalsis; on auscultation, hyperactive bowel sounds can be heard.

The goals for the care of a patient with GI bleeding include control of the hemorrhage, achievement and maintenance of hemodynamic stability, control of gastric acid secretion, observation for complications, preparation for surgical interventions if necessary, and patient and family education about the treatment and control of GI bleeding.

TAKE HOME POINTS

- It is important to take a focused patient history concerning factors pertaining to GI bleeding.
- Physical assessment findings can indicate certain underlying conditions that are the cause of the GI bleed.

FIRST-LINE AND INITIAL TREATMENTS FOR DECREASING GI BLEED

- Provide oxygen (O_2).
- Monitor vital signs and hemodynamic readings.
- Ensure IV access.
- Administer fluids (crystalloids, colloids) and blood.
- Insert nasogastric (NG) tube.
- Consider possible gastric lavage.
- Prepare for endoscopy.

To achieve hemodynamic stability, venous and arterial lines are inserted to allow access for volume infusion and continuous monitoring of hemodynamic parameters such as pulse, blood pressure (BP), mean arterial pressure (MAP), and central venous pressures (CVPs). A pulmonary artery catheter may be inserted to monitor pulmonary capillary wedge pressure (PCWP) and cardiac output (CO).

TAKE HOME POINTS

The treatment for hemorrhagic shock is volume replacement.

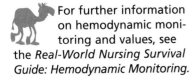

For further information on hemodynamic monitoring and values, see the *Real-World Nursing Survival Guide: Hemodynamic Monitoring.*

TAKE HOME POINTS

If massive volume replacement is required, the replacement products should be warmed to prevent hypothermia.

TAKE HOME POINTS

- Abuse of antacids can cause metabolic alkalosis.
- Misoprostol is an agent used in the prevention of ulcers specifically caused by the use of NSAIDs.

Volume should be administered to the patient in the form of crystalloids, colloids, and blood (the best form of volume replacement), as well as packed red blood cells (RBCs) and coagulation factors. RBCs promote O_2-carrying capacity, whereas coagulation factors promote hemostasis. O_2 therapy should be initiated to compensate for the decrease in O_2-carrying capacity of the blood associated with the loss of RBCs and hemoglobin; O_2 saturation should be assessed via pulse oximetry. An NG tube should be inserted to remove blood from the upper GI tract and to allow for an assessment of the amount of blood lost. Gastric lavage may be used to cleanse the stomach in preparation for endoscopy. A Foley catheter should be inserted to evaluate renal perfusion and urine output. The electrocardiogram (ECG) tracing should be assessed for any signs of myocardial ischemia that could be associated with decreased coronary perfusion, often associated with hemorrhagic shock.

Once hemodynamic stability is achieved in patients with peptic ulcer disease, gastritis, stress ulcerations and esophagitis, control of gastric acid secretion and pepsin action is accomplished through pharmacologic agents to promote healing. H_2-receptor antagonists, proton pump inhibitors, antacids, and mucosal protective agents are examples of the medications commonly used.

H_2-receptor antagonists act on the H_2-receptor antagonists found on the gastric parietal cell and decrease acid production. Examples of H_2-receptor antagonists include cimetidine (Tagamet), ranitidine (Zantac), famotidine (Pepcid), and nizatidine (Axid).

Proton pump inhibitors suppress gastric acid secretion by inhibition of the $H^+K^+-ATPase$ enzyme. This category of drugs is thought to be the most effective in the suppression of gastric acid secretion. The $H^+K^+-ATPase$ enzyme is responsible for the production of gastric acid in the parietal cell. Examples of proton pump inhibitors include omeprazole (Prilosec), lansoprazole (Prevacid), pantoprazole (Protonix), and rabeprazole (AcipHex).

Mucosal protective agents create a protective barrier around a known ulcer against the acid and pepsin action of the stomach and promote healing. Mucosal protective agents are activated in the presence of the acidic environment of the stomach. If used in combination with antacids, the mucosal protective agents should be administered 30 to 60 minutes before antacids. An example of the mucosal protectant is sucralfate (Carafate).

Antacids are used to neutralize stomach acid, inactivate the effects of pepsin by raising the pH of stomach contents, and stimulate the production of prostaglandins that can enhance the mucosal barrier. Antacids come in four forms: (1) magnesium hydroxide (milk of magnesia), (2) aluminum hydroxide (Amphogel), (3) calcium carbonate (Caltrate, Tums), and (4) sodium bicarbonate. Magnesium and aluminum hydroxide preparations are most commonly used. Antacids should be taken on a regular schedule after meals and at bedtime.

Patients with documented *Helicobacter pylori* infection are treated with combination antibiotics. Clarithromycin (Biaxin), tetracycline, amoxicillin (Amoxil), and metronidazole (Flagyl) are the most common.

The patient should be assessed for complications associated with GI bleeding with specific emphasis on hemodynamic status. If surgical intervention is required, the patient should be monitored for postoperative complications such as infection, peritonitis, fluid and electrolyte disturbances, and hemodynamic complications.

The nurse should also assess patency of the NG tube to ensure decompression of the upper GI track and prevent vomiting. Patients who are experiencing GI bleeding should receive nothing by mouth, and gastric or enteral feeding should be discontinued until the source of bleeding is identified. When recovering from a bleeding episode, the patient's diet is increased and prescribed as tolerated. The nurse should ensure patient comfort throughout the course of treatment. Comfort measures include both pharmacologic and nonpharmacologic measures.

In situations where medical management cannot stop GI bleeding, surgical intervention is indicated. Such situations would include hemorrhagic shock unresponsive to medical treatment, the need to transfuse a patient with more than eight units of blood in a 24-hour period and the presence of GI perforation.

The patient and family must receive education throughout the course of an episode of GI bleeding. Patients who require transfer to an intensive care unit (ICU) need an explanation of why the transfer is occurring. Once in the ICU, the patient and family should be oriented to the environment, including an explanation of equipment and procedures. Once a source of bleeding is identified, the treatment plan should be reviewed with the patient and family and they should be given an opportunity to ask questions and voice concerns. As the patient is recovering, the nurse should review and reinforce the treatment plan for the underlying cause of the bleeding.

 The head of the bed should be elevated to prevent aspiration in the presence of vomiting.

 TAKE HOME POINTS

No specific diet prescriptions are available for a patient who is recovering from GI bleeding. The diet should be geared to the treatment of the disease that is the underlying cause of the bleeding.

 TAKE HOME POINTS

The purpose of surgical intervention in a GI bleed is to prevent the patient from exsanguination.

 # Do You UNDERSTAND?

DIRECTIONS: **Select the best answer, and place the appropriate letter in the space provided.**

1. The nurse is reviewing the ABG results for a patient admitted for GI bleeding who is in hypovolemic shock. The patient ABG results are pH, 7.27; pCO_2, 38; pO_2, 78; HCO_3, 14; and O_2 saturation, 94%. The nurse understands that the **MOST** probable cause of the ABG result is the result of the following:
   a. Tachypnea associated with compensatory mechanisms in response to shock
   b. The conversion from aerobic to anaerobic metabolism caused by cellular injury and damage
   c. The increased production of bicarbonate by the kidney as a compensatory mechanism by the body in response to the shock state
   d. Cellular destruction releasing excessive amount of potassium into the vascular space

DIRECTIONS: **Match the treatment in Column A with the appropriate disease process in Column B.**

Column A

_____ 2. Balloon tamponade tube such as a Sengstaken-Blakemore is used to place direct pressure on the site of bleeding.

_____ 3. Surgical intervention is used to repair this arterial tear.

_____ 4. Antibiotic combinations are used to treat the inflammation caused by *Helicobacter pylori*.

_____ 5. Pharmacologic agents such as vaso-pressin and octreotide acetate are used to decrease portal pressures.

_____ 6. The patient is instructed not to eat immediately before bedtime to prevent pressure on the lower esophageal sphincter.

Column B

a. Chronic gastritis
b. Gastro-esophageal reflux
c. Mallory-Weiss tear
d. Esophageal varices
e. Peptic ulcer disease

What IS Bowel Obstruction?

Bowel or intestinal obstruction is a partial or complete obstruction of the small or large bowel that impedes the natural progression of digestive processing. Early recognition and appropriate management can prevent life-threatening complications for many patients. Despite dramatically decreased mortality rates over the past 2 decades, this disorder is still associated with significant morbidity. The clinical features of intestinal obstruction provide information about the characteristics of the obstruction and are the basis of medical and nursing interventions.

What You NEED TO KNOW

Bowel obstructions are classified descriptively by cause (nonmechanical or mechanical), location (small or large bowel), degree of lumen occlusion (partial or complete), onset (acute or chronic), type of lesion (intrinsic or extrinsic), and effects on the bowel (simple, closed loop, or strangulated). Nonmechanical obstructions are caused by neurologic or vascular defects that reduce peristalsis and allow for accumulation of bowel contents. Inflammation may accompany these processes and enhance the risk of complete obstruction. Mechanical obstructions occlude the bowel lumen because of their size or involvement of the bowel wall. The four primary pathophysiologic effects of bowel obstruction are (1) electrolyte and nutrient imbalances, (2) retention of bowel contents, (3) accumulation of gases, and (4) fluid shifts.

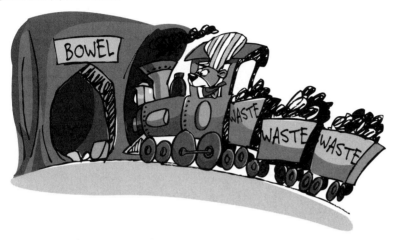

One of the most significant events that occur during obstruction is loss of fluid and electrolytes through increased bowel wall permeability. As the intestine distends with trapped fluids and gases, the intraluminal pressure exceeds the surrounding abdominal pressure and results in intestinal fluid leaking into the peritoneum. Electrolyte disturbances such as hypokalemia, hypocalcemia, hypomagnesemia, and hypophosphatemia occur because of decreased absorption. Obstructive processes also interfere with normal digestion and absorption, resulting in malabsorption syndromes.

Peristalsis is the normal rhythmic contractions of the bowel muscles to propel food substances and GI secretions forward through the bowel. When an obstructive mass is encountered, the digestive contents back up and adhere to each other. Normal bowel function is lost as air and digestive wastes accumulate behind the obstructed section of bowel. The location of the obstruction predicts the nature of the gas that accumulates and is transmitted to the blood. Normal digestive processes in the small intestine cause production of carbon dioxide (CO_2) and nitrogen, resulting in metabolic acidosis. In colonic obstruction, the normal GI flora produce methane, leading to increased serum ammonia levels and alkalosis.

The two significant life-threatening complications of bowel obstruction related to high intraluminal pressure are bowel perforation or rupture. These occur as the obstructing mass either erodes through the bowel wall (perforation) causing peritonitis or explodes from excessive intraluminal pressures (rupture).

At-Risk Populations

Risk factors for bowel obstruction include both GI disorders and external factors. Each potential causative factor occurs more commonly in specific patient age groups and affect either the small or large bowel.

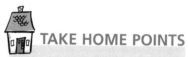

TAKE HOME POINTS

The nature and severity of fluid, electrolyte, and nutritional disturbances will vary with the location and completeness of the obstruction.

Risk Factors for Bowel Obstruction

SMALL INTESTINE	LARGE INTESTINE	EITHER SMALL OR LARGE INTESTINE
Crohn's disease (A,E)	Endometriosis (A)	Abdominal trauma (N,P,A,E)
Diaphragmatic hernia	Hirschsprung's disease (A,E)	Adhesions, postoperative
Esophageal stent (A,E)	Malposition of the colon (N,P)	Adhesions, radiation
Duodenal/pyloric ulcer (A,E)	Meckel's diverticulum (N,P)	Acariasis (N,P,A,E)
Intestinal ischemia (N,P,A,E)	Megacolon	Cystic fibrosis (N,P,A)
Intussusception (N,P,A,E)	Multiple sclerosis (A,E)	Cytomegalovirus (N,P,A,E)
	Ulcerative colitis (A,E)	Foreign body in the gastrointestinal (GI) tract (N,P,A,E)
	Volvulus (N,P,A,E)	Myasthenia gravis (A,E) Pregnancy (A) Tuberculosis (A,E) Tumors (P,A,E)

N, Neonates; *P,* pediatric; *A,* adults; *E,* elderly.

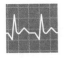

TAKE HOME POINTS

Current mortality from bowel obstruction ranges between 3.5% and 6%, but may be higher (7% and 14%) in older patients, those with concomitant mesenteric thrombosis, and when the large bowel is obstructed.

Emesis and stool characteristics provide clues to the location of the obstruction.

Across all age groups, the greatest risk for development of obstruction is abdominal adhesions, with most involving the small intestine. Abdominal adhesions can occur any time after abdominal or pelvic surgeries. They are the result of an inflammatory response to injury or particulate matter within the peritoneum. Three variables identified as enhancing the risk of postoperative obstruction caused by adhesions are (1) small bowel manipulation more than large bowel, (2) invasiveness or repetition of abdominal surgery, and (3) use of powdered gloves for surgical procedures.

Clinical Manifestations

The clinical findings of bowel obstruction are primarily related to the obstructive process, although the secondary complications of altered bowel function may contribute to the overall symptomatology. Primary effects include abdominal discomfort, distention, and alterations in bowel sounds. Secondary signs and symptoms include vomiting, malnutrition, hypotension, and fever.

The pain associated with bowel obstruction is moderate to severe, crampy, crescendo-decrescendo pain that is more severe when the small intestine is involved. Crampy periumbilcal pain is associated with jejunal obstruction. Severe and unremitting pain may signal strangulation with ischemic bowel, and rebound tenderness signifies progression to perforation (complications associated with higher mortality rates). Abdominal pain in partial obstruction often occurs after eating and is separated by times of no pain.

GI secretions are created continuously, and large amounts can collect above the area of obstruction. Because of the high volume of fluid, obstructions high in the small bowel cause vomiting, although abdominal distention is a more common finding in other locations of obstruction. Accumulation of fluid proximal to the obstruction also enhances peristaltic activity.

The increased peristalsis associated with this disorder is noted as hyperactive bowel sounds proximal to the site of obstruction, accentuated even more when complete obstruction is present. Bowel sounds are absent over the area of obstruction. The lack of intestinal contents distal to the obstruction produces hypoactive, quiet, or absent bowel sounds.

Inflammation as a result of the obstructive process or high intraluminal pressures causes compensatory fluid leakage from the bowel into the peritoneum. This fluid subsequently irritates the peritoneum, causing vascular fluid shifts into the peritoneum and accompanying hypotension and hypovolemia.

Characteristics of the GI fluid drained during management of small bowel obstructions reveal the location of the obstruction or unique features of the obstruction. Secretions may be clear, green, bilious (golden), bloody, or feculent. Obstructions of the high small bowel produce clear secretions, those of the middle small bowel are bilious secretions, and those of the low small bowel are green secretions. Feculent drainage in small bowel obstruction is a poor prognostic sign. With obstruction, stagnant intestinal drainage and ischemia to the bowel causes an overgrowth of bacteria that produce fecal-appearing and odorous drainage. Bloody drainage may signify ischemic bowel with mucosal sloughing.

Small bowel obstructions may not initially alter stool output, but often later cause absent stool. Stool characteristics are a direct reflection of the severity of large bowel obstruction. Partial or early symptoms of lower GI tract obstructions may include thin ribbonlike stools or watery stool. Complete obstruction causes acute and severe obstipation.

After evaluation of the patient's history and clinical findings, laboratory and radiologic studies confirm the likely location and cause of an obstruction. All patients with potential intestinal obstruction will have frequent measurement of their hematocrit, sodium, potassium, magnesium, calcium, BUN, amylase, and osmolarity. Electrolytes such as potassium, calcium, and magnesium are more deficient in small bowel obstruction. The CBC is monitored for anemia that may signal bleeding or an elevated hematocrit when dehydration occurs. The severity of leukocytosis is used to help differentiate simple, strangulated, and perforated obstructions. Simple obstruction causes mild elevations in the WBC count (10.0 to 15.0/mm^3), strangulation causes moderate elevations (15.0 to 25.0/mm^3), and mesenteric occlusion or perforation produce high WBC counts (>25.0/mm^3). Large bowel obstructions cause hypophosphatemia. Amylase levels are elevated when peritonitis complicates the bowel obstruction. Loss of vitamins and minerals can cause poor wound healing and various types of anemia. Low small bowel or high large bowel obstruction interfere with vitamin K

TAKE HOME POINTS

Abdominal pain occurs with bowel obstruction, and its characteristics must be assessed to assist with the identification of the type of bowel obstruction occurring.

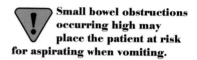

Small bowel obstructions occurring high may place the patient at risk for aspirating when vomiting.

TAKE HOME POINTS

Assessment of GI fluid drainage may reveal the location of the obstruction.

absorption and deficient production of coagulation proteins with subsequent coagulopathy.

Radiologic tests are the standard for diagnosis of intestinal obstruction, although the emerging role of helical computed tomography (CT) to replace traditional radiologic tests is still inconsistent. Most clinicians still use an abdominal flat plate radiograph to screen for obvious candidates for surgical interventions. The CT scan is most useful in differentiating the specific cause and location of mechanical obstructions, making it most useful when symptoms are severe and surgical intervention is being considered but not clearly indicated. Barium tests (enema or swallow) have been compared with standard radiology and CT scans and show 100% sensitivity for complete obstructions, but they are an added danger when adding substances to an obstructed bowel. Magnetic resonance imaging (MRI) and ultrasonography are currently under study for use in diagnosing this disorder. When noninvasive diagnosis remains inconclusive in confirming bowel obstruction, exploratory laparoscopy is used to evaluate the abdomen for causative factors and ascertain whether laparotomy is indicated.

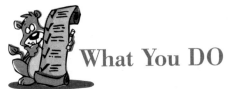 # What You DO

The first approach to treatment of possible intestinal obstruction is to identify potential risk factors, because some causes are clear indications for surgical therapy. After risk factors are defined, signs and symptoms are evaluated for peritoneal signs such as rebound tenderness and hypotension that indicate the need for immediate surgery. Determination of whether an obstruction is partial or complete will also be important for defining a treatment plan.

Prevention

Although intestinal obstruction may often be unavoidable, specific operative precautions are taken to reduce the incidence of postoperative adhesions. Preventive strategies used include glove washing, nonlatex surgical environments, and avoidance of suturing the peritoneal lining. In other patients, obstruction may not be prevented, but the progression from partial to complete obstruction may be abrogated. Medications that enhance GI motility (e.g., erythromycin, metoclopramide, neostigmine, octreotide) may be used to treat functional obstruction (e.g., paralytic ileus) or prevent the progression to complete obstruction.

Treatment

Intestinal obstructions are managed both medically and surgically, depending upon the severity of symptoms and reversibility of the underlying cause. When obstruction is thought to be reversible or when the patient is not a safe surgical candidate, conservative medical management with gut rest and intestinal tube decompression is implemented. NG or intestinal tubes drain GI fluids, reducing fluid at the site of obstruction, and are an extremely important aspect of medical management for small bowel obstruction. Mercury-weighted intestinal tubes may be used in partial mechanical obstructions of the proximal small bowel, although at least one study comparing both methods of GI drainage shows no advantage of these tubes over standard NG tubes. When large bowel obstruction is present, or trapped large bowel air is evident, a rectal tube is also used to reduce dangerous bowel dilatation that can lead to perforation.

Palliative interventions for patients with terminal disease associated with bowel obstruction are aimed at alleviating discomfort with the least invasive therapy possible. Intravenous (IV) fluids and nutrition, with pain medications, and drugs affecting GI motility are the most common interventions used. Palliative surgical procedures such as distal gastric and jejunal tubes, colonic dilatation, and intestinal stents have also been used to enhance quality of life.

While attempting to alleviate the obstruction, medical therapy must also allocate clinical priority to fluid and electrolyte balance. Extravasation of large amounts of fluid causes hypovolemia, but the infusion of replacement fluid often continues to leak interstitially. Intake and output measurement, CVP measurement, and evaluation for orthostasis are performed to maintain a plan for fluid balance. Continual electrolyte assessment and replacement reduce the incidence of arrhythmias, seizures, or other neuromuscular complications.

Surgical treatment of an obstruction is indicated when threatening perforation or bowel rupture occurs. Large, immovable masses such as tumors are almost always viewed as appropriate surgical indications. Common criteria defined as indications for surgical intervention in suspected bowel obstruction include (1) progression of pain, (2) lack of pain improvement after decompression, (3) tachycardia, (4) fever, and (5) leukocytosis. Laparoscopic management of small bowel obstruction rather than laparotomy is gaining popularity as advantageous in small bowel obstruction. Creative laparoscopic or endoscopic surgical placement of endoprostheses and stents have been used successfully in situations where a temporary colostomy would be required, as well as palliative care. In small bowel disease, particularly involving inflammatory disorders such as Crohn's disease, stricturoplasty has been successfully used to relieve partial small bowel obstruction. Whenever possible, a bowel resection with end-to-end anastomosis is performed. When distal ischemic bowel or extensive intestinal damage is present, a temporary or permanent colostomy is performed.

Nursing Responsibilities

Major areas of responsibility include the assessment of patient history, clinical findings, and laboratory and diagnostic test results. The nurse caring for a patient at risk for bowel obstruction must carefully evaluate all complaints of abdominal pain and perform frequent, focused assessment of the abdomen. Patients at risk or experiencing some degree of bowel obstruction must be questioned about the presence and nature of symptoms such as abdominal pain, nausea, early satiety, episodes of emesis, and the frequency or characteristics of stool output. Abdominal assessment aimed at detecting evidence of bowel obstruction

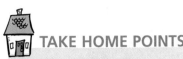

TAKE HOME POINTS

Always auscultate the abdomen before percussion or palpation to avoid altering bowel sounds.

or its complications includes listening to bowel sounds, palpation of the abdominal quadrants, notation of abdominal distention, or measurement of abdominal circumference.

In most circumstances, pain medication is administered sparingly so that changing abdominal pain can be assessed more thoroughly. Medications intended to aid peristalsis and prevent partial obstruction from progressing to complete obstruction may also worsen abdominal discomfort in near total obstruction. When palliative symptom management is the desired objective, medications that slow peristalsis may be administered for their ability to decrease abdominal discomfort.

Bowel Obstruction: Nursing Responsibilities

HISTORY	CLINICAL FINDINGS	LABORATORY TESTS	DIAGNOSTIC TESTS
Abdominal surgery, note adhesions	Abdominal distention	Serum electrolytes decreased: Na^+, Cl^-, Mg^+, K^+, Ca^+, P	Abdominal films
Change in bowel habits	Bowel sounds absent or diminished	CBC and differentials for anemia and infection	Barium enema or barium swallow
Blood in stool	Abdominal pain	Increased BUN because of blood in GI tract or renal dysfunction	CT of abdomen with or without contrast
History of inflammatory bowel disease	Rebound tenderness	Osmolality is decreased in over-hydration and increased in dehydration	Doppler ultrasound
	Vomiting	Increased serum amylase	MRI of abdomen
	Constipation or obstipation	Increased serum alkaline phosphatase	
	Hypotension	Increased serum creatinine kinase	
	Fever	Increased lactate dehydrogenase	

Na^+, Sodium; Cl^-, chloride; Mg^+, magnesium; K^+, potassium; Ca^+, calcium; P, phosphorus; CBC, complete blood count; GI, gastrointestinal; BUN, blood urea nitrogen; CT, computed tomography; MRI, magnetic resonance image.

Patients with suspected bowel obstruction are assessed often to detect signs or symptoms of bowel perforation, rupture, or intraabdominal sepsis. Unremitting and severe pain or rebound tenderness are immediately reportable symptoms of these life-threatening crises. Most patients with intraabdominal crisis also experience rapid and extreme fluid shifts into the peritoneum causing hypotension, dizziness, altered level of consciousness, and oliguria.

Patients with bowel obstruction are unable to eat or drink, so they require IV fluids, and electrolyte and nutrient replacement. Interventions for maintaining fluid and electrolyte balance are both metabolic and patient specific. Many clinical settings have standing orders for electrolyte replacement and follow-up blood drawing. For many patients with chronic obstruction, long-term parenteral nutrition is necessary. Because they are unable to eat or drink, they often complain of a dry mouth. It is important for nurses not to provide ice or candies normally used to treat dry mouth, because these strategies increase GI secretions. Frequent oral care is an acceptable alternative.

NG tubes are used for removal of retained upper GI tract secretions or air. Nursing management of NG tubes include assessment of correct placement, monitoring of straight or suctioned drainage, and nares care. Some clinicians advocate periodic assessment of NG aspirant for blood or pH, although this practice is guided by the intent to provide treatments such as blood product replacement or proton pump inhibitors. Rectal tubes may be used to remove large bowel air.

Nursing care of patients with bowel obstruction requires an integrated multidisciplinary approach of assessment and interventions. Nurses are essential coordinators of care and can advocate for care consistent with the patient's personal objectives and realistic prognosis. A thorough understanding of the pathophysiologic findings, common clinical presentation, diagnosis, and management enhance their ability to perform this role.

For further information on ECG interpretation, see the *Real-World Nursing series book: Fluids and Electrolytes.*

Do You UNDERSTAND?

DIRECTIONS: **Match the classification of bowel obstruction in Column A with the description in Column B.**

Column A	Column B
_____ 1. Cause	a. Intrinsic
_____ 2. Location	b. Mechanical
_____ 3. Type of lesion	c. Strangulated
_____ 4. Effects on the bowel	d. Small bowel

DIRECTIONS: **Circle all the electrolytes that are decreased as a result of decreased absorption by the intestines for intestinal obstruction.**

5. Helium   Magnesium   Potassium

   Hydrogen   Calcium   Phosphorus

Answers: 1. b; 2. d; 3. a; 4. c; 5. potassium, calcium, magnesium, phosphorus.

DIRECTIONS: **After each risk factor, write in either the words** *small intestine* **or** *large intestine* **as it relates to a true statement associated with bowel obstruction.**

6. Peptic ulcer   _____

7. Endometriosis   _____

8. Multiple sclerosis   _____

9. Crohn's disease   _____

DIRECTIONS: **Identify the following statements as** *true* **(T) or** *false* **(F) as it relates to bowel obstruction.**

_____ 10. Rebound tenderness in the abdomen can be a sign of bowel obstruction.

_____ 11. Ice chips are an appropriate interventions for persons with complete bowel obstruction.

_____ 12. Rectal tubes are used to remove air from the large bowel.

_____ 13. An NG tube can be used to remove upper GI tract air.

What IS Pancreatitis?

Pancreatitis is a serious illness caused by the inflammation of the pancreas. An episode of pancreatitis may be identified as either an acute or chronic condition. Acute pancreatitis may be severe, causing life-threatening conditions. The sudden onset of symptoms resulting in an acute situation may last for a short time, and if promptly treated the patient will have a full recovery. The severity is usually unpredictable and affects all age groups. The most common causes of acute pancreatitis include alcoholism, drug toxicity, abdominal trauma, or biliary duct obstruction. Viral infections may also contribute to inflammation of the pancreas.

Alcohol-related pancreatitis may develop in young patients in their thirties after 4 to 7 years of drinking, whereas biliary pancreatitis usually occurs in an older adult population.

TAKE HOME POINTS

Chronic pancreatitis progresses slowly and does not resolve itself. Chronic pancreatitis severely impairs the function of the pancreas and causes permanent damage to the gland.

What You NEED TO KNOW

The pancreas is a large gland located behind the stomach close to the duodenum (the first part of the small intestine). The pancreas' tadpole shape is divided into three parts: (1) head, (2) body, and (3) tail. The head of the pancreas is located right of the midline of the abdominal cavity with the body and tail pointing upward so that the tail is found lying close to the edge of the left side of the ribs.

The head of the pancreas is attached to the duodenum and shares this space with the liver. The bile duct from the liver drains bile into the bowel at the same place that pancreatic fluids enter the bowel from the head of the pancreas via the pancreatic duct. Because of the many blood vessels behind the pancreas and the general positioning of the pancreas in the body, any surgical procedure involving the pancreas is difficult and challenging for the surgeon.

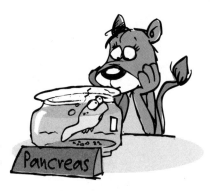

The pancreas is considered a gland because of its unusual combination of endocrine and exocrine functions. Endocrine cells, found in the islets of Langerhans, produce several hormones that pass directly into the blood stream. These hormones include insulin, glucagon, and vasoactive intestinal polypeptide (VIP). The pancreas also produces a variety of chemical digestive enzymes that pass into the duodenum, thus the label, *exocrine*. Exocrine secretions are produced by the acini cells. The most commonly known digestive enzymes produced by the pancreas include trypsin, chymotrypsin, lipase, and amylase.

The main function of the pancreas is to aid in food digestion and maintain a balance of sugar in the blood. Pancreatic enzymes remain inactive until they pass into the bowel, where they mix with bowel juices, become activated, and assist with digestion of carbohydrates, protein, and fats. Bile from the liver assists lipase in fat digestion by breaking the fat into tiny pieces. In pancreatitis, these powerful enzymes become activated prematurely and the pancreas begins digesting itself (autodigestion), resulting in bleeding. As the blood vessels are digested, they leak pancreatic chemicals into the abdominal cavity. When pancreatic blood vessels begin to erode, activated enzymes may gain access to the bloodstream where they begin circulating throughout the body.

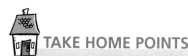

TAKE HOME POINTS

- A gland is any organ that produces chemicals for transport into either the bloodstream or another organ.
- In pancreatitis, the pancreas auto-digests itself.
- Pain is usually the main symptom in pancreatitis.

It is very easy to misdiagnose an acute case of pancreatitis because of vague patient complaints of fever, malaise, nausea, vomiting, and steady epigastric pain. However, one in four patients may have severe acute pancreatitis where the pain may become intense, radiating to the patient's back and flank, because the pancreas is located in the retroperitoneal space. The pain may lessen when the patient is sitting up and bending forward. Eating will exacerbate the pain by stimulating secretion of prematurely activated enzymes that promote autodigestion of the gland. Pain is usually increased after vomiting, rather than decreased, because of an increase in intraductal pressure caused by retching that allows further obstruction of the outflow of pancreatic secretions causing more damage to the organ.

One important note: No specific laboratory test is used to diagnose acute pancreatitis. Although increases in amylase, lipase, and trypsin serum levels may appear elevated early in the disease, only to return to normal values in cases of chronic pancreatitis.

Additional symptoms may include fever, tachycardia, low BP, and jaundice. Nausea, vomiting, and abdominal swelling are common symptoms as well. A rare sign, found in pancreatic hemorrhage, is the appearance of a reddish-purple or greenish-brown color located on the flank area (Turner's sign), a bluish color around the navel (Cullen's sign), or both.

⚠️ **Turner's and Cullen's signs are evidence of necrotizing pancreatitis, where bleeding into the abdomen is caused by death of pancreatic tissue.**

Pancreatitis

COMPLICATION	SIGNS/SYMPTOMS
Shock	Low blood pressure (BP) Increased heart rate (HR) Cold extremities Changes in mental status
Hypovolemia (secondary to internal and external bleeding and fluid loss)	Shock symptoms
Acute respiratory distress syndrome	Dyspnea Tachypnea Hypoxemia (Despite oxygen therapy)
Sepsis	Symptoms of shock with fever
Circulatory shock	Symptoms of shock
Pleural effusion	Respiratory distress Hypoxemia
Circulation of pancreatic enzymes throughout the body	Damage to kidneys, heart, liver, eyes, bone, skin, lining of gastrointestinal tract

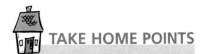

TAKE HOME POINTS

A pseudocyst, a severe complication of pancreatitis, is filled with pancreatic enzyme exudates.

A common cause of death in acute pancreatitis is secondary pancreatic infection. After the pancreatitis decreases, the pancreas becomes susceptible to infection because of extensive cell death caused by pancreatic necrosis. Prophylactic antibiotics are used to prevent potential septic complications. A pancreatic abscess may develop, causing a return of fever and pain, and is treated with broad-spectrum antibiotics.

A pancreatic pseudocyst is a very severe complication of pancreatitis that can appear weeks after the illness begins. A pseudocyst is an encapsulated saclike structure that forms on or around the pancreas and lacks the epithelial lining of a true cyst. The cyst may contain several liters of pancreatic enzyme exudates that may appear straw colored or dark brown. A pseudocyst may resolve spontaneously or may rupture, and death may occur if bleeding is a complication.

Loss of pancreatic function occurs in chronic pancreatitis as the gland begins to lose exocrine and endocrine functions. Though causes of chronic pancreatitis can rarely be identified, factors that produce the acute form can also cause the chronic form. In chronic pancreatitis, cells found in the islets of Langerhans that produce insulin to maintain proper sugar levels begin to malfunction and the patient may develop diabetes. As chronic pancreatitis continues and insulin levels drop, a patient may require insulin injections to be able to process sugars. A further complication of chronic pancreatitis is pancreatic insufficiency. This insufficiency is caused by the malabsorption of nutrients in the small intestine because of the formation of fibrous tissue that replaces healthy acinar tissue. When acini are no longer able to produce necessary enzymes needed to digest proteins, carbohydrates, and fats, patients may complain of bulky, fatty, foul-smelling stool (steatorrhea), weight loss, fever, malaise, and nausea and vomiting. The inability to digest nutrients may also lead to muscle wasting, weakness, and malnutrition.

Several options are available to aid the physician in diagnosing pancreatitis. A contrast-enhanced CT scan provides the best image of the pancreas and surrounding structures. A CT scan of the abdomen may reveal fluid accumulation and noted inflammation of the pancreatic gland.

Endoscopic retrograde cholangiopancreatography (ERCP) allows the physician to view magnified images of the pancreas via a fiber-optic camera. ERCP is primarily indicated when patients have severe disease symptoms and are suspected to have biliary pancreatitis. During the ERCP procedure, the physician is able to remove impacted stones from the bile duct.

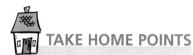
It is important to closely monitor blood glucose levels in patients with pancreatitis.

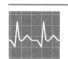
TAKE HOME POINTS

In pancreatitis a malfunction of insulin production occurs; therefore insulin will need to be administered.

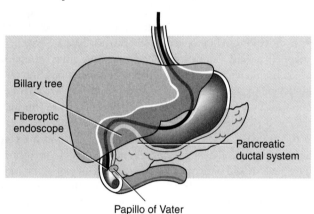

Billary tree

Fiberoptic endoscope

Pancreatic ductal system

Papillo of Vater

Ultrasonography is a noninvasive procedure acceptable for initial evaluation of the pancreas when biliary causes are suspected.

Plain radiographic studies are helpful in revealing gallstones that may be blocking the pancreatic duct. Calcification of the pancreas becomes present when previously healthy tissue is destroyed and is replaced by nonfunctioning scar tissue. These areas of calcification can be seen on radiographs.

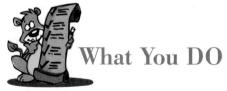

What You DO

Management of the patient with pancreatitis focuses on the rest of the pancreas, supportive care, relief of symptoms, and management of complications. Treatment includes maintenance of circulatory volume, pain relief, and decreasing pancreatic secretions.

Trousseau's sign

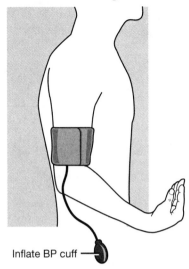

Inflate BP cuff

Chvostek's sign

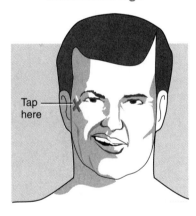

Tap here

🏠 **TAKE HOME POINTS**

- Demerol is the drug of choice for managing the pain in pancreatitis.
- It may be necessary to replace the pancreatic enzymes to promote the GI digestion process in patients with pancreatitis.

Vigorous IV replacement of electrolytes and proteins helps maintain circulatory volume and provides emergency treatment for shock. During IV rehydration, the nurse should pay close attention to BP and cardiac and pulmonary status. Nurses should monitor and report abnormalities in patient's electrolyte profiles, including signs of tetany (a positive Trousseau's sign, carpopedal spasm, Chvostek's sign, and paresthesias of fingers and around the oral cavity). IV calcium gluconate should be readily available for the patient who experiences tetany.

Pain management is achieved by administering Demerol (meperidine), rather than morphine, because morphine may cause spasm of the sphincter of Oddi, which increases bile obstruction. The nurse should monitor for signs of analeptic activity (central nervous system [CNS] stimulation) caused by the metabolite of meperidine, normeperidine, with prolonged use of Demerol. The nurse should assess pain levels before and after the administration of analgesics.

To decrease vagal stimulation, pancreatic secretion, and ampullary spasm, anticholinergics, such as atropine and propantheline (Propanthel), may be prescribed. Cimetidine (Tagamet) and aluminum-magnesium may also be ordered to decrease hydrochloric acid production and further decrease pancreatic secretions. Acinar cell activity can be inhibited by administering octreotide acetate to suppress GI hormones that stimulate pancreatic secretions. In cases of pancreatic insufficiency, pancrelipase may be prescribed to replace enzymes.

NG suction is an option for the patient with consistent vomiting, gastric distention, or ileus. Suctioning also reduces stimulation of pancreatic secretions by decreasing the contents that enter the small intestines. Nursing care should include the use of water-soluble lubricant around the nares to prevent irritation. Good oral hygiene should promote clean mucous membranes and decrease irritation of the oropharynx and dryness. The patient should discontinue oral intake until symptoms subside. For those patients who do not recover quickly, or who may have a complicated clinical course, total parenteral nutrition (TPN) therapy may be initiated to support nutritional status. Careful monitoring of laboratory studies will help prevent potential complications of hyperglycemia and hypoglycemia. Hyperglycemia will require an increase in IV insulin administration. In contrast, an IV bolus of dextrose 50% will reverse hypoglycemia if the solution contains excessive amounts of insulin.

Surgical intervention is usually a risky option because of the acutely ill presentation of the patient. A diagnostic laparotomy may be performed to débride a necrotic pancreas. Postoperative care includes management of several sump tubes that are placed to provide irrigation, air venting, and drainage. In severe cases the surgical incision may remain open and require irrigation and repacking every 2 to 3 days to remove necrotic tissue. A cholecystectomy should be performed if gallstones or gallbladder disease (GBD) are causative factors.

Patients who survive an episode of pancreatitis will be weak and debilitated for weeks or months after hospitalization. Because patients may not recall instructions during the acute phase, a home care referral would be appropriate so that the nurse can continue patient and family education. Written and verbal instructions should be included with dietary information, including the need to avoid high-fat foods, heavy meals, and alcohol. Information regarding resources and support groups are made available to the patient who is suspected to return to previous alcoholic habits.

Nursing goals for the patient experiencing pancreatitis include pain relief, decreasing pancreatic stimulation, relieving discomfort associated with NG drainage, improved nutritional status, maintenance of respiratory function, improvement of fluid and electrolyte status, and prevention of shock.

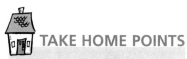

TAKE HOME POINTS

Foods to avoid include high fat, and drinks to avoid include alcohol in patients with pancreatitis.

Do You UNDERSTAND?

DIRECTIONS: Complete the crossword puzzle on page 226 using the clues listed below.

Down

1. Endocrine cells that produce insulin, glucagon, and VIP are found in the islets of _____.
3. This drug may be prescribed to replace enzymes that are suppressed in cases of pancreatic insufficiency.
5. This takes place when pancreatic enzymes become prematurely activated while still inside the pancreas.
6. Pancreatic fluids enter the bowel from the head of the pancreas via the _____ _____ (two words).
11. The trade name of the drug of choice for pain control.

Across

2. Signs and symptoms of the severely ill patient that may include low BP, increased heart rate (HR), cold extremities, and changes in mental status.
3. The main symptom in pancreatitis.
4. The abbreviation for therapy that supports nutritional status.
7. Pancreatic cells that produce exocrine secretions.
8. Describes the bulky, fatty, foul-smelling stool caused by the lack of enzymes needed to digest proteins, carbohydrates, and fats.
9. An anticholinergic used to decrease vagal stimulation, pancreatic secretion, and ampullary spasm.
10. Pancreatic _____ is caused by the malabsorption of nutrients in the small intestine.
12. Bleeding into the abdomen, caused by the death of pancreatic tissue, characterizes this type of pancreatitis.
13. A severe complication of pancreatitis that can appear weeks after the illness begins.
14. A common cause of death in acute pancreatitis.

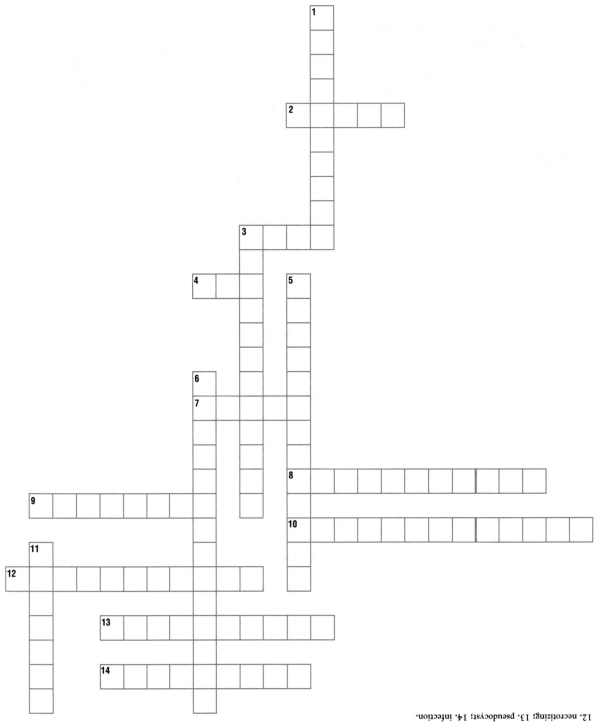

What IS Liver Failure?

Liver failure, also known as *hepatic failure*, is a condition in which the organ fails to fulfill its functions or is unable to meet the demands placed upon it. Acute diseases that cause sudden, massive hepatic destruction or chronic diseases that progressively cause hepatic damage can result in liver failure. Viral hepatitis, cirrhosis, benign or malignant neoplasms, biliary atresia, and primary or secondary cholangitis are examples of diseases that can lead to liver failure if their progression is not slowed or reversed. Liver failure can also be caused by the ingestion of toxic substances such as chemicals or overdoses of medications. Liver disease and subsequent liver failure can occur at any age from the neonate to the geriatric patient.

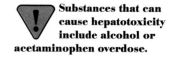

Substances that can cause hepatotoxicity include alcohol or acetaminophen overdose.

What You NEED TO KNOW

The first step in caring for a patient with liver disease is to understand the liver's functions. This foundational knowledge can assist the nurse with understanding why clinical signs and symptoms occur and the rationale for treatment.

The liver is the largest solid organ in the body. The organ is located primarily in the right upper quadrant of the abdomen. A portion of the liver's left lobe extends into the left upper abdominal quadrant. The liver functions as a digestive, endocrine, hematologic, and excretory organ. The liver carries out more than four hundred (400) functions. Primary functions of the liver include storage and filtration of blood; bile production and metabolism; bilirubin elimination; carbohydrate, fat, and protein metabolism; storage of glycogen and fat; conversion of ammonia to urea; production of clotting factors and removal of activated clotting factors; metabolism of sex hormones; inactivation of aldosterone and antidiuretic hormones (ADHs); detoxification of drugs and foreign substances; and vitamin and mineral storage. The architecture of the liver is composed of five parts: (1) the circulatory system, (2) the lobule and hepatocytes, (3) the reticuloendothelial system (RES), (4) the hepatobiliary system, and (5) the connective tissue structure.

The liver has a dual blood supply. Both the hepatic artery and portal vein supply the liver. Arterial flow enters the hepatic artery via the celiac trunk of the aorta. The portal vein carries blood, enriched with nutrients and metabolic products, from capillaries in the stomach, small and large intestines, pancreas, and spleen to the liver. Blood is removed from the liver via the hepatic veins. The hepatic veins empty into the inferior vena cava. The liver is a highly vascular organ and contains about 25% of the body's total CO. Normal blood flow through the liver approximates 1500 ml/min.

The work of the liver is accomplished in the functional unit, the *lobule*. The lobule is composed of hepatocytes, arterioles and venules, sinusoids, Kupffer's cells, and bile canniculi. The liver's dual blood supply comes together in the sinusoid. Here the oxygenated arterial blood and the metabolic enriched venous blood are processed by the hepatocytes and the many functions of the liver are carried out. Kupffer's cells, which are a part of the reticuloendothelial system, line the walls of the sinusoids. The function of the Kupffer's cells is to phagocy-tize bacteria, foreign materials, and toxins. The bile canniculi are responsible for the transport of bile salts and pigments through the liver lobule to the gallblad-der where the substances are stored.

The second step in caring for a patient with liver disease is to understand the diseases, both acute and chronic, that can lead to liver failure. Hepatitis is an inflammation of the liver cells caused by a viral or bacterial infection or toxic substances. If the inflammatory process is not reversed, liver cells are damaged and die. Hepatitis can be an acute or chronic disease. Chronic hepatitis is an inflammation of the liver that lasts 6 months or longer. The mode of transmis-sion, symptoms, and treatment differ among the types of hepatitis.

Biliary diseases that can lead to liver failure include biliary atresia and scle-rosing cholangitis. Biliary atresia is a pediatric disorder characterized by the con-genital absence or underdevelopment of one or more of the biliary structures. As the condition progresses, jaundice, portal hypertension, biliary cirrhosis, and liver failure can result. Surgery is the recommended treatment for atresia. Sclerosing cholangitis is an inflammation of the bile ducts. The inflammation is brought about by a bacterial infection or an obstruction of the bile ducts from tumor or stones. If allowed to go untreated, the problem can lead to liver failure. Sclerosing cholangitis is treated with antibiotics and surgical intervention for obstruction.

Cirrhosis is a chronic, progressive, irreversible disease. The progression of cir-rhosis can be slowed by treatment of the causative factors. Four classifications of cirrhosis exist that are based on the various causative agents. The classifications are alcoholic (Laennec's), biliary, cardiac, and postnecrotic. A chronic inflam-matory process causes disruption in the liver's blood and biliary flow, which results in hepatocyte damage and the formation of fibrotic tissue. The normal liver architecture is replaced with fibrotic, nodular scar tissue. The fibrosis and cellular damage of cirrhosis can lead to subsequent liver failure.

Other diseases that can lead to liver failure include Budd-Chiari syndrome, Crigler-Najjar syndrome, and cystic fibrosis. Budd-Chiari syndrome is character-ized by obstruction of the hepatic vein, preventing outflow of blood from the liver. Cystic fibrosis is a genetic disease that can result in pancreatic fibrosis, bil-iary obstruction, hepatitis, and cirrhosis, all of which can lead to liver failure. Crigler-Najjar syndrome is a genetic disease characterized by severe unconjugat-ed hyperbilirubinemia in the neonate that can lead to severe neurologic conse-quences and liver failure if not treated.

FIRST-LINE AND INITIAL TREATMENTS FOR LIVER DISEASE

- Understand the liver's functions.
- Understand the underlying diseases.
- Understand the clinical manifestations.

The third step in providing care for the liver failure patient is to understand the clinical manifestations of the liver failure. Initial symptoms of liver failure are vague. Initial symptoms include malaise, weakness, fatigue, exhaustion, loss of appetite, weight loss, abdominal discomfort, nausea, and vomiting. Progression of the disease brings about more severe, specific symptoms with systemic effects. These symptoms include jaundice, coagulopathies, fluid and electrolyte imbalances, nutritional deficiencies, portal hypertension, varices, ascites, hepatic encephalopathy, infections, and hepatorenal syndrome.

The pathway for the development of jaundice is a complex one. It begins when old or damaged RBCs are broken down by the reticuloendothelial system. Bilirubin is a product of hemoglobin breakdown. Bilirubin is released into the circulation and binds to albumin. In this form, bilirubin is called *unconjugated bilirubin*. Unconjugated bilirubin enters the liver via the general circulation. In the liver, bilirubin undergoes a process called *conjugation*. Conjugation changes bilirubin from a lipid-soluble product to a water-soluble product. In this form, bilirubin can be excreted. The liver then excretes conjugated bilirubin through the bile ducts. Bilirubin is moved through the biliary system as a component of bile to the small intestine, where enzymes act upon it and urobilinogen is formed. A large portion of urobilinogen is excreted in the feces. A smaller portion is reabsorbed into the circulation. Liver failure results in high levels of bilirubin in the general circulation. Jaundice occurs because of increased bilirubin levels deposited from the circulation into the tissues.

Acute renal failure can occur in association with liver failure. A decrease in renal blood flow and GFR and increased levels of aldosterone are thought to be the underlying causes. Hepatorenal syndrome is characterized by progressive azotemia, elevated serum creatinine levels, and oliguria. Treatment includes the administration of fluids and diuretics to improve renal blood flow, GFR, and urine output. Hemodialysis may be needed to support the kidneys while the underlying cause of the liver failure is treated.

Ascites is the accumulation of fluid within the peritoneal cavity. It is complicated by portal hypertension, hypoalbuminemia, and the inactivation of the hormones aldosterone and ADH. With liver failure, aldosterone and ADH are inactivated. The inactivation of aldosterone signals the kidneys, via the renin-angiotensin system, to hold on to sodium and water and excrete potassium. The inactivation of ADH results in additional fluid retention. The excess volume in the vascular space results in a hyperdynamic state. The excess volume cannot be maintained in the interstitial space because of the kidneys' inability to metabolize proteins. Albumin is responsible for maintaining colloid osmotic pressure in the vascular system. In the absence of albumin, fluids from the vascular system cross over into the interstitial space. The result is edema and ascites. With the

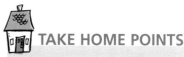

TAKE HOME POINTS

Signs and symptoms of liver failure are seen when the liver's functions cannot be carried out or are impaired.

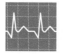

Bilirubin stains the tissues and causes a yellowish discoloration of the skin, mucous membranes, and sclera. Excess bilirubin in the general circulation is also filtered out by the kidneys and results in brownish, yellow-colored urine.

TAKE HOME POINTS

Hepatorenal syndrome is renal failure that occurs in conjunction with liver failure.

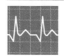

Monitoring of renal function via diagnostic tests and urine output is needed for persons in liver failure.

loss of fluid from the vascular space, the kidneys sense a decreased blood volume and through the renin-angiotensin system signal the release of aldosterone. A problematic cycle is established through fluid retention in the vascular space (inactivation of aldosterone and ADH), loss of fluid into the interstitial space (inability of liver to metabolize protein resulting in hypoalbuminemia), fluid collection in the interstitial space (edema and ascites), and the body's own homeostatic mechanisms (renin-angiotensin system), which senses the loss of fluid from the vascular space and signals the kidneys to hold on to more sodium and water. Significant accumulation of ascitic fluids in the peritoneal cavity can cause abdominal organ compression and discomfort, respiratory compromise because of pressure on the diaphragm, and impaired skin integrity. The treatment of ascites involves the restriction of sodium, bed rest, and pharmacological therapy with diuretics. Abdominal paracentesis is another treatment modality.

Paracentesis is accomplished by the insertion of a needle into the peritoneal cavity. Peritoneal (ascitic) fluid is then withdrawn. Abdominal paracentesis is used for the analysis of ascitic fluids and as a temporary relief measure for worsening or severe symptoms. LeVeen and Denver shunts have also been used for the treatment of ascites that has been refractory to medical management. The shunts use a pressure gradient or pump pressure to move ascitic fluid from the peritoneum into the general circulation. The excess fluid is then excreted via the kidneys.

Leveen shunt

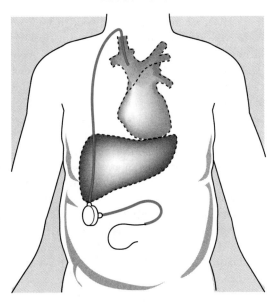

Portal hypertension is a result of impaired blood flow caused by tissue damage and fibrosis. Increased pressure within the portal circulation; impaired blood flow to the liver; and slowed, congested circulation from the portal vein are the results. Splenomegaly can be a consequence of the increased pressure.

Esophageal, anterior stomach veins, and rectal veins are also affected. The veins become engorged, distended, and susceptible to hemorrhage as result of the increased pressure within the portal circulation. The distended veins are known as *varices*. Distended esophageal veins result in esophageal varices, whereas distended rectal veins produce hemorrhoids. Rupture of the friable veins can result in life-threatening GI hemorrhage. Treatment of varices focuses on the reduction of portal pressures through the use of pharmacological therapy, endoscopic procedures, and balloon tamponade.

If the treatment modalities do not effectively manage the esophageal varices, then radiographic or surgical intervention is considered. The radiographic procedure involves the placement of a stent that creates a portosystemic shunt. Surgical techniques to reduce portal hypertension include the placement of portacaval, mesocaval, or splenorenal shunts. The shunts divert blood flow and result in a reduction of portal pressures.

Hepatic *encephalopathy* is a term used for the CNS manifestations of liver failure. A range of symptoms from confusion to coma is seen. The cause of encephalopathy is not known. The cause is thought to be the inability of the liver to convert ammonia to urea. Protein is broken down in the GI tract. Ammonia is a product of protein metabolism. Ammonia ions diffuse from the GI tract into the circulation and are transported to the liver for conversion to urea. When the liver cells are unable to perform the conversion, ammonia levels build up. Elevated ammonia levels in the circulation have a neurotoxic effect on the CNS. The clinical signs of hepatic encephalopathy are defined in four, progressively worsening stages.

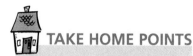

TAKE HOME POINTS

All treatment modalities for varices are not without side effects and potential complications that can worsen or complicate the liver failure condition.

Stages of Hepatic Encephalopathy

STAGE	SYMPTOMS
Stage I	Tremors
	Slurred speech
	Impaired decision making
Stage II	Drowsiness
	Loss of sphincter control
	Asterixis
Stage III	Dramatic confusion
	Somnolence
Stage IV	Coma
	Unresponsiveness

Asterixis

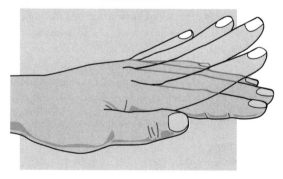

Treatment of hepatic encephalopathy involves the reduction of ammonia levels. This is accomplished by dietary and pharmacological means. Protein intake is reduced to 20 to 40 grams per day. Pharmacological agents, neomycin and lactulose, are used to reduce the breakdown of protein by bacteria. Neomycin reduces the normal bowel flora. Lactulose creates an acidic environment in the bowel that prevents ammonia from leaving the colon and entering the bloodstream. Lactulose also exhibits a laxative effect and eliminates ammonia from the GI tract.

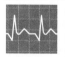
Asterixis is a hand-flapping tremor induced by extending the arm and dorsiflexing the wrist.

Carbohydrate, fat, and protein metabolism are affected by liver failure. When the blood glucose level exceeds the body's needs, excess glucose is converted to glycogen and stored in the liver. This is a process called *glycogenesis*. When the body needs glucose, glycogen is released from storage and used for energy. This is called *glycogenolysis*. If glycogen levels are used up, then the liver uses amino acids and fats for energy via a process called *gluconeogenesis*. In liver failure the organ is unable to effectively convert glucose to glycogen and use fats for gluconeogenesis; thus the body has no means for creating energy stores, and problems associated with meeting cellular energy needs develop. The clinical result is hypoglycemia, fatigue, weight loss, and malnutrition. The liver also metabolizes fats. The end results of fat digestion are fatty acids, glycerol, and cholesterol. In the liver the metabolic substances are converted to the lipoproteins (LDL, HDL, and VLDL). When the process is interrupted, as with liver failure, fat accumulates in the liver. The condition is known as *fatty liver*. The fat accumulation impairs the liver's ability to carry out its functions. The liver produces three major plasma proteins: (1) albumin, (2) globulin, and (3) fibrinogen. Albumin is responsible for maintaining plasma oncotic pressure. Oncotic pressure helps to hold fluids in the vascular space and prevent them from leaking out into the interstitial space, causing edema. Globulins promote cellular enzyme reactions, and fibrinogen plays an important role in coagulation and the establishment of hemostasis. Additional protein clotting factors II, V, VII, VIII, IX, and X are not synthesized by the failing liver. Liver failure patients who are unable to metabolize fibrinogen and synthesize clotting factors will have a range of symptoms from petechiae, ecchymosis, bleeding from oral mucous, and nosebleeds to massive hemorrhage. Disseminated intravascular coagulation (DIC) is also a complication that may result from the inability of the liver to metabolize fibrinogen and other clotting factors. In the presence of liver failure, the lack of plasma protein production and metabolism can lead to edema, loss of certain cellular enzyme reactions, and coagulopathies.

Another problem with protein metabolism is the failed liver's inability to convert ammonia, an end product of protein metabolism, into urea. Ammonia levels increase and result in subsequent effects on the nervous system and skin. The effects are discussed in depth in the section on hepatic encephalopathy. A sign of abnormal protein metabolism is fector hepaticus, which is characterized as a very sweet, acetone-like breath.

The liver also metabolizes and is a storage bank for vitamins A, B, D, K, and E. Vitamin K is necessary for the synthesis of clotting factors II, VII, VIII and X. Vitamin deficiencies and subsequent nutritional problems result from liver failure.

The liver plays a role in protecting the rest of the body from bacterial invasion, toxic substances, and poisons. Enzymes found in the liver metabolize a high percentage of drugs. Liver failure slows or stops the ability to filter medications from the blood and results in a prolonged duration of action or a potentiated action. Kupffer's cells filter out bacteria. The loss of Kupffer's cell function can result in infection and sepsis.

The liver's inability to metabolize hormones can result in dermatologic lesions and changes in sexual characteristics or function. Dermatologic lesions such as vascular nevi (spiders), telangiectasias, and spider angiomas can be seen on the upper part of the body. Changes in male sexual characteristics such as testicular

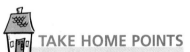

Liver failure patients may exhibit problems with clotting abnormalities because the liver produces clotting factors.

TAKE HOME POINTS

- Bile is a necessary component of fat digestion and absorption. The liver is responsible for bile synthesis. When the liver is unable to synthesize bile, fats are excreted and unable to be used as an energy source.
- The skin becomes itchy because of ammonia irritation of the skin cells.

atrophy, gynecomastia, and decreased pubic or facial hair are seen. Sexual dysfunction in the form of impotence can also occur.

The liver is a highly vascular organ and, as previously mentioned, the inactivation of aldosterone and ADH results in a hyperdynamic state because of an increased intravascular volume. Palmar erythema, redness of the palms of the hands, may be seen in association with a high CO and the hyperdynamic state. It is also thought to be associated with increased levels of circulating estrogens.

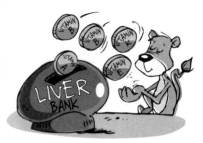

Diagnostic Tests

A number of diagnostic tests are used to determine the cause of liver disease, the range of complications, and the extent of organ damage. In liver failure the liver enzymes, alkaline phosphatase, aspartate transaminase, and alanine transaminase, are elevated. Serum protein levels such as albumin are decreased. Clotting factors including prothrombin time (PT) and partial thromboplastin time (PTT) are elevated and prolonged. Serum ammonia, total bilirubin, and conjugated and unconjugated bilirubin levels are elevated. Urine bilirubin and urobilinogen elevations will also occur. Electrolytes are monitored for alterations in blood sugar, sodium, and potassium. The CBC is assessed for anemia and infection. ABGs are obtained to assess the patient's acid-base status and for potential ventilatory problems. Stools and gastric samples should be assessed for the presence of blood (guaiac positive). Liver biopsy, ultrasound, CT scans, and MRI may be prescribed to determine the underlying cause of liver failure. A combination of history, clinical signs and symptoms, and diagnostic tools will assist the medical team in the diagnosis of liver disease and whether or not the disease has progressed to the point of organ failure.

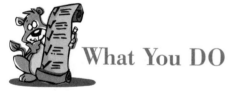

What You DO

The treatment of liver failure centers on the identification of the cause of liver disease, interventions to correct the cause or slow progression, and the provision of supportive therapy. Supportive therapy includes the correction of fluid and electrolyte abnormalities, nutritional support, elimination of hepatotoxins, and prevention and treatment of complications.

Patients diagnosed with end-stage liver disease have few treatment options for cure. Transplantation is one possible option. Transplant criteria include the presence of an acute or chronic liver disease for which all forms of therapy have failed. Potential transplant candidates must undergo physiologic and psychologic evaluation to determine whether or not transplant is a viable treatment option. Survival rates are 85% at the end of 1 year and 70% at 5 years. Limitations of this treatment modality are the shortage of organs.

Clinical trials are in process to determine if extracorporeal liver assist devices can maintain a patient while the underlying cause of liver failure is treated, or whether the device can be used as a bridge to support the patient until a donor organ can be found.

The care of a patient with liver failure presents a clinical challenge for the nurse because of the complexity of liver functions and the systemic ramifications of liver failure. The nurse's role in the care of a patient with liver failure includes patient assessment, monitoring, documentation, reporting of patient responses to diagnostic and treatment plans, observation for complications, supportive care, and patient and family teaching. Consistent systems assessments; monitoring of vital signs, intake, and output; measurement of hemodynamic parameters; and documentation of findings to identify complications or a worsening condition are the foundations of care. Laboratory values are obtained, assessed, and monitored. Nutritional assessment and support is necessary. Dermatologic assessment should include observing for bruising, petechiae, itching, spider angiomas, edema, and pressure ulcer formations. Pressure reduction measures should be prophylactically established. For patients with ascites, the head of the bed should be elevated to reduce fluid pressure exerted on the diaphragm and to promote lung expansion. The patient should be assessed for any signs and symptoms of the development of pleural effusions and monitored for signs of inadequate hemostasis. Testing of stool and gastric contents by guaiac should occur. Bleeding precautions should be implemented because of the coagulopathies associated with liver failure. Neurologic assessments are needed to identify hepatic encephalopathy and whether the condition had progressed. Medications that are metabolized by the liver should be minimized. If these medications cannot be eliminated and are necessary for the patient, then the multidisciplinary team should be consulted for dose review and adjustment. Discussion with the patient, family, or both on the treatment plan and options for treatment is required. The establishment of advanced directives should be accomplished and possible end-of-life decisions discussed.

Do You UNDERSTAND?

DIRECTIONS: **Match the descriptions in Column A with appropriate symptoms of liver failure in Column B.**

Column A

_____ 1. Progressive azotemia, elevated serum creatinine levels, and oliguria

_____ 2. A yellowish discoloration of the skin, mucous membranes, and sclera

_____ 3. Fluid accumulated within the peritoneal cavity

_____ 4. Engorged, distended veins caused by increased pressure within the portal circulation

_____ 5. Coma caused by inability of liver to convert ammonia to urea

Column B

a. Hepatorenal syndrome

b. Ascites

c. Jaundice

d. Varices

e. Hepatic encephalopathy

Answers: 1. a; 2. c; 3. b; 4. d; 5. e.

DIRECTIONS: **Identify the following statements as *true* (T) or *false* (F).**

_____ 6. Cirrhosis is a reversible disease process.

_____ 7. Stage IV of hepatic encephalopathy is characterized by coma and unresponsiveness.

_____ 8. The functional unit of the liver is the hepatocyte.

_____ 9. Alcohol and acetaminophen are substances that can cause hepatotoxicity.

_____ 10. In a patient with hepatic encephalopathy, the nurse would expect to find an elevated serum ammonia level.

_____ 11. Liver transplant survival rates are 50% or less at the end of 1 year.

8 Renal System

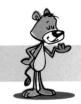

What IS Acute Tubular Necrosis?

The term *acute tubular necrosis* (ATN) is frequently used to identify common renal injuries that are results of nephrotoxic and ischemic renal injuries. *ATN* is one term to describe acute renal failure (ARF). Two types of pathologic changes occur in ATN: (1) necrosis of the tubular epithelium leaving the basement membrane intact after an acute ischemic or toxic event, and (2) necrosis of both the tubular epithelium and basement membrane that is associated with tubular ischemia. The cause of ATN is variable because of the types of insults that lead to tubular necrosis, and the prognosis varies. The classification of ARF may be specified by the cause of the ATN, which may be prerenal (before the kidney), intrarenal (inside the kidney), and postrenal (after the kidney). Another way to classify ATN is by identifying what the result of the cause was, such as ischemic or nephrotoxic ATN.

TAKE HOME POINTS

ATN is a type of ARF that follows a sequence of events.

What You NEED TO KNOW

ATN usually occurs after an acute ischemic or toxic event such as untreated prerenal failure (hypoperfusion), nephrotoxic medications (aminoglycosides), and contrast agents, and it has a well-defined sequence of events. The onset of this phase is characterized by an acute decrease in glomerular filtration rate (GFR), the amount of blood that circulates through the kidneys, and is the key component of urine production. Normal GFR for the average adult is 125 ml/min. In ATN, the GFR drops to very low levels that leads to a decline in urine production below

400 ml in 24 hours. Sudden increases in serum creatinine and blood urea nitrogen (BUN) concentrations occur during this phase. Creatinine and BUN are by-products of protein breakdown and become nitrogenous waste, which is retained in the body; this is referred to as *azotemia*. This phase is followed by the maintenance phase, which is characterized by continued reduction in GFR; it continues for approximately 1 to 2 weeks but can be variable. The BUN and creatinine continue to rise as a result of the sustained decrease GFR; however there may be a slight production in urinary output. The recovery phase is the final phase (in which tubular function and GFR is restored) and is characterized by an increase in urine volume and gradual decrease in BUN and serum creatinine to their preinjury levels. The following table summarizes the GFR, BUN, and creatinine levels occurring in each phase.

Summary of the Stages of Acute Tubular Necrosis

INITIAL PHASE	MAINTENANCE PHASE	RECOVERY PHASE
• Acute ischemic toxic effect • Acute decreased GFR • Urine production <400 ml per 24 hours • Increased BUN and creatinine	• GFR continues to decrease • Increased BUN and creatinine continues • Increased urine production	• Tubular function and GFR are restored • Increased urine production • Gradual decrease in BUN and creatinine

Ischemic Acute Tubular Necrosis

Ischemic ATN may be considered part of the spectrum of prerenal azotemia and risk factors. Specifically, these risk factors include the following:
- Hypovolemic states—hemorrhage, volume depletion from GI or renal losses, burns, fluid sequestration
- Low cardiac output states—congestive heart failure (CHF) and other diseases of myocardium, valvulopathy, arrhythmia, pericardial diseases, or tamponade
- Systemic vasodilatation—sepsis, anaphylaxis
- Disseminated intravascular coagulation (DIC)
- Renal vasoconstriction—cyclosporine, amphotericin B, norepinephrine, epinephrine, hypercalcemia

Nephrotoxic Acute Tubular Necrosis

The kidney has a rich blood supply, receiving 25% of cardiac output, which makes it easily assessable to toxins. This is a necessary function of the kidney to excrete these toxins. These toxins may be exogenous or endogenous nephrotoxins.

Exogenous Nephrotoxins

ATN occurs in 10% to 30% of patients receiving aminoglycosides, even when blood levels are in apparently therapeutic ranges. Risk factors for the development of aminoglycoside-induced ATN include preexisting liver disease, preexisting renal disease, concomitant use of other nephrotoxins (e.g., amphotericin B,

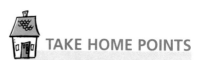

TAKE HOME POINTS

Any event or disease process that contributes to a decrease in renal blood flow can result in ischemic ATN.

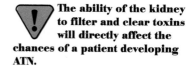

The ability of the kidney to filter and clear toxins will directly affect the chances of a patient developing ATN.

The older one is, the greater chance one has of ATN developing when receiving aminoglycosides.

radiocontrast media, cisplatin), advanced age, shock, female sex, and a higher aminoglycoside level 1 hour after dose. A high trough level has not been shown to be an independent risk factor.

Aminoglycosides preferentially affect the proximal tubular cells. These agents are freely filtered and quickly taken up by the proximal tubular epithelial cells, where they are incorporated into lysosomes after first interacting with phospholipids on the brush border membranes. They exert their main toxic effect within the tubular cell by altering phospholipid metabolism. In addition to their direct effect on cells, aminoglycosides cause renal vasoconstriction. Aminoglycoside uptake by the tubules is a saturable phenomenon, so uptake is limited after a single dose. Not surprisingly, a single daily large dose is preferable to three doses per day. One dose per day presumably causes less accumulation in tubular cells once the saturation point is reached. In fact, clinical nephrotoxicity develops much more commonly with three doses per day than with one dose per day; 24% of patients receiving three daily doses developed clinical nephrotoxicity, compared with only 5% of the one daily dose group in one study. However, other studies comparing a single daily dose to multiple daily doses have failed to find a difference in the incidence of nephrotoxicity.

Amphotericin B: The likelihood of nephrotoxicity from amphotericin B increases in direct proportion to the total dose administered. Nephrotoxicity is more likely to occur if greater than 3 grams total is administered.

Contrast-induced nephrotoxicity has become a frequent occurrence because of the demand for diagnostic tests that require these substances in susceptible patients. Iodinated contrast media causes vasoconstriction and also has a direct toxic effect on tubular cells. Certain patients are at an increased risk of developing contrast-induced nephropathy. Diabetes mellitus and baseline renal insufficiency are particularly important risk factors. Others include history of hypertension, large contrast load, older age, and presence of proteinuria.

The prevention of contrast nephrotoxicity has received attention. In susceptible patients, the use of nonionic contrast media reduces the likelihood of clinical nephrotoxicity. In all patients, saline infusion (e.g., 1 L of half-isotonic sodium chloride solution) before and during the study, and discontinuation of diuretic therapy, effectively minimizes nephrotoxicity. Studies have also suggested that pretreatment with oral N-acetylcysteine, which acts as an antioxidant, reduces the nephrotoxicity of contrast media.

- **Cyclosporine and tacrolimus:** These drugs induce renal vasoconstriction and can cause ARF and chronic interstitial nephritis.
- **Sulfa, acyclovir, and indinavir:** These drugs cause ARF by tubular obstruction as a result of crystal formation in the tubular urine.
- **Others:** Cisplatin, methotrexate, and foscarnet are other causes of drug-induced tubular toxicity.

Endogenous Nephrotoxins

The breakdown of muscle (i.e., rhabdomyolysis), leading to myoglobinuria, occurs in many clinical settings, including exercise, crush injuries, alcoholism, viral illnesses, as well as with the use of certain medications, cocaine, and in

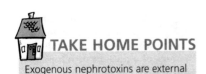

TAKE HOME POINTS

Exogenous nephrotoxins are external substances taken in by the patient.

patients who have seizures. In a small number of patients with myoglobinuria, ATN develops.

Risk factors for development of ATN in the setting of rhabdomyolysis include extracellular fluid (ECF) volume depletion, liver dysfunction, seizures, and hypotension.

- **Hemoglobinuria:** ARF is a rare complication of hemolysis and hemoglobinuria. Most often it is associated with transfusion reactions. In contrast to myoglobin, hemoglobin has no apparent direct tubular toxicity, and the ARF in this setting is probably related to hypotension and decreased renal perfusion.
- **Crystals:** Acute crystal-induced nephropathy is encountered in conditions where the crystals are generated endogenously because of high cellular turnover (i.e., uric acid, calcium phosphate), as observed in certain malignancies or the treatment of malignancies. However, this condition is also associated with ingestion of certain toxic substances, such as ethylene glycol, or nontoxic substances such as vitamin C.
- **Multiple myeloma:** Multiple myeloma causes renal failure by several mechanisms: prerenal azotemia because of volume contraction, cast nephropathy because of increased light chain proteins precipitated into the tubular lumen, hypercalcemia, uric acid nephropathy, and drug-induced interstitial nephritis.

Diagnostics

Acute Tubular Necrosis Laboratory Values

LABORATORY STUDY	CHARACTERISTICS
Serum chemistries	• BUN increased • Creatinine increased • Hyponatremia • Hyperkalemia • Hypermagnesemia • Hypocalcemia • Hyperphosphatemia • Metabolic acidosis
CBC	• Anemia
Urinalysis	• Sediment: pigmented, muddy brown granular casts • Urine electrolytes

BUN, Blood urea nitrogen; *CBC,* complete blood count.

Imaging Studies

- An abdominal radiograph is of limited benefit in ARF, with the exception of diagnosing (or helping to exclude) nephrolithiasis.
- Ultrasound, computed tomography (CT) scan, and magnetic resonance imaging (MRI) are extremely useful, both to exclude obstructive uropathy and to measure renal size and cortical thickness. Renal ultrasound is a simple procedure that should be undertaken in all patients with ARF.

TAKE HOME POINTS

The exact mechanism of renal failure is not clearly understood, but several theories include direct toxic injury, development of DIC, mechanical tubular obstruction by the pigment, and intrarenal ischemia from vasomediator release.

TAKE HOME POINTS

Endogenous nephrotoxins are internally occurring substances.

TAKE HOME POINTS

- Hypercalcemia and hyperuricemia may suggest a malignant condition as a cause of ATN.
- Erythroprotein production is not only decreased in ARF but bleeding is also made more likely because of dysfunctional platelets (from uremia).
- Casts in the urine may be absent in 20% to 30% of patients with ATN.
- Urine electrolytes may help differentiate ATN from prerenal azotemia.

Procedures

Biopsy is rarely necessary and only performed when the exact renal cause of ARF is unclear and the course is protracted. Prerenal and postrenal causes must be ruled out first. The diagnosis of ATN is made on a clinical basis with the help of detailed and accurate history, thorough physical examination, and pertinent laboratory examinations and imaging studies. A more urgent indication for renal biopsy is in the setting of clinical and urinary findings that suggest renal vasculitis rather than ATN; this diagnosis needs to be established quickly so that appropriate immunomodulatory therapy can be initiated. The biopsy is performed under ultrasound or CT scan guidance after ascertaining the safety of the procedure. A biopsy may also be more critically important in the renal transplant patient to rule out rejection.

Prognosis

As mentioned earlier, the mortality rate of ATN is about 50%. However, this is probably related more to the severity of the underlying disease than to ATN itself. For example, the mortality rate in patients with ATN after sepsis or severe trauma is much higher (about 60%) than the mortality rate in patients with ATN that is nephrotoxin related (about 30%). However, the nurse should remember the following points:

- Patients with oliguric ATN have a worse prognosis than patients with non-oliguric ATN. This is probably related to more severe necrosis and more significant disturbances in electrolyte balance.
- A rapid increase in serum creatinine (i.e., >3 mg/dl) probably indicates a poorer prognosis. Again, this probably reflects more serious underlying disease.
- Of the survivors of ATN, approximately 50% have some impairment of renal function. About 5% continue to undergo a decline in renal function, and another 5% never recover kidney function and require dialysis.

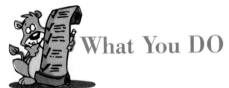 **What You DO**

Nursing Care

- Assessment (history): When obtaining a patient's history, the nurse should look for disorders that can lead to ischemic or nephrotoxic ATN. The patient should be asked about any recent illnesses, past illnesses, medications, and over-the-counter (OTC) medications. The nurse should determine the patient's urinary status and document any urgency, hesitancy, urine stream force, and volume of urine. The patient should be asked if he or she is experiencing any signs and symptoms of a urinary tract infection (UTI). The nurse should have the patient explain his or her fluid intake during a typical 24-hour period and evaluate the patient's weight status, focusing on any recent weight gain that would support fluid retention.
- Assessment (physical examination): The nurse should obtain data that will support fluid volume excess such as hypertension, tachycardia, peripheral

edema, and basilar crackles. If patients are in the diuretic phase, they may appear dehydrated, with dry mucus membranes, poor skin turgor, negative jugular vein distention (JVD), and orthostatic hypotension. Patients can be very drowsy, confused, irritable, and even combative as a result of the accumulation of metabolic waste products.

- During a psychologic assessment, patients tend to be very anxious because of the unknown outcome. The nurse should keep an open communication pattern with the patient and significant others and reinforce the good prognosis without giving false hope.

Recognizing the clinical signs and symptoms of ATN can mean the difference between life and death of the patient. Identifying these important signs will have the largest impact on the patient's prognosis. The nurse should assess for a drop in urine production accompanied with pruritus, poor skin turgor, anorexia, nausea, vomiting, weight loss (because of decreased food intake or increased catabolism) or weight gain (because of edema or ascites), and complaints of generalized weakness and fatigue. Confusion and lethargy should alert the nurse to possible renal failure in high-risk patients.

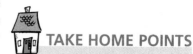

TAKE HOME POINTS

Usually patients who experience ATN are previously healthy and may have developed renal failure as a result of an iatrogenic problem.

FIRST-LINE AND INITIAL TREATMENTS FOR ACUTE TUBULAR NECROSIS

- Assess and recognize the signs of ATN.
- Assess fluid volume.
- Weigh patient each day.
- Monitor urine output.
- Restrict fluids.
- Restrict intake of sodium, phosphorous, potassium, magnesium, and protein.
- Monitor serum electrolyte lab values.
- Administer ordered medications.

- Conduct and document a complete fluid volume excess assessment, which should include auscultation for basilar crackles, jugular distention, tachycardia, increased blood pressure (BP), peripheral edema, and shortness of breath.
- Remember that rest and recovery are important goals of nursing care for the patient with ATN. The need is to reduce the metabolic rate, to limit tissue breakdown, and to decrease nitrogenous waste production.
- Be creative in assisting the patient who has been ordered to restrict fluids to quench his or her thirst by using ice chips, gum, or hard candy between fluid allotments. Give medications during meals to decrease using up the fluid allotment.
- Incorporate continuous assessment of the patient's skin into the nursing care plan. ATN patients are at an increased risk for skin breakdown as a result of uremia accumulation under the skin. The accumulation of uremia leads to dryness and itching of the skin. Instruct patients on ways to use distraction to decrease itching. Keep the fingernails trimmed and smooth. Apply skin emollients liberally, avoid harsh soaps, and bathe patient only when needed.

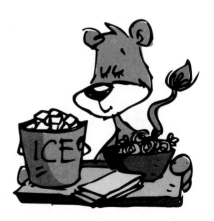

Frequent turning and repositioning helps to prevent skin breakdown. Good peritoneal hygiene should be a standard.

- Remember that nutritional interventions involve restricting intake of sodium, phosphorous, potassium, magnesium, and protein. Monitor serum electrolyte laboratory values, remembering that these numbers may be normal or decreased as a result of hemodilution. Documentation of intake and output should be kept hourly to monitor the urinary output. Weigh the patient daily at the same time of day to assess for significant weight gain 1.5 kg/24 hrs. Notify the physician if urinary output drops below 30 ml/hr. The patient's fluid intake should be restricted to approximately 1200 to 1500 ml/24 hrs.

The following formula should be used to calculate the fluid intake for the next 24 hours:

Urinary output (previous day or nondialysis day if on dialysis) – 500 to 800 (insensible water loss) = Amount of intake

 If the cause of ATN is a nephrotoxic agent, preventing further exposure to the agent should be a primary nursing goal.

If the patient developed ischemic ATN as a result of hypotension or CHF, these pathologies must be managed to prevent further renal damage. Administering such medications as antihypertensive drugs will control hypertension, thus decreasing renal damage. Medications such as digoxin (Lanoxin) and dopamine (Intropin) may be needed to prevent renal hypoperfusion by increasing the cardiac output, thus decreasing renal damage. All medications that require kidney excretion need to be assessed for dose alterations.

Discharge and Home Health Guidelines

All patients who experienced an ATN episode should be discharged with an understanding of renal function, signs and symptoms of impending renal failure, and how to monitor their own renal functions. Being followed by a nephrologist for at least 1 year is the current recommendation. Daily weight checks and daily rest periods to prevent overexertion should be encouraged. The nurse should explain the dietary and fluid restrictions, emphasizing the importance of follow-up and compliance in the treatment and recovery of renal failure.

TAKE HOME POINTS

Prevention of infection is crucial in preventing further complications. Therefore the nurse should avoid urethral catheters if possible. If a urethral catheter must be used, then meticulous catheter care must be provided.

Do You UNDERSTAND?

DIRECTIONS: Identify the following statements as *true* (T) or *false* (F).

_____ 1. The BUN and creatinine should decrease in the initial phase of ATN.

_____ 2. The GFR is approximately 125 ml/hr.

_____ 3. In ATN, one of the first signs is a decrease in urine production below 400 ml/24 hrs.

_____ 4. Fluid volume excess should be the focus of the nurse's assessment and physical examination when caring for patients at risk for ATN.

_____ 5. When caring for patients with ATN, the nurse needs to use the following formula to calculate fluid allotment: Urinary Output (previous day/nondialysis day if on dialysis) – 500 ml to 800 ml (insensible water loss) = Intake in Next 24 Hours.

DIRECTIONS: Match the following incident with the appropriate cause of ATN (each can be used more than once).

_____ 6. Patient overdoses on a nephrotoxic drug   a. Prerenal

_____ 7. Patient has hypertension   b. Intrarenal

_____ 8. Patient develops ATN because of enlarged   c. Postrenal
         prostate

_____ 9. Patient experienced a hypotension episode

_____ 10. Patient is diagnosed with renal artery stenosis

What IS Chronic Renal Failure?

Chronic renal failure (CRF) is a gradually progressive disorder characterized by an irreversible loss of renal function and reduction in the GFR, resulting in the development of the clinical syndrome called *uremia*. GFR is the rate at which the kidneys produce waste products (ultrafiltrate). *Uremia* is the term used to describe the cluster of signs and symptoms brought about by renal excretory dysfunction. These signs and symptoms include azotemia, fluid and electrolyte disturbances, acid-base imbalances, anemia, fatigue, anorexia, nausea, vomiting, and pruritus, as well as cardiovascular and neurologic manifestations. Azotemia and uremia both result from the inability of the kidney to excrete nitrogenous waste products from the body.

TAKE HOME POINTS

- *Azotemia* refers to the elevation of BUN and creatinine levels related to a decrease in GFR.
- Before a change in the BUN is detected, you already have 60% renal dysfunction.

Pathogenesis

CRF is the end result of all the chronic renal disorders. Common causes include diabetes mellitus, hypertension, atherosclerotic renovascular disease, chronic ingestion of nephrotoxic drugs, chronic glomerulonephritis, and ureteral or prostatic obstruction. Damage occurs in the renal parenchyma with the destruction of individual nephrons. As diseased nephrons become dysfunctional, the remaining healthy nephrons hypertrophy and hyperfiltrate to maintain adequate GFR and renal function. It is thought to be the decrease in the number of properly functioning nephrons, rather than an increase in the number of dysfunctional nephrons, that eventually leads to renal impairment. The loss of renal function is gradual because of the ability of the kidneys to compensate until the GFR (most frequently measured by urine creatinine clearance) drops to <10 ml/min. At this point a loss of more than 90% of functioning nephrons has occurred—a level simply too great to maintain renal homeostasis. The pattern of progression from normal renal function to end-stage renal disease (ESRD) involves four stages: (1) diminished renal reserve, (2) renal insufficiency, (3) renal disease, and (4) ESRD.

Pattern of Progression of Renal Disease

DISEASE STAGES	CHARACTERISTICS
Diminished renal reserve	• GFR is reduced to 50% of normal. • Serum BUN and creatinine levels remain normal. • Patient is asymptomatic.
Renal insufficiency	• GFR is reduced to 20% to 50% of normal. • Azotemia is present, usually in conjunction with anemia and hypertension. • Decreased ability of the kidney to concentrate urine may lead to the development of polyuria and nocturia.
Renal disease	• Reduction in GFR to less than 20% to 25% of normal. • Edema, metabolic acidosis, and hypocalcemia occur. • Patient may exhibit overt uremia with cardiovascular, gastrointestinal, and neurologic complications.
End-stage renal disease	• Reduction in GFR to less than 10% of normal. • Represents the terminal stage of uremia.

GFR, Glomerular filtration rate; *BUN*, blood urea nitrogen.

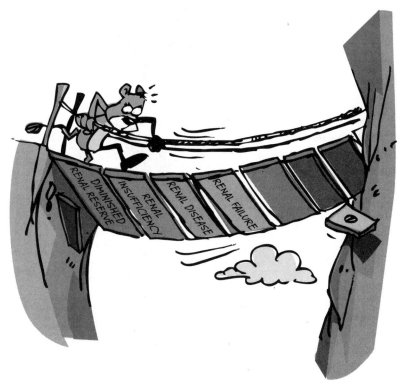

At-Risk Populations

Diabetic nephropathy is the leading cause of CRF in the United States. Patients with diabetes mellitus represent one third of those who develop CRF. Hypertension is another leading risk factor accounting for approximately one fourth of all cases. Occlusive renovascular disease, which tends to occur more frequently in men over the age of 50 with existing atherosclerosis, also increases risk.

Although unclear why, African-American men experience a higher incidence of renal dysfunction as a result of hypertension than Caucasians.

What You NEED TO KNOW

Signs and symptoms of CRF occur late in the course of the disease. By the time they present, significant permanent damage has already occurred. The delay between the occurrence of damage to the nephrons and the onset of symptoms is due to the ability of the kidney to compensate until approximately 90% of renal function is lost. At this point, uremia sets in and the patient is said to be in ESRD.

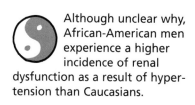
Older adults are at increased risk for CRF because of a decrease in the number of functioning nephrons, the volume and rate of blood flow, and the GFR that occurs as part of the aging process.

Clinical Manifestations of Chronic Renal Failure

Fluid and electrolyte imbalances	• Edema • Hyperkalemia
Acid-base imbalance	• Metabolic acidosis
Abnormalities of calcium, phosphate, and bone metabolism	• Hyperphosphatemia • Hyperparathyroidism • Renal osteodystrophy
Cardiovascular disease	• Hypertension • Dysrhythmias • Uremic pericarditis • Congestive heart failure • Edema
Hematopoietic disorders	• Anemia • Bleeding tendencies
Gastrointestinal effects	• Anorexia • Nausea and vomiting • Diarrhea or constipation • Weight loss • Gastrointestinal bleeding • Uremic esophagitis • Uremic gastritis • Uremic colitis • Uremic fetor
Integumentary manifestations	• Sallow complexion • Pruritus • Uremic frost
Neuromuscular complications	• Headache • Altered mental status • Peripheral neuropathy • Restless leg syndrome • Encephalopathy • Myopathy • Seizures • Coma

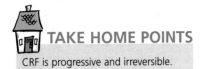

TAKE HOME POINTS

CRF is progressive and irreversible.

CRF is a progressive, irreversible condition. The rate of progression varies among individuals. If left untreated, electrolyte imbalance and fluid overload eventually lead to cardiac dysrhythmias, pulmonary edema, cerebral edema, and death. Renal replacement therapy (RRT) and renal transplant provide the only means of prolonging life once the patient has reached end-stage renal failure.

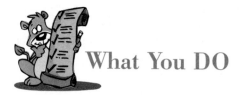

What You DO

Treatment of CRF includes interventions aimed at slowing the progression of the disease, managing symptoms, and providing for the removal of waste products once the kidneys can no longer support this process.

- Management of fluid overload includes adherence to a regimen consisting of a diet low in protein and sodium, fluid restriction, diuretics, and daily weight monitoring.
- Management of electrolyte and acid-base imbalances includes assessing for elevations in sodium, potassium, chloride, and phosphorus and a decline in calcium. Potassium levels should be carefully monitored as hyperkalemia can lead to life-threatening dysrhythmias. Dietary intake of potassium should be restricted as needed.

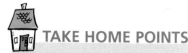

TAKE HOME POINTS

Fluid management and dietary control can be used to slow the progression of CRF for several years.

FIRST-LINE AND INITIAL TREATMENTS FOR CHRONIC RENAL FAILURE

- Dialysis may be needed to treat severe hyperkalemia.
- Management of abnormalities of calcium, phosphate, and bone metabolism consists of the administration of calcium supplements or an active form of vitamin D (calcitriol) to treat hypocalcemia and prevent severe bone loss leading to renal osteodystrophy. Phosphate-binding agents such as calcium acetate are used to treat hyperphosphatemia.
- Management of cardiovascular effects begins with the treatment of hypertension. Treatment usually requires the administration of antihypertensive medications such as an angiotensin-converting enzyme (ACE) inhibitor. Other effects on the cardiovascular system include the development of CHF and pulmonary edema because of fluid overload. Dialysis may help treat both these effects.
- Management of hemopoietic effects focuses on treating anemia that results from diminished renal secretion of erythropoietin. Epoetin alfa (Epogen or Procrit) may be prescribed when hematocrit levels fall below 30%.

The only effective treatments for ESRD are RRT and renal transplant. *RRT* is a term used to describe a variety of techniques used to remove excess fluid, electrolytes, and metabolic waste products from the body when the kidneys are no longer able to do so. These techniques include traditional intermittent hemodialysis (IHD), peritoneal dialysis (PD), and continuous renal replacement therapy (CRRT). Each of these techniques involves the movement of molecules in and out of blood across a semipermeable membrane. When this process occurs using an artificial membrane outside of the body, it is termed *hemodialysis* or *hemofiltration*. If the exchange takes place in the body across the peritoneal membrane, it is termed *PD*. (See center insert in Figure 8-6 for the process of osmosis and diffusion across a semipermeable membrane.)

Hemodialysis is accomplished using a dialyzer and a dialysate solution composed of an isotonic solution of water and electrolytes. These electrolytes may include sodium, potassium, calcium, magnesium, chloride, and bicarbonate. During dialysis, this solution allows for the movement of molecules across an artificial membrane based on the principles of diffusion and filtration. This results in the equilibration of electrolytes and removal of metabolic waste products in the blood. Hemodialysis requires vascular access. Access may be temporary or permanent and may take the form of a central venous catheter, arteriovenous fistula, or arteriovenous graft. A major concern is the loss of vascular access because of clot formation, infection, or inadequate blood flow. Interventions designed to maintain access include careful assessment of the site for the presence of a thrill and bruit, avoiding compression or restriction of blood flow to the site, and avoiding invasive procedures near the site. If the access site becomes occluded, an attempt to salvage it may be tried using embolectomy, angioplasty, or thrombolysis.

Hemodyalisis circuit

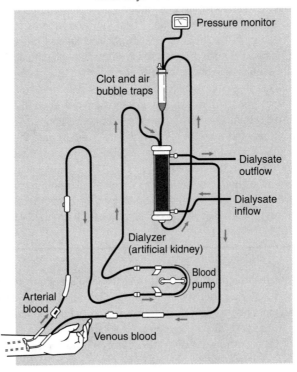

PD uses the same principles of diffusion and filtration as hemodialysis to achieve elimination of excess fluid, electrolytes, and waste products. PD involves the use of a catheter placed in the peritoneal cavity, allowing the peritoneal membrane to function as the semipermeable membrane across which dialysis occurs. One method, known as *continuous ambulatory peritoneal dialysis* (CAPD), involves the use of manual exchanges that are performed at various intervals throughout the day. A sterile dialysate solution is infused into the peritoneal cavity, allowed to remain for a prescribed period of time (usually several hours), and then drained out into a collection bag. Thus an exchange consists of a cycle of fill, dwell, and drain. Another method is the use of a programmable cycler that provides for automated multiple overnight exchanges. Complications of PD include infection at the catheter insertion site, peritonitis, and occlusion of the catheter because of fibrin deposition. Sterile technique must be observed when performing PD. Additional interventions include careful assessment of the catheter insertion site and inspection of the drained dialysate for color, clarity, and presence of fibrin aggregates.

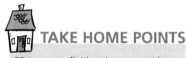

TAKE HOME POINTS

PD removes fluid and waste products from the body using the peritoneal cavity as the dialysate membrane.

Peritoneal dialysis

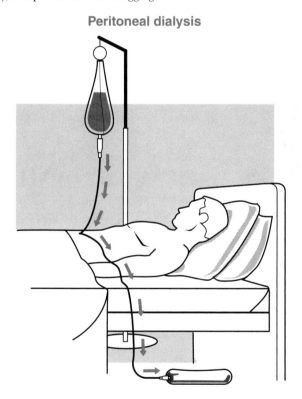

Nursing Responsibilities

- The patient should be educated regarding the importance of complying with dietary restrictions of fluids, protein, sodium, and phosphate.
- The patient should be instructed to avoid ingestion of nephrotoxic substances, including over-the-counter medications such as acetaminophen (Tylenol).

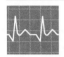

TAKE HOME POINTS

One pound of weight gain represents approximately 500 ml of fluid retention.

The nurse should assess for the presence of a thrill and bruit every 4 to 6 hours in the patient with an arteriovenous (AV) fistula or graft.

• **The nurse should never compromise the vascular access—it is the patient's lifeline.**
• **The nurse should never perform venipuncture, administer an injection, or inflate a BP cuff on the extremity where the fistula or graft is located.**

TAKE HOME POINTS

The nurse should instruct the CRF patient to avoid tight or restrictive clothing around the affected arm and to not rest the head on the affected arm while sleeping.

• Fluid intake, urine output, and daily weight should be monitored.
• Serum electrolytes, BUN, and creatinine should be monitored.
• Hemoglobin and hematocrit should be monitored.
• The nurse should assess for signs and symptoms of disease progression, such as anorexia, nausea and vomiting, edema, fatigue, or weakness.
• Any signs of infection such as fever or productive cough should be reported to the physician.
• Patients experiencing pruritus should be instructed to avoid the use of strong soaps, to always rinse thoroughly, and to shower rather than bathe when possible.
• Psychosocial support should be provided to the patient. As the disease progresses, the patient should be educated regarding renal replacement therapies, kidney transplant, and his or her right to refuse treatment.
• If the patient is receiving hemodialysis, the nurse should assess and protect the vascular access site.
• If the patient is receiving PD, the nurse should assess for signs and symptoms of peritonitis such as abdominal pain, rebound abdominal tenderness, and fever.
• The nurse should assess returned dialysate for clarity, color, and presence of clots.
• Temperature and white cell count should be monitored.
• The use of strict sterile technique should be ensured when performing exchanges.

Do You UNDERSTAND?

DIRECTIONS: **Select the best answer, and place the appropriate letter in the space provided.**

_____ 1. Compensatory mechanisms that allow normal renal function to be maintained for long periods of time despite renal injury include:
  a. Hyperfiltration
  b. Vasodilation
  c. Atrophy
  d. Homeostasis

_____ 2. ESRD is said to have occurred when kidney function is reduced to:
  a. 10%
  b. 50%
  c. 75%
  d. 90%

Answers: 1. a; 2. a.

_____ 3. The potential life-threatening electrolyte imbalance most common in the patient with ESRD is:
   a. Hyponatremia
   b. Hypercalcemia
   c. Hypophosphatemia
   d. Hyperkalemia

_____ 4. For each pound a patient gains, the nurse can estimate the patient is retaining fluid of approximately:
   a. 100 ml
   b. 250 ml
   c. 500 ml
   d. 1000 ml

What IS Continuous Renal Replacement Therapy?

CRRT refers to a variety of techniques used to provide extracorporeal fluid or solute removal on a continuous basis (typically for persons with renal failure). CRRT may be used in the management of patients with ARF, fluid overload, or metabolic or hemodynamic instability. Specific indications for CRRT include oliguria, anuria, hyperkalemia, severe acidosis, azotemia, pulmonary edema, uremic encephalopathy, uremic neuropathy, uremic myopathy, uremic pericarditis, severe hyponatremia or hypernatremia, hyperthermia, diuretic-resistant cardiac failure, and drug overdose with a filterable toxin.

 TAKE HOME POINTS

CRRT provides a means of dialyzing a critical care patient who is hemodynamically unstable.

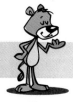

What You NEED TO KNOW

CRRT relies on the principles governing fluid and solute transport across a semipermeable membrane. These include diffusion, convection, and ultrafiltration. Diffusion describes the passage of solutes across a semipermeable membrane from an area of higher concentration to one of lower concentration. In convection, a solvent carries solutes. As the solvent is pushed across a semipermeable membrane, in response to a transmembrane pressure gradient, solutes are dragged along. Ultrafiltration describes the process in which plasma water and crystalloids are separated from whole blood across a semipermeable membrane in response to a transmembrane pressure gradient.

 TAKE HOME POINTS

Diffusion is the process of solutes moving across a semipermeable membrane from an area of higher concentration to one of lower concentration.

Answers: 3. d; 4. c.

Diffusion

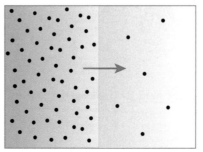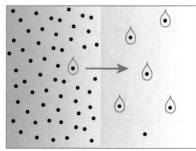

Modes of Continuous Renal Replacement Therapy

All forms of CRRT rely on an extracorporeal circuit with a semipermeable membrane and some form of arteriovenous or venovenous access. Arteriovenous modes require cannulation of both an artery and a vein. No blood pump is needed because this method relies on the force of the arteriovenous pressure gradient to push blood through the circuit. In contrast, venovenous modes require no arterial cannulation. Instead, vascular access is most commonly achieved by inserting a double lumen catheter into a central vein. One lumen then functions as an arterial (or outflow) line and the other as the venous (or inflow) line. Blood is circulated through this system by use of a roller pump in the prefilter line segment and a drip chamber in the line returning the blood from the filter.

Modes of CRRT include continuous arteriovenous hemofiltration (CAVH), continuous arteriovenous hemodialysis (CAVHD), continuous venovenous hemofiltration (CVVH), continuous venovenous hemodialysis (CVVHD), continuous venovenous hemodifiltration (CVVHDF), and slow continuous ultrafiltration (SCUF). The newer venovenous modes are gradually replacing the older arteriovenous modes of CRRT.

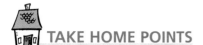

TAKE HOME POINTS

To operate, CRRT needs an arterial outflow line and a venous inflow line.

Modes of Continuous Renal Replacement Therapy

CAVH	• Is the original and simplest form of CRRT.
	• Requires cannulation of both an artery and vein (usually femoral).
	• Blood flow through the system depends on a mean arterial pressure 60 mm Hg.
	• Advantages include that CAVH is relatively simple to use.
	• Disadvantages include the following:
	  • Arterial bleeding if disconnections or leaks in circuit occur
	  • Poor clearance rates in patients with low or unstable blood pressure
	  • Risk of clot formation in extracorporeal circuit as a result of low blood flow

CAVH, Continuous venovenous hemodialysis; *CRRT,* continuous renal replacement therapy.

Modes of Continuous Renal Replacement Therapy—cont'd

CAVHD	• Is used when CAVH cannot provide adequate waste removal. • Uses the principle of diffusion. • Dialysate delivered to an extracorporeal compartment is used to remove solutes, resulting in more rapid reduction in BUN and creatinine. • Similar to CAVH, mean arterial pressure must be maintained above 60 mm Hg to ensure proper blood flow through the system. • Decreases blood flow, resulting in the same disadvantages as CAVH.
CVVH	• Relies on the principle of convection. • Replacement solution is added to the extracorporeal circuit to enhance convective transport; fluid removal can occur if desired. • Major feature of this mode is that it does not require arterial access. CVVH relies on a pump to control blood flow rather than arterial pressure. • The venovenous modes incorporate safety devices to detect low pressures and presence of air in circuit.
CVVHD	• Works by diffusion and can be understood as simply a slow form of dialysis. • Use of dialysate increases the clearance rate of small solutes. • Like CVVH, this mode of CRRT uses a pump rather than relying on arterial pressure. Potential complications associated with arterial cannulation are avoided.
CVVHDF	• Uses both convection and diffusion to remove fluid, metabolic waste, inflammatory mediators, and other toxins. • Diffusion occurs as dialysate is run counter to the blood. • Convection occurs as an electrolyte replacement fluid is pumped into the blood.
SCUF	• Form of CRRT used to treat refractory fluid overload. • Works by convection to remove ultrafiltrate in a controlled manner that allows for slow fluid removal. • Fluid replacement is unnecessary because of the slow rate of fluid removal.

CAVH, Continuous arteriovenous hemofiltration; *CRRT,* continuous renal replacement therapy; *CAVHD,* continuous arteriovenous hemodialysis; *BUN,* blood urea nitrogen; *CVVHD,* continuous venovenous hemodialysis; *CVVH,* continuous venovenous hemofiltration; *CVVHDF,* continuous venovenous hemodifiltration; *SCUF,* slow continuous ultrafiltration.

CRRT provides a slow, gentle method of fluid and solute removal that helps to maintain homeostasis and prevent complications in critically ill patients with ARF, multiorgan failure, and hemodynamic instability associated with other forms of RRT.

PD is considered a form of RRT. PD, however, is limited by insufficient solute clearance, inability to correct hyperkalemia quickly, a high risk of peritonitis, hyperglycemia, poor fluid removal, and respiratory difficulty because of large volumes of fluid instilled in peritoneal cavity. In addition, because it requires an intact peritoneal membrane, it is contraindicated for patients with abdominal wounds, infections, or scar tissue. These limitations prevent the use of PD in the management of most ARF patients.

The most commonly used RRT is IHD. The usefulness of IHD is limited, however, in the unstable or critically ill patient. IHD may result in severe hemodynamic instability that forces the therapy to be discontinued and is associated with several complications. The most significant complication is hypotension, especially in the critically ill patient with multiorgan dysfunction. Other complications of IHD include dysrhythmias, hypoxemia, hemorrhage, infection, dialysis dysequilibrium syndrome, and seizures.

CRRT provides better azotemic and uremic control than IHD, enhances fluid volume removal without compromising intravascular volume, and improves both electrolyte balance and nutritional support in the critically ill patient. Specific benefits may be seen in patients who cannot tolerate the intermittent fluid overload occurring between dialysis, such as those with acute respiratory distress syndrome (ARDS) and pulmonary edema. In addition, CRRT improves oxygenation and respiratory function in such patients. CRRT is useful in optimizing nutritional status. Because CRRT provides a mechanism for the continuous removal of water and sodium, adequate amounts of parenteral nutrition may be delivered without the fear of fluid overload. CRRT reduces energy expenditure in febrile patients. Patients with CHF resistant to diuretics respond favorably to CRRT, because it contributes to hemodynamic stability by generating a rise in cardiac index without a fall in arterial pressure. CRRT is also the treatment of choice in patients with or at risk for cerebral edema. Unlike IHD, which can increase intracranial pressure by rapid solute movement causing herniation and death, CRRT maintains cerebral pressure perfusion and does not induce such surges in intracranial pressure.

IHD can cause an increase in intracranial pressure from the rapid solute movement and can contribute to the development of massive cerebral edema causing herniation and death.

TAKE HOME POINTS

Dialysis dysequilibrium syndrome occurs when hemodialysis causes a rapid decrease in BUN, which results in the development of cerebral edema.

TAKE HOME POINTS

CRRT assists in maintaining hemodynamic stability during fluid removal process.

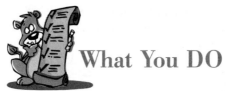

What You DO

CRRT is performed in the critical care unit. The critical care nurse is responsible for caring for the patient and managing the equipment. Before beginning CRRT, the nurse should be sure to note baseline vital signs, cardiac rhythm, hemodynamic parameters, and current weight and laboratory values. The nurse should assess the physician's prescriptions to determine mode; type of replacement fluids and dialysate (if used); the flow rates for blood, fluids, and medications; and parameters for the amount of fluid to be removed. The CRRT machine should be set up according to the manufacturer's directions. This includes hanging fluids, priming the tubing, and adding an anticoagulant to the system if prescribed (usually heparin or trisodium citrate). The patient should be connected to the machine via the established vascular access. Blood leaves the body through the red-colored line and returns through the blue-colored line. The nurse should check to be sure all connections are secure and press start when ready to begin.

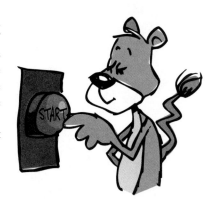

Nursing Responsibilities

The nurse should do the following:

- Assess hemodynamic status including BP, heart rate (HR), and rhythm. Transient hypotension sometimes occurs just after beginning therapy and may be corrected by decreasing the rate of blood flow to the machine. In some cases, it may be necessary to treat hypotension with fluid replacement and vasopressors, as prescribed.
- Assess fluid volume status, including central venous pressure (CVP), pulmonary artery pressure (PAP), and pulmonary artery wedge pressure (PAWP). Assess breath sounds, skin turgor, edema, and weight.
- Assess hourly and cumulative ultrafiltrate rate and note the color of the ultrafiltrate.
- Measure hourly and cumulative intake and output. The nurse should be sure to include all forms of intake such as medications, blood products, and enteral, or parenteral feedings, as well as output such as chest tube or nasogastric (NG) drainage.
- Administer fluid replacement based on hourly fluid balance goal as determined by the physician.
- Assess electrolyte and acid-base balance every 4 to 6 hours. The nurse should administer supplements as needed.
- Assess for bleeding. The nurse should ensure the entire circuit is always visible, secure all connections, and position carefully to avoid disconnection. Sedation may be needed for agitated or restless patients.
- Assess temperature. The patient may become hypothermic because of the cooling effects of extracorporeal circulation. Use an in-line fluid warmer attached to the return (blue) line. Warming blankets should be used with caution to avoid concealing the circuit.
- Assess for infection. The nurse should monitor for fever and elevated white cell count, assess catheter insertion site, use sterile technique when accessing lines, and perform sterile dressing changes in accordance with institution policy.
- Assess coagulation status of the patient. Partial thromboplastin time (PTT) should be monitored.
- Assess and maintain patency of the circuit. The nurse should flush the system with saline or heparin according to policy.
- Assess the system for air and blood leakage. System and alarms should be monitored and fixed as needed.

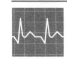

Once CRRT has begun, the nurse must monitor the patient and assess for any complications. Complications may include hypotension, hemorrhage, hypothermia, infection, and air embolism.

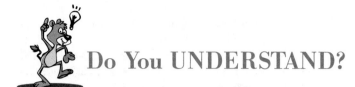

Do You UNDERSTAND?

DIRECTIONS: **Select the best answer, and place the appropriate letter in the space provided.**

_____ 1. Principles governing fluid and solute transport across a semipermeable membrane in CRRT include diffusion and:
   a. Conversion
   b. Convection
   c. Active transport
   d. Capillary membrane permeability

_____ 2. The type of vascular access required for a patient undergoing CVVHDF is:
   a. Arterial
   b. Venous
   c. Arteriovenous
   d. Venovenous

_____ 3. SCUF is a form of CRRT used to treat:
   a. Azotemia
   b. Dehydration
   c. Fluid overload
   d. Uremia

_____ 4. IHD may be unsuitable for the critically ill patient because it can result in:
   a. Fluid overload
   b. Hypertension
   c. Multiorgan failure
   d. Severe hemodynamic instability

Answers: 1. b; 2. d; 3. c; 4. d.

9 Endocrine System

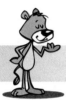

What IS Diabetes Mellitus?

Diabetes mellitus is a disorder of the endocrine system that causes alterations in glucose metabolism. Two primary classifications of diabetes exist: type I and type II. Both classifications of diabetes result from dysfunctional pancreatic cells.

What You NEED TO KNOW

Pancreas

The pancreas is an organ with both endocrine and exocrine functions. The exocrine function is to release a juice full of enzymes and other components that helps with the process of digestion. One of the functions of this juice is to adjust the pH of the contents of the duodenum, so the pancreatic enzymes can work efficiently. Pancreatic enzymes include proteases, amylases, and lipases to facilitate the breakdown of proteins, starches, and fats. Tissue exists in the pancreas called the *islets of Langerhans*. This tissue contains the primary endocrine cells referred to as *alpha*, *beta*, and *delta* cells.

ALPHA, BETA, AND DELTA CELLS

- Alpha cells produce glucagon which helps maintain normal blood sugar levels through the breakdown of glycogen (glycogenolysis) and the formation of glycogen from fats and proteins (gluconeogenesis). Hypoglycemia stimulates the release of glucagon, and hyperglycemia inhibits glucagon release.

257

For further information on type I or type II diabetes, see *Real-World Nursing Series: Pathophysiology.*

TAKE HOME POINTS

In type I diabetes:
If an absolute lack of insulin exists, then the patient will require exogenous administration of insulin.

In type II diabetes:
If a relative lack of insulin exists, a proper diet and exercise, as well as oral hypoglycemic agents, may be used to manage the patient.

- Beta cells produce insulin, which is the key that allows cells to be permeable to glucose along with amino acids, potassium, magnesium, and phosphate. Insulin assists in carbohydrate, protein, and fat metabolism and in the formation of new proteins. Patients who are insulin deficient have depleted protein and decreased glucose in muscle cells. An abnormal release of stored body fat occurs because of a shift from carbohydrate to fat metabolism. Ketone formation results from the metabolism of fats; if left untreated it results in ketoacidosis and coma.
- Delta cells secrete somatostatin, which inhibit growth hormone, thyroid-stimulating hormone, insulin, glucagon, and other gastrointestinal (GI) hormones.

Complications

Many acute and chronic complications are associated with type I and type II diabetes. Other complications often are a result of chronic hyperglycemia and alterations in metabolism. Serious complications result from vascular and neuropathic alterations. Diabetes is the leading cause of end-stage renal failure and new blindness in adults.

What IS Diabetic Ketoacidosis?

Approximately 15% of patients with type I diabetes die by the age of 40.

DKA occurs in the type I diabetic and results in total body dehydration, disturbances in electrolyte balance, and an acidosis.

Diabetic ketoacidosis (DKA) is one of the more serious metabolic crises that can result from hyperglycemia in patients with uncontrolled diabetes mellitus. The incidence of DKA occurs most frequently in adolescents and older adults with type I diabetes. DKA results from a deficiency of insulin, which leads to four life-threatening metabolic derangements. First, because the beta cells in the pancreas have the inability to produce insulin, the ensuing hyperglycemia causes a hyperosmolar state. This hyperosmolarity results in fluid shifting from inside the cell to the serum; eventually this fluid is lost in the urine, causing electrolyte shifts and total body dehydration. Other metabolic derangements occur because no insulin exists to allow glucose to enter the cells; therefore cells begin to break down fats and proteins to use for fuel. This process causes the formation of ketones. Ketones decrease the blood pH and the bicarbonate concentration causing a ketoacidosis.

What You NEED TO KNOW

Clinical Manifestations

DKA can be the initial presentation of an undiagnosed type I diabetic or can appear when patients have missed or reduced insulin doses. Glucoregulatory hormone excess promoting hyperglycemia occurs with illness, stress, growth spurts, and pregnancy. Medications that interfere with insulin secretion or action include thiazide diuretics, Dilantin, sympathomimetics, and glucocorticoids. The result of excess glucose (hyperglycemia) and insufficient insulin can lead to DKA.

The hallmark symptoms of DKA include dehydration, ketosis, metabolic acidosis, and ketonuria. The patient may also exhibit weakness, anorexia, vomiting, abdominal pain, altered mental status, tachycardia, orthostatic hypotension, poor skin turgor, dry mucous membranes, and Kussmaul respirations (the attempt of the body to eliminate ketones through respirations, giving the breath a fruity, sweet odor).

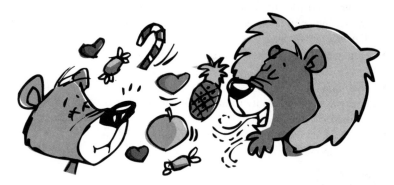

In DKA, diagnostic findings may include serum glucose levels of >250, often >500 mg/dl, glycosuria, increased serum osmolarity, serum acidosis, elevated blood urea nitrogen (BUN), and initially a hyperkalemia.

Serum Osmolality

Serum osmolality is the concentration of solute particles in the blood. It is possible to calculate serum osmolality by using the serum measurements of sodium, glucose, and BUN. Serum osmolality is increased in patients with acidosis, DKA, hyperglycemia, hyperglycemic hyperosmolar nonketotic coma, hypernatremia, methanol poisoning, and nephrogenic diabetes insipidus. The serum osmolality formula is the following:

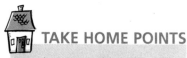

TAKE HOME POINTS

Normal serum osmolality: 280 to 300 mOsm/kg

$$\text{Serum osmolality} = (2 \times \text{Serum sodium}) + \frac{\text{Serum glucose}}{18} + \frac{\text{BUN}}{2.8}$$

Anion Gap

The anion gap is a calculation of the difference between the major positively charged electrolytes (cations) and the major negatively charged electrolytes (anions) in the serum. It helps determine the cause of metabolic acidosis. the anion gap formula is the following:

$$\text{Anion gap} = \frac{(\text{Serum sodium [Na}^+] + \text{Serum potassium [K}^+])\ -}{(\text{Serum chloride [Cl] + Serum bicarbonate [HCO}_3])}$$

Causes of DKA:
- Initial presentation in undiagnosed type I diabetic
- Missed or reduced insulin doses
- Illness, particularly infection and stress hormone excess, that increases blood sugar levels
- Stress
- Growth spurts
- Pregnancy

Medications that interfere with insulin secretion or action include glucocorticoids (hydrocortisone, prednisone, dexamethasone), phenytoin (Dilantin), thiazide diuretics (hydrochlorothiazide), sympathomimetics (albuterol, dobutamine, dopamine, epinephrine, norepinephrine, phenylephrine).

DKA laboratory values:
- Serum glucose levels elevated (usually >250 mg/dl)
- Elevated BUN
- Glucosuria
- Elevated serum osmolality (usually >300 mOsm/L)
- Arterial pH: <7.35
- Hyperkalemia (often, initially): >5.4 mEq/L
- Anion gap: >20 mEq/L

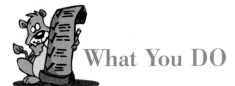 **What You DO**

Goals of treatment include correction of the acidosis, correction of the electrolyte and fluid disturbances, insulin to lower serum glucose levels, prevention of ketosis, and prevention of complications. When treating patients with DKA, the medical team should do the following:

FIRST-LINE AND INITIAL TREATMENTS FOR DKA

- Closely monitor blood glucose levels and acidosis (arterial blood gasses [ABGs]).
- Replace fluids and electrolytes.
- Administer insulin.
- Monitor cardiac, pulmonary, and neurologic systems.
- Identify and correct precipitating event.
- Educate the patient and the patient's family.

Medical Interventions and Nursing Responsibilities

When treating patients with DKA, the medical team should do the following:
- Monitor serum glucose levels at least every 2 hours. Serum glucose levels should be monitored every 1 to 2 hours while the patient is receiving a continuous insulin infusion.

- Replace life-threatening fluid and electrolyte deficits. The fluid of choice is usually 0.9% normal saline (NS), which allows for replacement of extracellular fluid (ECF) volume deficits. Initial replacement is usually rapid; then, when the patient's blood pressure (BP) is normal, hypotonic saline (0.45% NS) can be used.
- Monitor acidosis by assessing ABGs. Correction of fluid and electrolyte imbalance will allow the kidneys to conserve bicarbonate and restore acid-base balance. Acidosis is usually treated with bicarbonate when the serum pH is 7.10 or less. In this setting bicarbonate is added to hypotonic NS and replaced slowly.
- Administer rapid-acting insulin. Administration of regular intravenous (IV) insulin at a rate of 0.1 to 0.2 U/kg/hr is recommended via continuous infusion to accomplish a gradual decrease in serum glucose.
- Monitor cardiac, pulmonary, and neurologic status.
- Monitor and correct electrolyte imbalances. IV replacement of potassium, chloride, phosphate, and magnesium may be required. Osmotic diuresis may result in a major potassium deficit. If no contraindication such as renal disease exists, potassium replacement usually begins with fluid therapy but should be based on serum and urine laboratory values. Phosphate depletion may result in impaired cardiac and respiratory function.
- Correct underlying, precipitating events (usually infection).
- Provide patient and family support and education. Education is essential in prevention of further episodes of diabetic crisis. Emphasis should be placed on glucose monitoring and regulation, eating schedules, diet, exercise, and rest.
- Avoid complications of therapy.

Do You UNDERSTAND?

DIRECTIONS: After reviewing the following results of a patient's physical examination, calculate serum osmolarity and anion gap.

A 34-year-old woman has a 4-year history of insulin-dependent diabetes. A recent episode of influenza has led to her admission to the intensive care unit (ICU). A physical examination reveals the following:

Respiratory rate: 40 (respirations deep and rapid)
Heart rate (HR): 118 bpm
BP: 88/50 mm Hg
Temperature: 101.8° F, rectally
Skin: Dry, with poor turgor (patient is lethargic but responsive to simple commands)
Admission laboratory data:
- Serum glucose: 540 mg/dl
- BUN: 70

Lowering glucose levels too rapidly can cause cerebral edema, resulting in seizures, coma, or both. ANY change in level of consciousness in a patient on an insulin drip should include the intervention of seizure precautions and having an immediate blood glucose level assessed.

TAKE HOME POINTS

Total body water deficit may be 3 to 4 L in hyperglycemia.

Rapid correction of acidosis may result in severe hypoxemia at the cellular level.

TAKE HOME POINTS

- The goal of treating hyperglycemia is to prevent complications of excess insulin administration and to restore normal uptake of glucose by the cells.
- Potassium phosphate may be used to treat a potassium deficit in hyperglycemia.

- Hemoglobin (Hgb): 14 g/dl
- Hemocrit (HCT): 48%
- Serum sodium: 129 mEq/L
- Serum potassium: 5 mEq/L
- Serum chloride: 94 mEq/L
- pH: 7.23
- Partial pressure of carbon dioxide (pCO_2): 22
- HCO_3: 8

1. Calculate the serum osmolarity.

_____

2. Calculate the anion gap.

_____

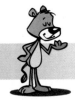

What IS Hyperosmolar Nonketotic Coma?

Hyperosmolar nonketotic (HHNK) coma is also a serious metabolic complication of diabetes, but it is usually seen in patients with type II diabetes. Because type II diabetes is a problem of relative insulin deficiency rather than an absolute deficiency, the cells are able to use some glucose. However, not enough glucose is available for cellular metabolism because of the insulin deficiency, so hyperglycemia develops. This promotes cellular dehydration, osmotic diuresis, and fluid and electrolyte disturbances, but ketosis and acidosis are minimal or absent. These patients are profoundly dehydrated with blood glucose levels typically exceeding 600 mg/dL or greater. Marked hyperosmolarity and elevated BUN levels also exist.

TAKE HOME POINTS

HHNK occurs in the type II diabetic and results in total body dehydration and disturbances in electrolyte balance, without acidosis.

What You NEED TO KNOW

HHNK usually occurs in individuals with type II diabetes who have omitted or reduced their hypoglycemic agent. Other precipitating causes include drugs, enteral feedings, hyperalimentation, and peritoneal dialysis.

Answers: 1. serum osmolarity = 313 mOsm/L = (2 × 129) + (540 ÷ 18) + (70 ÷ 2.8); 2. anion gap = 32 mEq/L = (129 + 5) − (94 + 8).

Clinical manifestations include:
- Profound dehydration
- Hypotension
- Tachycardia
- Diminished central venous pressure (CVP)
- Dry mucous membranes
- Poor skin turgor
- Neurologic impairments including confusion, seizures, and coma

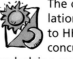 The older adult population is predisposed to HHNK, and a concurrent illness or underlying cause usually exists.

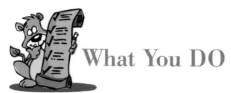

What You DO

The treatment goals for HHNK are similar to the interventions for DKA. Rapid replacement of fluids to correct dehydration is one of the most important interventions. Often, physicians use isotonic fluids to replace half of the estimated fluid deficit within the first 12 hours and the remainder within 24 hours.

A fast-acting form of insulin is typically administered by IV infusion to closely control blood glucose levels. When the blood glucose level approaches 300 mg/dl, addition of dextrose into the IV infusion should be considered, because the blood glucose level can precipitously drop and the patient can become hypoglycemic. The patient's cardiovascular and neurologic status should be monitored, along with monitoring for embolic complications. The nurse should remember that HHNK and DKA are precipitated by underlying problems, often infection, so it is essential to treat the underlying problem. In addition, to prevent future recurrences, patient and family education should be reinforced.

When treating DKA or HHNK patients, the nurse should closely monitor serum potassium levels! Because patients with DKA or HHNK are hyperosmolar, dehydrated, and depleted of potassium intracellularly, rehydration by replacement fluids alone can decrease serum potassium levels. In addition, insulin therapy causes potassium to move into the cell along with glucose, further decreasing serum potassium levels.

Do You UNDERSTAND?

DIRECTIONS: **After reviewing a patient's history and results of laboratory studies, provide short answers to the two following questions.**

RK is a 76-year-old woman who lives alone. Her medical history includes twice-daily diuretics for the treatment of hypertension and a recent complaint of thirst and urination over the past month. Her daughter took her to the emergency department because she was lethargic and difficult to arouse. Her skin and mucous membranes appeared dry. She was in a sinus tachycardia. Laboratory studies disclosed the following values:

Blood glucose level: 1230 mg/dl
Serum sodium: 144 mEq/L
Serum potassium: 5.5 mEq/L
BUN: 79 mg/dl

Creatinine: 2.8 mg/dl
Serum osmolarity: 361 mOsm/kg
pH: 7. 35
HCO$_3$: 18 mEq/L
Urine: Positive for glucose
Serum and urine ketones: Negative

1. Is RK more likely to have DKA or HHNK? Why?

_____

_____

_____

_____

2. What are some important nursing and medical interventions for RK?

_____

_____

_____

_____

What IS Hypoglycemia?

Acute hypoglycemia occurs when the blood sugar (glucose) levels drop rapidly. Without enough glucose, brain cells cannot use adenosine triphosphate (ATP) for energy, and this causes cerebral dysfunction. This process causes sympathetic nervous system (SNS) stimulation and increased levels of epinephrine, glucagons, growth hormone, cortisol, and adrenocorticotrophic hormone. These hormones suppress the secretion of insulin and act to increase blood sugar levels by gluconeogenesis and glycogenolysis. Epinephrine and cortisol also inhibit glucose use in muscles.

Answers: 1. RK is more likely to have HHNK. RK's laboratory values reflect a glucose level of >1000, no acidosis, and no urine and serum ketones; 2. RK's serum osmolarity and BUN reflect dehydration. RK needs IV replacement of fluids and rapid-acting insulin to reduce the glucose levels (usually in an insulin drip, so glucose levels can be closely controlled and monitored). RK also needs close monitoring of serum electrolyte levels. RK should be frequently assessed for changes in heart rhythm, respiratory rate and rhythm, and alterations in levels of consciousness.

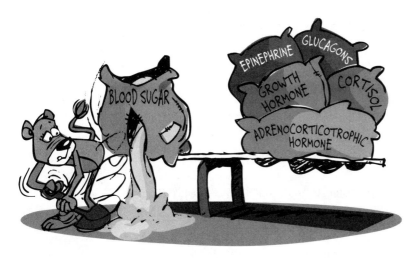

What You NEED TO KNOW

The following are clinical manifestations of hypoglycemia:
- Sweating, tremors
- Blurred vision, hunger, weakness
- Behavior changes and confusion
- Anxiety, paresthesias, and poor coordination
- Slurred speech, headache
- Palpitations, nausea
- Seizures, stupor, coma

 TAKE HOME POINTS

- Nocturnal hypoglycemia may present as night sweats, nightmares, and a morning headache.
- It is important to do a complete assessment and history of the hypoglycemic patient, because the hypoglycemia might be a symptom of another health problem such as myxedema coma (complication of hypothyroidism).

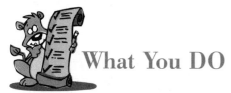

What You DO

It is essential to identify patients at risk for prevention of hypoglycemic episodes and monitor these patients for manifestations of hypoglycemia. If the patient has a blood glucose level above 80 mg/dl with symptoms, fast-acting carbohydrates (FACs) are typically not administered. A diet drink should be administered, and the blood glucose level rechecked in 15 minutes. If the patient's blood glucose level has dropped below 80 mg/dl at recheck, the nurse should assess the patient's ability to swallow and administer FACs.

FACs include **ANY ONE** of the following:
- 4 oz ($^1/_2$ cup) of apple juice
- 4 oz of orange juice
- 4 oz of cranberry juice
- 4 oz of cola
- 8 oz of skim milk

! **Severe, prolonged hypo-glycemia can cause brain damage. Any abnormal behavior in a patient taking insulin should be considered a hypoglycemic reaction until proven otherwise.**

If the patient has a blood glucose level of <60 mg/dl, the nurse should assess the patient's ability to swallow and immediately administer FACs. The patient and blood glucose level should be assessed every 15 minutes until the blood glucose level is >70 mg/dl. If the patient has not been placed on nothing by mouth (NPO) status, a complex carbohydrate snack may be given. If the patient is unable to swallow, NPO, or unresponsive, glucagon can be given intramuscularly or subcutaneously or Dextrose 50 (D50) can be given through an established IV site.

Differences Among Diabetic Ketoacidosis, Hyperosmolar Nonketotic Coma, Hypoglycemia

	DKA	HHNK	HYPOGLYCEMIA
Symptoms	• Confusion, lethargy • Warm, dry, flushed skin • Weakness • Anorexia, nausea • Abdominal pain • Tachycardia • Fruity, acetone breath • Deep rapid respirations • Thirst	• Confusion, lethargy • Warm, dry flushed skin • Weakness • Tachycardia • Rapid respirations • Acetone breath absent • Thirst	• Cold, clammy skin • Pallor • Profuse sweating • Normal mucous membranes • Irritability, tremors • Poor concentration • Tachycardia • Bradycardia (in coma) • Normal-to-rapid respirations • Acetone breath absent • Hunger
Laboratory values			
Blood glucose	Elevated	Significantly elevated (may be >1000 mg/dl)	Below normal
Serum sodium	Normal to decreased	Variable	Normal
Serum potassium	Variable	Variable	Normal
Serum osmolarity	Elevated but usually <330 mOsm/L	Significantly elevated >350 mOsm/L	Normal
Arterial blood gases	Decreased pH Metabolic acidosis with compensatory respiratory alkalosis	Normal-to-mild acidosis	Normal-to-slight respiratory acidosis
Serum ketones	Positive	Negative	Negative
Urine	Positive for glucose or ketones	Negative for glucose or ketones	Negative for glucose or ketones
Interventions	Insulin, fluid and electrolyte replacement	Insulin, fluid and electrolyte replacement	Glucose, glucagon

DKA, Diabetic ketoacidosis; *HHNK,* hyperosmolar nonketotic coma.

Diabetic Crises

```
            ┌─────────────────┐
            │  Unresponsive   │
            │    patient      │
            └────────┬────────┘
                     │
            ┌────────▼────────┐
            │  Blood glucose  │
            └────────┬────────┘
          High │           │ Low
       ┌────────▼──────┐  ┌─▼──────────────┐
       │   Diabetic    │  │  Hypoglycemia  │
       │ ketoacidosis  │  └────────────────┘
       │    (DKA)      │
       │ or hyperglycemic │
       │ hyperosmolar  │
       │ nonketotic coma │
       │    (HHNK)     │
       └───────┬───────┘
       ┌───────▼───────┐
       │ Arterial blood │
       │   gases (pH)  │
       └───────┬───────┘
    Normal │        │ Acidosis
    ┌───────▼─┐   ┌──▼──────────┐
    │  HHNK   │   │   Ketones   │
    └─────────┘   └──┬──────────┘
              Negative │      │ Positive
          ┌───────────▼──┐  ┌─▼────────┐
          │ Another type │  │   DKA    │
          │  of acidosis │  └──────────┘
          └──────────────┘
```

Do You UNDERSTAND?

DIRECTIONS: **Identify the following statements as *true* (T) or *false* (F).**

_____ 1. The key to identifying hypoglycemia is the presence of acidosis.

_____ 2. Any abnormal behavior in patients taking insulin should be considered a hypoglycemic reaction until proven otherwise.

_____ 3. A hypoglycemic patient will have positive serum ketones.

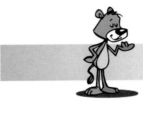

What IS Syndrome of Inappropriate Antidiuretic Hormone?

TAKE HOME POINTS

In SIADH an excessive amount of ADH is released, which results in water being reabsorbed, which contributes to fluid and electrolyte imbalances.

Syndrome of inappropriate antidiuretic hormone (SIADH) is caused by excessive release of antidiuretic hormone (ADH). The syndrome is characterized by increased water reabsorption in the kidneys, serum sodium dilution (hyponatremia), and elevated serum levels of ADH. Symptoms associated with SIADH-related hyponatremia include lethargy, confusion, and in extreme cases, coma and death. SIADH is strongly associated with neoplasm, particularly small-cell carcinoma of the lung. Nursing care focuses on improving fluid and electrolyte balance and neurologic status.

What You NEED TO KNOW

Under normal conditions, ADH, also called *vasopressin*, is secreted by the posterior pituitary gland in response to increased osmolarity. ADH regulates osmolarity by increasing the permeability of distal tubules and collecting ducts in the kidney to water. Large amounts of water are reabsorbed, diluting solutes, lowering serum osmolarity, and concentrating urine.

In SIADH, ADH levels are increased several fold, causing an excessive increase in water reabsorption. An increase of water in the ECF dilutes sodium. As water is reabsorbed, small increases in BP cause loss of sodium from the ECF in the urine through pressure natriuresis.

The following place a person at high risk for developing SIADH:
- Neoplasm—specifically small-cell lung cancer
- Central nervous system (CNS) disorders—head trauma, stroke, tumor
- Postoperative patients—especially after pituitary surgery
- Antineoplastic agents—cisplatin, vincristine, cyclophosphamide, vinblastine
- Nicotine use
- Medications—tranquilizers, barbiturates, anesthetics, thiazide diuretics

The symptomology depends on the severity of the hyponatremia and the length of time the patient has been hyponatremic.

Clinical Manifestations Associated with Hyponatremia

SERUM SODIUM LEVELS	ASSOCIATED SYMPTOMS
130-140 mEq/L	Impaired taste, anorexia, dyspnea with exertion, fatigue, dulled sensorium
120-130 mEq/L	Severe gastrointestinal symptoms including vomiting and abdominal cramps
<115 mEq/L	Confusions, lethargy, muscle twitching, convulsions

Other syndromes can be associated with hyponatremia and increased urine sodium levels; these include hypothyroidism, adrenal insufficiency, metabolic acidosis associated with vomiting, osmotic diuresis, diuretics, and renal failure. In addition, during pregnancy women may develop hyponatremia as low as 130 mEq/L because of the release of the hormone relaxin. This is a normal change. A thorough history of illness and medication use is instrumental in diagnosis.

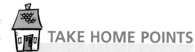

TAKE HOME POINTS

Symptoms of SIADH may be the presenting symptom in patients with small-cell lung cancer.

Comparison of Laboratory Values: Normal vs SIADH

NORMAL LABORATORY VALUES OF ADULTS	SIADH DIAGNOSTIC EVALUATION
Serum sodium (137-145 mEq/L)	Serum hyponatremia (<137 mEq/L)
Urine sodium (40-220 mEq/L/day)	Urine hypernatremia (>40 mEq/L)
Urine osmolality (50-1200 mOsm/kg)	Urine hyperosmolarity (>100 mOsm/kg)
Uric acid (2-7 mg/dl)	Low uric acid concentration (<4 mg/dl)
Serum potassium (3.5-5.0 mEq/L)	Normal serum potassium
pH (7.35-7.45)	Normal pH
Urine specific gravity (1.002-1.028)	Elevated urine specific gravity
ADH level (0-4.7 pg/mL)	Elevated ADH level

SIADH, Syndrome of inappropriate antidiuretic hormone; *ADH,* antidiuretic hormone.

Prognosis

The prognosis of SIADH depends on the cause. In ectopic ADH secretion, SIADH normally resolves with tumor regression. Any neurologic deficit is usually reversible. In transient SIADH after surgery, ADH levels gradually return to normal within 5 to 7 days.

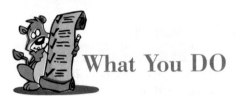

What You DO

Treatment for SIADH is primarily focused on elimination of the cause. Water restriction (500 to 1000 ml/day) is instituted. The patient may be placed on a high-salt, high-protein diet, and any medications that might potentiate ADH are discontinued. In severe hyponatremia, IV hypertonic saline is administered and may be given with diuretics such as furosemide (Lasix) or mannitol (Osmitrol). Medications that interfere with the action of ADH on the kidney may be initiated, including lithium carbonate (Lithobid, Lithonate) or demeclocycline (Declomycin). No drug therapy is available to suppress ectopic release of ADH.

If the cause is unknown, the medical history may provide clues. A history of stroke, cancer, pulmonary disease, or head injury should be particularly considered as significant in the diagnosis of SIADH.

The patient should be assessed for symptoms of hyponatremia, including neurologic status. The level of consciousness should be determined, and any change should be noted. The patient's safety should be protected at all times, and the nurse should assist with ambulation. Fall precautions and seizure precautions should be initiated as appropriate. Frequent neurologic checks should be performed and daily electrolyte laboratory results monitored.

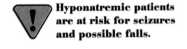

Hyponatremic patients are at risk for seizures and possible falls.

Fluid restrictions should be maintained and input and output documented. The patient should be weighed daily, and comfort measures for thirst should be provided, such as lozenges, swabs, or ice chips. Water or ice chips should not be kept at the bedside. The nurse should help the patient and family understand the importance of fluid restriction and monitoring daily weights. In addition, the signs and symptoms of hyponatremia should be taught.

FIRST-LINE AND INITIAL TREATMENTS FOR SIADH

- Monitor electrolyte laboratory values.
- Restrict fluids.
- Infuse hypertonic saline.
- Administer prescribed medications, such as furosemide, mannitol, lithium carbonate, and demeclocycline.
- Protect the patient from possible injury (seizures).
- Ensure accurate intake and output.
- Weigh the patient each day.

Do You UNDERSTAND?

DIRECTIONS: Select the best answer, and place the appropriate letter in the space provided.

_____ 1. SIADH is most strongly associated with:
   a. Small-cell lung cancer
   b. Pregnancy
   c. Breast cancer
   d. Surgery

_____ 2. The symptoms of SIADH are most strongly associated with:
   a. Hypernatremia
   b. Hyponatremia
   c. Water intoxication
   d. Urine hyperosmolarity

_____ 3. The following are appropriate nursing actions associated with SIADH *except:*
   a. Monitor strict intake and output.
   b. Institute safety procedures.
   c. Keep water and ice chips at bedside.
   d. Weigh the patient each day.

What IS Diabetes Insipidus?

Diabetes insipidus (DI) is caused by a deficiency in the production or release of ADH by the posterior pituitary gland. The insufficient amount of circulating ADH results in the renal tubules being unable to conserve free water, which is clinically seen as polyuria.

Answers: 1. a; 2. b; 3. c.

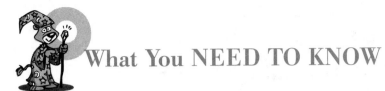

What You NEED TO KNOW

Normally, ADH is secreted by the posterior pituitary gland and regulates water balance and serum osmolality. In DI something is interfering with the production, transport, or release of ADH, which results in excessive water loss and the inability to dilute serum solutes. The following are common categories of DI:

Neurogenic

- Posterior pituitary region lesion (hypothalamus, pituitary, craniopharyngioma)
- Congenital defect
- Severe head trauma
- Intracranial surgery (especially region of pituitary)
- Increased intracranial pressure (ICP)
- CNS infections (meningitis, encephalitis)
- Metastatic malignancies
- Autoimmune response
- Granulomatous disease (tuberculosis [TB], sarcoidosis)
- Idiopathic diseases and conditions

Nephrogenic

- Renal disease (pyelonephritis, polycystic disease, obstructive uropathy)
- Decrease or absence of ADH receptors
- Cellular damage to loop of Henle nephrons
- Drugs (lithium, ethanol, amphotericin, demeclocycline, phenytoin)
- Hypokalemia
- Hypercalcemia

Psychogenic

- Water intoxication
- Excessive IV fluid administration
- Drugs (anticholinergics, tricyclic antidepressants)

Clinical Manifestations

- Polyuria (30 to 40 L/24 hr)
- Polydipsia
- Hypotension (systolic blood pressure [SBP] in adult <90 mm Hg)
- Tachycardia (HR >100 beats per minute)
- Weight loss
- Dehydration (decreased skin turgor, dry mucous membranes)
- Mental status changes (confusion, restlessness, irritability, lethargy, coma)
- Seizures
- Constipation
- Diagnostic evaluation includes serum and urine laboratory tests

Serum Findings

- Serum sodium >145 mEq/L
- Serum osmolality >300 mOsm/kg
- Serum ADH decreased in neurogenic DI, may be normal with nephrogenic or psychogenic diabetes insipidus

Urine

- Urine specific gravity (USG) <1.005
- Urine osmolality <300 mOsm/kg

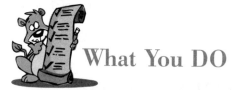

What You DO

Treatment for DI is focused on correcting the underlying cause, as well as restoring and maintaining fluid volume. To restore and maintain fluid volume, the patient will require volume replacement. Depending upon the mental status of the patient and whether he or she is able to drink enough fluid, the patient should be able to drink enough water to maintain fluid volume. However, for patients who are unable to orally take in adequate amounts of fluid, they will most likely require IV administration of fluids. In either case it is important that the patient be adequately hydrated, otherwise he or she will exhibit signs and symptoms of fluid volume loss (hypotension, tachycardia). If the DI is psychogenic, then the management is to remove the causative agent, which in this case would be by restricting fluid intake.

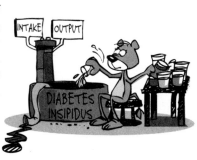

Medications Used to Treat Diabetes Insipidus

DRUG	DOSE	LIMITATIONS	SIDE EFFECTS
Desmopressin (acetate)	**Intranasally** 10-40 mg (micrograms) at bedtime or in divided doses **Parenteral** 2-4 mg twice daily	High cost ($2000/yr)	• Nasal congestion • Headache • Flushing • Hyponatremia (overtreatment)
Vasopressin (Pitressin)	**IM or SC** 5-10 units every 6-12 hours **IV** 0.2-0.4 units/min up to 0.9 units/min	Very short duration (1-2 hours)	• Sweating • Tremor • Pounding in head • Abdominal cramps • Nausea • Angina • Increased blood pressure • Water intoxication

IM, Intramuscular; *SC,* subcutaneous; *IV,* intravenous.

Medications that are used in the management of DI include replacing the ADH with an exogenous hormone supplement. For the initial management of the patient in DI, the medication of choice is vasopressin (Pitressin) and for the patient with a chronic neurogenic DI the medication of choice is desmopressin acetate (DDAVP).

Nursing management of the patient with DI includes astute assessment skills of fluid volume and neurologic status. Monitoring a patient's intake and output, weight, vital signs, laboratory values, and treatment outcomes are crucial in effectively managing the patient with DI. In addition, patient and family education is important in assisting the patient and family to understand the disease process of DI, the importance of drinking fluid, and the importance of the medication regimen prescribed.

Do You UNDERSTAND?

DIRECTIONS: Select the best answer, and place the appropriate letter in the space provided.

_____ 1. In which cause of DI would you implement fluid restriction?
  a. Neurogenic
  b. Psychogenic
  c. Anatomic
  d. Pleurogenic

_____ 2. Overmedication with an exogenous ADH medication in a person with DI can cause:
  a. Constipation
  b. GI hemorrhage
  c. Third spacing
  d. Dehydration

DIRECTIONS: Unscramble the italicized letters to complete each of the following statements.

3. The _____ _____ gland is

responsible for the production and release of ADH. (*ripseoort; rtiuyaipt*)

4. To maintain fluid volume, the patient will require _____

replacement. (*elvmuo*)

5. A medication that is given intranasally and is the exogenous replacement

of ADH is _____. (*sopsienemdsr*)

Answers: 1. b; 2. c; 3. posterior pituitary; 4. volume; 5. desmopressin.

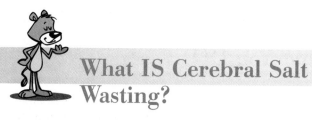

What IS Cerebral Salt Wasting?

Cerebral salt wasting (CSW) is defined as a condition in which the patient becomes both hypovolemic and hyponatremic. CSW is a different condition from SIADH, and the two should not be confused. Although both SIADH and CSW have hyponatremia, SIADH is dilutional because of the large amounts of water being reabsorbed. In contrast, CSW is primary because sodium is being lost through the large amount of urinary output.

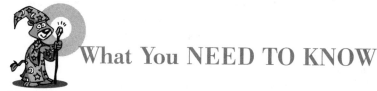

What You NEED TO KNOW

Many patients with neurologic disease (i.e. post craniotomy, pituitary tumor, head injuries) have difficulties with water and sodium regulation: DI, SIADH, and CSW. Therefore it is extremely important to determine which problem the nurse is dealing with so that it can be treated and managed correctly. CSW is attributed to the failure to regulate sodium absorption by the CNS.

Laboratory Value Comparison

	CSW	SIADH	DI
Serum sodium	<134 mEq/L (primary)	<134 mEq/L (dilutional)	>145 mEq/L
Serum osmolality	Hypoosmolality	<280 m/Osm/L	>295 mOsm/L
BUN	High	Normal or low	High
Urine-specific gravity	>1.010	>1.005	<1.005
Urine sodium (must compare with serum sodium)	High	High	Low
Weight	Decreased	Increased	Decreased

CSW, Cerebral salt wasting; *SIADH,* syndrome of inappropriate antidiuretic hormone; *DI,* diabetes insipidus; *BUN,* blood urea nitrogen.

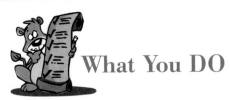

What You DO

Treatment for CSW is focused on fluid volume and sodium replacement. Usually, fluid volume replacement is done through IV administration of NS (0.9%) or hypertonic saline (3%) solution (or by administration of both). The goal of volume replacement is to match the volume out (urine output). Although the hypertonic saline solution aids in replacing sodium, the patient may also be prescribed oral salt. Careful attention must be given when administering hypertonic solutions, because they can cause volume expansion and create more urine loss of fluids. In addition, serum sodium should not be rapidly corrected, because it has been associated with pontine myelinolysis—a loss of myelin on the nerve fibers within the midbase of the pons of the brain. The patient should also be monitored for possible seizure activity, because the serum sodium is <134 mEq/L.

Nursing management of the patient with CSW includes astute assessment skills of fluid volume, laboratory values, and neurologic status. Monitoring a patient's intake and output, weight, vital signs, laboratory values, and treatment outcomes are crucial in effectively managing the patient with CSW.

TAKE HOME POINTS

Treating CSW like SIADH with fluid restrictions could be fatal.

Do You UNDERSTAND?

DIRECTIONS: **Match the following laboratory finding treatments in Column A with the correct endocrine abnormality in Column B.**

Column A	Column B
_____ 1. Administration of DDAVP	a. CSW
_____ 2. USG: 1.020	b. SIADH
_____ 3. Serum sodium: 158 mEq/L	c. DI
_____ 4. Fluid restriction	
_____ 5. USG: 1.001	
_____ 6. Weight gain	
_____ 7. Urine sodium: 120	
_____ 8. Administration of hypertonic saline IV	
_____ 9. Dilutional hyponatremia	
_____ 10. BUN: 8	

Answers: 1. c; 2. a; 3. c; 4. b; 5. c; 6. b; 7. c; 8. a; 9. b; 10. b.

CHAPTER

10 Hematologic System

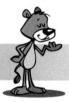

What IS Acute Sepsis?

At least two or more of the following signs and symptoms characterize acute sepsis:

- Temperature >38° or <36° C
- Tachypnea
- Tachycardia
- White blood cell count (WBC) >12,000 cells/mm
- WBC <4000 cells/mm, or differential >10% bands

The septic process is initiated by the launch of immune mediators that are part of the inflammatory reaction. This process starts a chain of complex inter-actions that are controlled by numerous feedback mechanisms. Eventually the immune system is overwhelmed, and the process actually harms the body. *Systemic inflammatory response syndrome* (SIRS) refers to a host's response to a variety of clinical insults, both infectious and noninfectious, and is part of the acute sepsis process.

FIRST-LINE AND INITIAL TREATMENTS FOR SEPSIS

- Eradicate the offending organism.
- Provide supplemental oxygen (O_2).
- Administer intravenous (IV) fluids.
- Administer appropriate medications.

Treatment of SIRS involves:

- Supportive measures: O_2 and fluids
- Immunotherapy (control the excessive host inflammatory response)

Lung, urinary tract, and venous access device infections are major sources of septic infections. Peritonitis is the most frequent source of sepsis in the surgical patient. The source of the infection has a major role in predicting mortality. For

TAKE HOME POINTS

- Acute sepsis patients have a microbial infection with a systemic response.
- *Bacteremia* refers to a patient's blood cultures being positive for any type of bacteria.

> A septic patient will have SIRS, but a patient with SIRS does not necessarily have sepsis.

Those most at risk for developing sepsis are the chronically ill, those who are immunocompromised, those with malignancies, the very young, and the very old.

example, the patient with urosepsis has a better prognosis for recovery than the patient with pulmonary sepsis. For this reason the prognosis related to sepsis may depend on its origin.

 # What You NEED TO KNOW

Sepsis is most often caused by gram-negative bacteria but can also be caused by gram-positive bacteria, fungi, or yeasts. There has been an increase in antibiotic-resistant sepsis over the past few years that is attributed to the use of broad-spectrum antibiotics. There have also been more reported cases of sepsis that may be attributed to the increasing use of invasive diagnostic tests and invasive monitoring devices. The general population is living longer with more chronic and immunocompromised illnesses, predisposing them to developing complications such as sepsis while they are hospitalized.

Presenting symptoms of infection may include fever, purulent drainage from incision or wound sites, respiratory infection with productive cough, wound erythema with tenderness, abdominal rigidity, or a number of other specific findings depending on the infection site. The best means of treatment for sepsis is dependent upon pinpointing the source of infection and diagnosis of the invading microorganism with laboratory confirmation, including cultures from urine, blood, sputum, wound surfaces, cerebrospinal fluid (CSF), and possibly cultures from the tips of invasive catheters.

TAKE HOME POINTS

A negative blood culture does not mean that someone does not have sepsis.

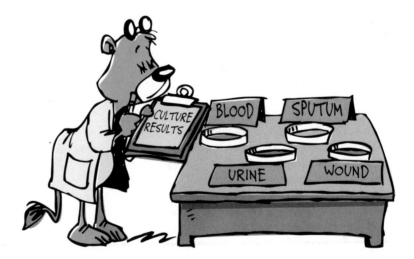

 If septic shock is not quickly identified and properly managed, then the patient can rapidly decompensate into respiratory failure, cardiovascular collapse, and death.

Septic shock is a major complication associated with sepsis; it is a distributive shock characterized by hypotension, tachycardia, tachypnea, and decreased level of consciousness. Because acute sepsis can be potentially fatal, the nurse must be vigilant in his or her assessment to identify the early signs and symptoms of shock.

Multiple-organ dysfunction syndrome (MODS) can occur if the progression of the inflammatory response is not addressed quickly or if the infectious process and resulting inflammatory response progresses rapidly. If the O_2 saturation of a septic patient continues to decline despite increasing the flow of inspired oxygen (FiO_2), then acute respiratory distress syndrome (ARDS) may be occurring. Yet another complication that can occur from sepsis is disseminated intravascular coagulation (DIC).

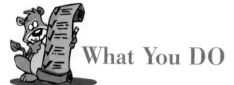

What You DO

It is important to identify patients early on that are at risk for sepsis, such as the elderly, the very young, the immunocompromised, the chronically ill, and those with malignancies. Another population at increased risk is that with indwelling catheters or invasive monitoring devices, such as indwelling urinary catheters or central venous lines. In the immediate postoperative patient, the nurse should expect a slight increase in body temperature. However, if the postoperative patient meets one or more of the previously mentioned criteria, the nurse should be more vigilant in assessing and reassessing the patient for signs and symptoms of sepsis.

One of the first signs of a patient becoming septic is the presence of confusion. Systolic pressures tend to increase somewhat and the pulse pressure may widen as long as intravascular volume is adequate. Tachypnea will be present along with tachycardia. Crackles may be present at bilateral lung bases, even in the absence of pulmonary infection.

Often the prognosis of the patient depends on early identification of the offending microorganism and treatment of the infection with appropriate antibiotic therapy. For this reason the nurse should place priority on obtaining cultures as prescribed by the physician before starting antibiotic therapy. Blood cultures can be drawn while initiating the patient's IV line. Often a physician will prescribe blood cultures "times two, same time, different sites." This direction means that the nurse should draw two different sets of blood cultures at the same time but from different sites on the patient according to institution protocol. This procedure is prescribed because a site can be contaminated if the skin is not prepped appropriately. Institution protocol dictates the skin preparation for a blood culture. Urine, wound, and sputum cultures should be obtained promptly and according to institution protocol before initiation of antibiotic therapy. Because the patient's recovery depends on eradication of the causative bacteria, it is important to initiate the prescribed antibiotic as soon as cultures are obtained. The physician may also prescribe a broad-spectrum antibiotic until the cultures isolate the offending microorganism. Once the microorganism is identified and isolated, the physician may change the prescription to a more specific antibiotic.

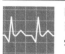
Because hypotension is a characteristic sign of sepsis, decreased renal perfusion may result in renal impairment, especially if left untreated.

If bleeding is seen at puncture sites, in urine collection bags, or on mucous membranes, this would prompt the nurse to suspect the threat of DIC.

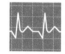
It is important to identify the signs and symptoms of sepsis early to prevent progression of sepsis into septic shock.

TAKE HOME POINTS

A blood culture positive for a microorganism is more reliable if it is positive from separate sites.

Septic patients will often require supplemental O_2. Infection causes increased metabolic demands, which causes an increased need for O_2. Initially the patient may be placed on O_2 at 5 to 6 L/min by nasal cannula. In more advanced stages, the patient may need O_2 delivered at 100% by a nonrebreather mask. Tachypnea in patients with and without fever may be a result of endotoxins released by the invading microorganisms or by defense mechanisms mediated by the body. As sepsis progresses, lung water increases because of the higher alveolar capillary permeability. This elevation of lung water increases the hypoxia, which results in an even higher respiratory rate. The higher respiratory rate leads to fatigue, which then leads to hypercapnia triggering the CNS to further increase the respiratory rate. This process continues to exhaustion. In this case the nurse needs to assist with ventilating the patient as needed and prepare for intubation.

Fluid replacement is important in the septic patient because of vasodilation, increased capillary permeability, and lost fluid in the interstitial space. Although blood volume is adequate in the septic patient, it is misplaced. There will be an expected decrease in systemic vascular resistance (SVR). An 18-gauge IV access site is essential. Often the condition of these patients will decline, and they will need central venous access. If the condition degenerates into septic shock, the physician may prescribe vasoactive and inotropic drugs.

The nurse should anticipate monitoring BP by means of an arterial catheter; the arterial line offers a more precise measurement than a noninvasive cuff pressure during hypotensive states. The patient should be observed for changes in level of consciousness to indicate hypoxia or decreased cerebral perfusion. Frequent vital sign monitoring helps the nurse assess the patient's response to therapy. Mean arterial pressure (MAP) should be monitored closely because of the variable pressures in the septic patient. The nurse should notify the physician promptly if a trend of decreasing MAP exists. Pulmonary artery pressures (PAPs) and central venous pressures (CVPs) enable the nurse to assess the effectiveness of the patient's treatment and help prevent fluid overload by allowing the nurse to monitor the patient's hydration status. It is also important to monitor urine output. A urine output of >30 ml/hr or >0.5 ml/kg/hr indicates adequate renal perfusion.

Arterial blood gas (ABG) diagnostics may be prescribed to assess for oxygenation status. WBC count will increase in response to infection but may decrease in later stages as the bone marrow stores become depleted. The nurse should monitor hemoglobin and hematocrit levels for decreasing red blood cells that limit the body's ability to transport O_2. In addition, he or she should monitor the indicators of renal function: trends in blood electrolytes, blood urea nitrogen (BUN) levels, and creatinine levels.

Hyperglycemia may be the first indication of sepsis in the diabetic patient. Control of hyperglycemia may be difficult until the infection is under control. For this reason the blood glucose of a diabetic patient admitted with an infection should be monitored very closely.

There has been some debate over the treatment of fever in the septic patient. Very few studies exist relating the control of temperature to the mortality rate, morbidity rate, or both. Many physicians do treat fever because of the increased

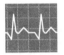

Acute sepsis patients can progress into ARDS very quickly because of the increased alveolar capillary permeability.

Close monitoring of the blood pressure (BP) and cardiovascular status of the patient is essential.

A MAP of <60 mm Hg negatively affects perfusion of the brain and kidneys. Thus a decreasing MAP should be addressed quickly.

TAKE HOME POINTS

Hypoglycemia is relatively uncommon in sepsis but does occasionally occur in patients with other underlying problems.

demands that the hypermetabolic state places on the body. Some studies show that decreasing fever also decreases O_2 demand for organs and tissues. Still others suggest that fever itself may provide some protection from the microbial pathogens. Patient comfort is clearly improved when fever is at least partially controlled.

Patient education involves informing the patient of the rationale for each intervention. The patient that has blood cultures prescribed "same time, different sites" will be more cooperative about having two needle sticks if the nurse first explains why the procedure is done this way and why it is in his or her best interest. Often the patients at greatest risk for developing sepsis are the very old, the very young, or the chronically ill. In this case it is appropriate to explain the nursing interventions to the family members.

Do You UNDERSTAND?

DIRECTIONS: Fill in the blanks to complete the sentences using the words listed on the following page. Words are used only once, and some words are not used at all.

1. Gram-negative or gram-positive bacteremia with SIRS is

   _____ _____.

2. People at increased risk for developing acute sepsis are

   _____.

3. Presenting symptoms of acute sepsis may include fever, tachycardia,

   tachypnea, widened pulse pressure, and _____.

4. Septic patients have fluctuating BPs, and a MAP <60 mm Hg can

   negatively affect _____ and

   _____ perfusion.

5. Urine output >30 ml/hr or >0.5 ml/kg/hr indicates

   _____ renal perfusion.

6. To counteract vasodilation caused by inflammatory mediators resulting in increased capillary permeability, _____ drugs may be ordered.

7. Often the prognosis of the patient depends on early identification of the offending organism and the treatment of it with appropriate

_____.

vasopressive	altered loc	adequate
chronotropic	cerebral and renal	suboptimal
inotropic	inadequate	cardiac and pulmonary
acute sepsis	antibiotics	erythema
hypovolemia	immunocompromised	

What IS Thrombocytopenia?

TAKE HOME POINTS

The breakdown, or lysis, of fibrin produces fibrin degradation products (FDP) in the blood.

Thrombocytopenia is a decrease in the number of platelets (disk-shaped cells that are formed when mature granular megakaryocytes shed their cytoplasm) that circulate through the body. Platelets function in helping blood to clot, supplying a phospholipid surface so that there can be an interaction between clotting factors in the blood, and in assisting in fibrinolysis that aids in lysis of fibrin clots and vessel repair. The two major emergencies associated with thrombocytopenia are (1) hemorrhage and (2) shock (septic or hypovolemic).

What You NEED TO KNOW

TAKE HOME POINTS

In patients with an enlarged spleen, the platelets become trapped in the spleen and cannot be released into the bloodstream, causing a decrease in the total platelet count on the laboratory report.

Platelets mature in the bone marrow of the pelvis, long bones, ribs, sternum, skull, and spleen and are regulated by the hormone called *thrombopoietin*. Approximately two thirds of all platelets are then released into the bloodstream, where they aid in the mechanism of clotting, and the remaining one third are stored in the spleen, where they are housed until the body calls for them to be released.

Three main causes of thrombocytopenia exist: (1) low production of platelets by the body (that is, decreased production of megakaryocytes, called *megakaryocytopoiesis*, because of cancer and its treatment, sex linked Wiskott-Aldrich syndrome, May-Hegglin anomaly, Fanconi's syndrome, neonatal rubella, nutritional deficiency of folate or vitamin B12); (2) abnormal distribution of platelets to where they are needed (i.e., hypersplenism, liver disease, hypothermia); and (3) increased destruction of platelets or coagulopathy dysfunction as the result of diseases and conditions, medications, or medical treatment.

Causes of Platelet Destruction

DISEASES AND CONDITIONS	MEDICATIONS	MEDICAL TREATMENT

• AIDS/HIV
• Cancer
  • Leukemia
  • Lymphoma
  • Hodgkin's disease
• Cirrhosis
• DIC
• Eclampsia
• Exanthema subitum
• HELLP syndrome
• Hepatitis C (chronic)
• Hyperthyroidism
• Inflammatory bowel disease
• ITP
• Leptospirosis
• Malaria
• Sepsis
• SLE
• TTP
• Typhoid fever
• Vitamin K deficiency
	• Alcohol
	• Amphotericin B
	• Aspirin
	• Beta-lactam antibiotics
	• Cephalosporin antibiotics
	• Cimetidine
	• Famotidine
	• Furosemide
	• Gold
	• H$_2$ antagonists
	• Heparin
	• Indomethicin
	• Isoniazid
	• MMR immunization
	• NSAIDs
	• Oral hypoglycemics
	• Penicillin
	• Phenytoin
	• Procainamide
	• Quinidine
	• Quinine
	• Ingestion of excessive tonic water
	• Rifampin
	• Thiazides
	• Tricyclic antidepressants
	• Vaccines
	• Valproic acid
		• Alpha-interferon therapy
		• Bone marrow transplant
		• Central venous catheters
		• Chemotherapy (especially platinum-based and alkylating agent therapy)
		• Postliver transplant
		• Radiation therapy

AIDS, Acquired immunodeficiency syndrome; *HIV,* human immunodeficiency virus; *DIC,* disseminated intravascular coagulation; *HELLP,* hemolysis, elevated liver enzymes, low platelets; *ITP,* idiopathic thrombocytopenic purpura; *SLE,* systemic lupus erythematosus; *TTP,* thrombotic thrombocytopenic purpura; *MMR,* measles (rubeola), mumps, rubella; *NSAIDs,* nonsteroidal antiinflammatory drugs.

 Thrombocytopenia can be seen in children with exanthema subitum (ES) with a positive herpesvirus 2.

Heparin-induced thrombocytopenia (HIT) occurs in 5% of patients and typically develops 5 to 14 days after initial heparin administration.

TAKE HOME POINTS

- Bone marrow infiltration by tumor cells replaces the normal platelet cells causing thrombocytopenia. Tumor cells also replace red cells causing anemia and WBCs causing granulocytopenia. A decrease in platelets, WBCs, and red blood cells is called *pancytopenia*.
- One 5-grain aspirin tablet can coat platelets so that blood does not clot for 9 to 12 days, the usual lifetime of a platelet.

• Panic value is <20,000 cells/μl or mm³ and exhibits petechiae of the skin, blood-filled mouth bullae, and mucous membrane bleeding from the oral cavity, nose, uterus, or gastrointestinal (GI), urinary, or respiratory tracts.
• In oncology, no relationship exists between platelet count and risk of hemorrhage; therefore transfusion support should be aggressive.

TAKE HOME POINTS

- Platelets, also called *thrombocytes*, are produced in the bone marrow and have an average life span of 10 days.
- The risk of hemorrhage is >50% when the platelet count is <20,000 cells/μl or mm³.

Normal total platelet laboratory values for adults include 150,000 to 400,000 cells/μl or mm³; cord blood 100,000 to 290,000 cells/μl or mm³; newborn 100,000 to 300,000 cells/μl or mm³, neonate 150,000 to 390,000 cells/μl or mm³; and 3 months to 10 years 100,000 to 473,000 cells/μl or mm³.

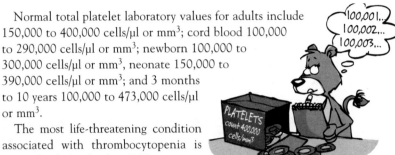

The most life-threatening condition associated with thrombocytopenia is septic shock that leads to DIC, intravascular clotting, and formation of micro-emboli in the capillaries. Once DIC develops, the body is continuously depleted of clotting factors; this leads to hemorrhage. Hemorrhage frequently occurs in the brain, and presentation of intracranial hemorrhage is associated with headache, diplopia, confusion, seizures, and changes in mental state.

What You DO

Care of the patient with potential or actual thrombocytopenia includes physical assessment and laboratory assessment, as well as interventions for prevention and actual hemorrhage and hypovolemic or septic shock. Hypovolemic shock consists of loss of blood volume, and septic shock consists of increased serum glucose, thrombocytopenia, hypoperfusion, hypotension, hyperglycemia, multisystem organ failure, or a combination of these symptoms.

Physical assessment includes assessment for bleeding from vital organs—brain, lungs, and GI tract. Neurologic assessment includes history of recent blow or fall to the head, headache, blurred vision, papillary changes, confusion, or disorientation. Respiratory assessment includes hemoptysis (coughing up blood), congestion, wet cough, and epistaxis (nose bleed). GI assessment includes hematemesis (vomiting up blood), blood found in stool, or nasogastric (NG) tube drainage with positive occult test. Genitourinary (GU) assessment includes testing for blood in the urine. Vital signs include hypotension and tachycardia. The skin, mucosa, and eyes should be assessed next. Assessment of the skin should include assessing for petechiae, purpura, and easy bruising. The oral mucosa should be assessed for bleeding gums, petechiae, and hemorrhagic blebs on the palate and oral mucosa. Retinas should be assessed for hemorrhage using an ophthalmoscope, and sclera should be assessed for bleeding and redness via observation.

Grading system for degree of platelets on laboratory tests:
0 = 100,000/μl or mm³
1 = 75,000 to 100,000/μl or mm³
2 = 50,000 to 75,000/μl or mm³
3 = 25,000 to 50,000/μl or mm³
4 = <25,000/μl or mm³

The nurse should assess total platelet counts 1 hour and 24 hours after platelet transfusions. Laboratory values should be assessed as prescribed, and the nurse should know the last two values for comparative data.

Laboratory Assessment for Thrombocytopenia

TEST NAME	DESCRIPTION	ADULT NORM VALUE	NORM
Platelet count, total	Actual number of circulating platelets per cubic millimeter of blood	150,000-400,000/mm^3	Decreased
PT	Amount of time for clot formation	10-15 seconds	Increased
aPTT	Measures how well the coagulation sequence is functioning for clotting ability	<35 seconds	Increased
INR	Calculated value that monitors response to anticoagulant therapy	≤3.0	Increased or normal
Capillary fragility test	Tourniquet test to measure platelet deficiency	Females ≤10 petechiae; Males ≤≤5 petechiae	Increased
FDP	Measures activity of the fibrinolytic system	2-10 µg/ml	Increased
Folic acid, serum	Measures amount of folic acid, folate, in bloodstream	<12 ng/ml or <27.2 nmol/L	Decreased
Vitamin B12	Water soluble vitamin used up in rapid cell turnover	100-1100 ng/ml	Increased in chronic granulocytic leukemia
Platelet antibody, blood	Detect platelet autoantibodies and isoantibodies to transfusion of blood products	Negative or <1000 molecules of IgG per platelet	Positive

PT, Prothrombin time; *aPTT,* activated partial thromboplastin time; *INR,* international normalized ratio; *FDP,* fibrin degradation products; *IgG,* immunoglobulin G.

Nursing Interventions

When treating patients with thrombocytopenia, the nurse should do the following:

- Try to avoid invasive procedures such as bone marrow biopsies (although this may be necessary for diagnosis), endoscopies, enemas and suppositories, intramuscular (IM) or subcutaneous (SQ) injections, and excessive venipunctures. Obtaining central or peripheral venous access will be necessary to infuse platelets and implement hemodynamic monitoring.
- If invasive procedures are necessary, infuse platelets during and after invasive procedures and apply pressure for at least 5 minutes to venipuncture and bone marrow aspiration sites. Use of topical thromboplastin, obtained from a pharmacy, may be necessary to halt bleeding from bone marrow aspiration sites.

Insertion of a balloon catheter into the bronchus or nares may also be necessary to create pressure to halt bleeding.

- For intubation with a cuff apparatus, deflate the cuff every 1 to 2 hours to avoid esophageal erosion or trauma leading to hemorrhage.
- Remember that constipation, nausea, and vomiting can raise intracranial pressure (ICP) and should be prevented by use of anticonstipation and antiemetic medications.
- Place a person with a nosebleed in high Fowler's position to avoid aspiration and lower anxiety. Apply ice, nasal packing, or topical epinephrine (or a combination of these therapies) to decrease bleeding. Apply direct pressure to the sides of nose just underneath the nose bone.
- Count the number of menstrual pads used to assess the amount of blood loss in females, and administer hormones to control bleeding if medically necessary.
- Avoid the use of straight razors (use an electric razor instead).
- Avoid use of hard toothbrushes. Instead, use a soft or sponge-type toothbrush.
- Transfuse platelets according to institutional protocol. The usual increase expected is 5000 to 10,000 cells/µl or mm^3 platelets per unit transfused. If the 1-hour posttransfusion platelet count shows less improvement than at least 5000 cells/µl or mm^3 per unit transfused, then the patient is considered to be alloimmunized. This means the patient has developed antibodies against HLA antigens transfused with the platelets. In this case the patient should be given HLA-matched platelets only for transfusion (usually obtained from a family member). If the platelet count continues to decrease 24 hours posttransfusion, then infection, fever, coagulopathy, and hepatosplenomegaly need to be considered as causes.
- Administer epinephrine as prescribed to release platelets from the spleen.
- Administer corticosteroids as prescribed to increase platelet production.
- Administer Lepirudin 0.4 mg/kg by IV bolus and follow with 0.15 mg/kg IV per hour to maintain the aPTT to 1.5 to 2.5 times the median normal.
- Administer immunosuppressive and other medication therapy as prescribed. This can include corticosteroids, vincristine, Rituximab (a monoclonal antibody), or alfa-2b interferon with ribavirin.
- Administer lithium carbonate or folate to stimulate production of platelets in the bone marrow.
- Remember that replacement therapy with fresh or frozen plasma transfusions or cryoprecipitate can be effective in augmenting the production of coagulation factors by the liver.
- Administer vitamin K (aquaMEPHYTON, Mephyton) IM in the dose prescribed (usually up to 25 mg for an adult and up to 5 mg for pediatric patients) to assist in hepatic synthesis of factors II, VII, IX, and X that aid in blood clotting.
- Prepare the patient for possible abdominal computed tomography (CT) scan and bone marrow aspiration.

TAKE HOME POINTS

- The platelets found in stored blood lose their effectiveness after 24 hours at the usual storage temperature of 4° C.
- Platelets are stored at room temperature and are effective for up to 5 days. Maximum effectiveness is found in transfusing platelets within 6 hours of obtaining them from a donor.
- All blood products should be exposed to irradiation before transfusion to severely immunocompromised patients, because this limits proliferation of lymphocytes. A label will be found on the transfusion bag saying "Irradiated blood product" or "Irradiated."

- **Complications of platelet transfusions include hemolytic and nonhemolytic transfusion reactions, graft versus host disease (GVHD), and transfusion-related acute lung injury (TRALI).**
- **The nurse should transfuse whole blood to restore and maintain blood volume during acute hemorrhage.**

- For septic shock associated with thrombocytopenia consider these areas for interventions in critical care: hemodynamic monitoring (CVP), pulmonary capillary wedge pressure (PCWP), PAP, cardiac output (CO), electrocardiogram (ECG); respiratory monitoring (ABGs, breath sounds); fluids and electrolytes; and neurologic (alert, oriented, confused) and hematologic monitoring (complete blood count [CBC], platelet count, D-dimer to assess for DIC, FDP, prothrombin time [PT], partial thromboplastin time [PTT]).

Do You UNDERSTAND?

DIRECTIONS: Circle the correct answers.

1. Circle all the places in the body where platelets mature.

pelvis	ribs	long bones	bladder
kidneys	sternum	skull	heart

2. Circle all the diseases that can be associated with thrombocytopenia.

AIDS	colitis	cirrhosis
scurvy	leukemia	stroke

DIRECTIONS: Match the body system in Column A with the appropriate nursing assessment in Column B for a patient with thrombocytopenia.

Column A

_____ 3. Neurologic
_____ 4. Respiratory
_____ 5. GI
_____ 6. GU

Column B

a. Blood in the urine
b. Hematemesis
c. Headache
d. Hemoptysis

DIRECTIONS: Choose the correct answer for each of the following statements from the two italicized options listed in the parentheses.

7. A thrombocytopenic patient with epistaxis should have his or her body

placed in high _____ position.

(*dorsal recumbent, Fowler's*)

8. Bleeding from the bronchus in a patient with thrombocytopenia can be

stopped by the use of _____.

(*a balloon catheter, topical dopamine*)

9. The patient has a total platelet count of 4000 cells/mm^3, and the nurse has

just discontinued one of the patient's peripheral IV sites. The nurse should

apply pressure to this IV site for at least _____.

(*1 minute, 5 minutes*)

10. The patient is thrombocytopenic and wants to brush his or her teeth. The

nurse should offer a _____ toothbrush.

(*hard bristle, spongelike*)

**DIRECTIONS: Match the medication or treatment in Column A with the
rationale in Column B associated with a patient with
thrombocytopenia.**

Column A	Column B
_____ 11. Epinephrine	a. Augments coagulation factors in the liver
_____ 12. Fresh frozen	b. Stimulates platelet production in the
plasma transfusion	bone marrow
_____ 13. Folate	c. Assists in hepatic synthesis of factors II,
_____ 14. Vitamin K	VII, IX, and X
	d. Releases platelets from the spleen

What IS Disseminated Intravascular Coagulation?

DIC is a condition that clinically ranges from an acute situation in which
excessive hemorrhaging and thrombosis occurs to a chronic presentation with
minor abnormalities of diffuse bleeding and thrombosis of generalized or local
organ infiltration. Stages of microvascular clotting followed by active hemorrhaging characterize DIC, because of two important factors: (1) consumption

of coagulation factors and platelets and (2) fibrinolysis. Underlying or associative causes for DIC include shock states (sepsis, anaphylactic, circulatory), blood transfusion reactions, neoplasms, vascular and hematopoietic disorders, obstetric complications (retained fetus, eclampsia, septic abortion, abruptio placentae), crush and tissue injury or necrosis, and liver disease.

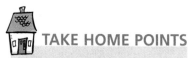

TAKE HOME POINTS

In DIC, diffuse bleeding and clotting occur.

What You NEED TO KNOW

Initiation of DIC results when tissue thromboplastin and tissue factor is liberated by tissue injury (resulting in activation of the extrinsic pathway) or with endothelial damage (thereby instigating the intrinsic pathway). Regardless of the causative and precipitating factor, widespread systemic hypercoagulation results in microvascular and macrovascular thrombosis. Vascular thrombosis interferes with blood flow and potentially results in peripheral ischemia and end-organ destruction. Because organ perfusion is severely hampered, clinical manifestations of multisystem organ dysfunction ultimately result. All organs are involved, but those most at risk include the skin, lungs, and kidneys.

After diffuse microvascular clotting, hemorrhage emerges as the next step in the evolution of DIC. Consumption of the clotting factors and platelets occurs because of systemic coagulation; therefore activation of the fibrinolytic system arises, producing disseminated fibrinolysis. The normal lysis of clots (fibrinolysis) is produced in the clotting cascade. Because of the overwhelming nature of thrombosis, subsequent lysis of clots is equally intense. (See diagram on the following page.)

Diagnosis

Diagnosis of DIC is most reliably based on clinical signs and symptoms. Laboratory evidence is very beneficial in confirmation of clinical manifestations. Often, abnormal clotting profiles in patients with DIC will demonstrate thrombocytopenia, prolonged clotting times (PT and activated partial thromboplastin time [aPTT]), and suppressed clotting factors. Another diagnostic test is the D-dimer, which is helpful in identifying the activity of thrombin and fibrinolysis, which are integral in the pathophysiology of DIC.

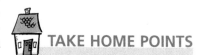

TAKE HOME POINTS

The D-dimer is the most reliable, specific diagnostic test for diagnosing DIC.

Clinical Manifestations

With two separate phases of DIC, clinical manifestations can be widespread, but overall they signify the lack of tissue perfusion, and ultimately, poor tissue oxygenation. With the development of microemboli in the vascular circulation, signs and symptoms reflect the lack of tissue oxygenation, which may vary from ischemia to total tissue infarction, ultimately resulting in cellular death. Ischemic changes affect all tissue and organ systems, leading to end-organ failure and possible multisystem organ dysfunction. Because of tissue ischemia and the normal process of clot formation, the body reacts with lysis of clots to increase perfusion to O_2- and nutrient-deprived areas. Because of the extent of

Pathophysiology of Disseminated Intravascular Coagulation

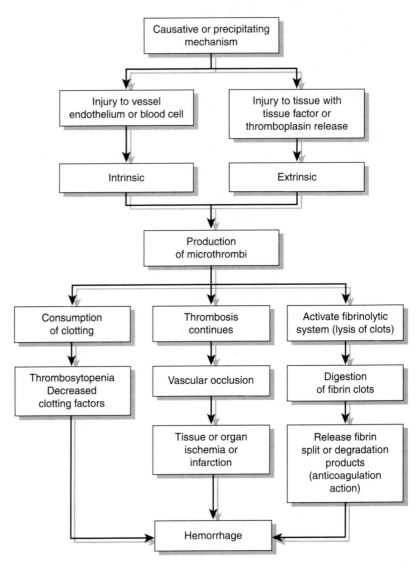

lysis of clot formation and consumption of coagulation factors with microemboli development, massive hemorrhage can occur throughout the systemic circulation. Hemorrhaging can further tissue ischemia and worsen possible existing shock states. Circulatory collapse, because of massive bleeding, can necessitate the further use of blood products and vasopressors to maintain tissue perfusion, end-organ perfusion, and oxygenation. Clinical manifestations in organ systems, including ischemic and hemorrhagic changes, are further detailed following:

Ischemic and Infarct Changes in Organ Systems in Disseminated Intravascular Coagulation

SYSTEM	ISCHEMIC	TISSUE INFARCTION
Skin	Pale Cyanosis	Necrosis Gangrene
CNS	Confusion Coma Transient ischemic attacks	Infarct Stroke (CVA)
Renal	Oliguria Azotemia	Acute renal failure Necrosis
Lungs	Hypoxia	Pulmonary embolism Pulmonary infarction
GI	Ulcers Decreased bowel sounds	Bowel necrosis Lack of bowel sounds

CNS, Central nervous system; *CVA*, cerebrovascular accident; *GI*, gastrointestinal.

Hemorrhage and Effects on Organ Systems in Disseminated Intravascular Coagulation

SYSTEM	EFFECTS
Skin	Bruising Bleeding from central lines and puncture sites
CNS	Cerebral bleeding Acute change in level of consciousness
Renal	Hematuria Oliguria
Lungs	Hemoptysis Hypoxia
GI	Distended abdomen Bloody emesis, stool

CNS, Central nervous system; *GI*, gastrointestinal.

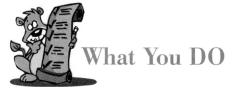

What You DO

Medical management of DIC is based on the individualized patient's condition and underlying cause. The first step is removal of the underlying pathology if possible. Generally treatment includes transfusion of blood products, such as packed red blood cells, platelets, fresh frozen plasma (to correct clotting factors consumption); as well as cryoprecipitate (factor VIII) to correct hypofibrinogenemia.

Heparin therapy continues to be a controversial treatment modality. Heparin inhibits the coagulation process by preventing tissue factor from initiating the extrinsic pathway, thus preventing consumption of coagulation factors and fibrin accumulation. However, heparin and other antifibrinolytic agents (especially when used concurrently) are generally contraindicated in patients at risk for severe bleeding dysfunctions and thrombotic complications.

To ensure optimal tissue and organ perfusion while maintaining BP, CO, and urine output, fluid resuscitation will be required with possible vasopressor therapy. Invasive hemodynamic monitoring may be used to provide further data about intravascular volume and perfusion. Hypoperfusion and organ ischemia necessitate the implementation of interventions to decrease O_2 demand and increase O_2 delivery. O_2 provision is accomplished through many avenues, which may include mechanical ventilation. Along with providing O_2, decreasing the demand is possible with sedation, decreased temperature (using antipyretics), pain control (using narcotics), and rest. Ensuring that O_2-carrying capacity is optimized requires assessing a patient's blood count and replacing blood products as necessary.

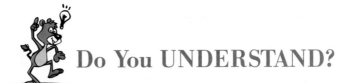

Do You UNDERSTAND?

DIRECTIONS: **Provide a short answer to each of the following questions.**

1. What are the two distinct stages that characterize DIC?

2. Hemorrhaging within DIC occurs mainly because of what two factors?

3. What are some precipitating mechanisms for DIC?

_____

_____

_____

_____

_____

4. What is the most important step in the medical management of DIC?

_____

_____

_____

5. What is the most reliable, specific laboratory test for diagnosing DIC?

_____

6. What monitoring skills are important to ensure optimal tissue and organ perfusion?

_____

_____

_____

_____

_____

_____

11 Integumentary System

What IS a Burn?

Burns are a group of conditions with outcomes that include the removal of skin by thermal (heat or radiation), chemical, or electrical means. Removal of skin can be planned, such as in electrodessication of warts or removal of pyogenic granulomas or skin cancers, or unplanned, such as in accidents or infliction by intentional harm.

What You NEED TO KNOW

More than 2 million cases of burns, including 440,000 children, are seen in the United States each year. Just over half of all fatalities occur at work. In addition, the report of sunburn by adult's ages 18 to 29 years is high at 57.5%. Burns in the elderly have a high mortality rate of about 59%. Those over 65 years include burns by scalding in 41%, flame burns in 53%, and electrical burns in 3%. Assessment of all burns includes the type of burn (thermal, electrical, or chemical) and severity (depth, extent, and co-morbid conditions).

- Burns in children are more severe than in adults because of their smaller body surface areas (BSAs) are less able to regulate temperature, skin thickness, and higher fluid volume needs.
- Dementia (44%), alcohol use (21%), and cigarette use (10%) account for the majority of burns in the older adult population.

The type of burn indicates the initial care implemented. The severity of the burn includes the depth of the burn (superficial, partial thickness, or full thickness) and the extent of the burn based on percent of body area burned (rule of nines).

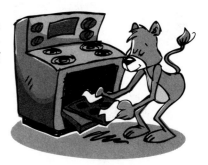

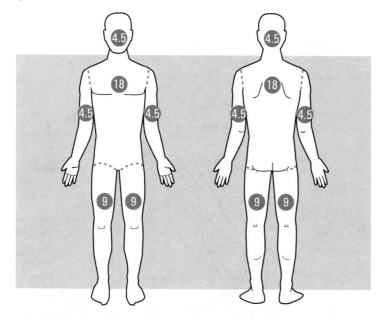

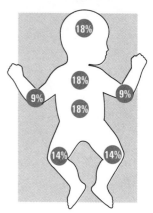

FIRST-LINE AND INITIAL TREATMENTS FOR ENSURING SAFETY AT THE BURN SCENE

- **Thermal.** Ensure scene safety for the nurse and the victim. Remove the victim from the unsafe area only if trained to do so.
- **Electrical.** Ensure scene safety. Do not touch the victim until a person trained to remove the electrical power source does so.
- **Chemical.** Ensure scene safety. A person knowledgeable in chemical fire should determine safety. Wear protective clothing.

Electrical burns are divided into high- and low-voltage burns. High-voltage electrical burns occur with 1000 volts or greater, and low-voltage electrical burns occur with <1000 volts. Tissue injury resulting from electricity is the result of electric energy being converted into heat, and the greatest heat is at the contact points. Four types of injuries are associated with an electrical burn:

Entrance wounds. Caused by entry of electric current into the body and might appear as flat, black or depressed

Exit wounds. Caused by electric current exiting the body and might appear as black, charred, and "blown out" as the current exits the body

Arc wounds. Caused by the electric current crossing a specific body part (e.g., knee, elbow, axilla) and an increase in temperature occurs that elicits a "petechiae-type" appearance

Thermal wounds. Caused by electrical current that ignites a person's clothing, resulting in a thermal burn

Superficial burns. Epidermis only—pain and redness (average recovery time is 1 week)

Partial-thickness burns. Epidermis plus dermis—pain and blistering (average recovery time is 2 months)

Full-thickness burns. All skin layers involved; may include subcutaneous tissue, bones, muscles, and organs (painless if nerves are burnt; average recovery time is 6 months to 1 year)

Depth of Burn Injuries

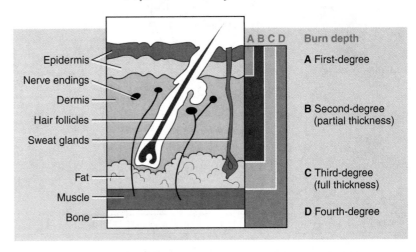

The co-morbidities to assess for in patients with burns include the following:

- Age <5 years old or >55 years old
- Burns to joints, face, genitals, feet, or hands
- Burn encircles body
- Preexisting organ illness: lung disease, heart disease, liver disease, kidney disease
- Preexisting immunosuppression as a result of cancer or acquired immunodeficiency syndrome (AIDS)
- Neurologic trauma such as cervical spine fracture

The physiologic response of the body to a burn has three phases:

1. During the first phase, initially (and up to 48 hours later) a shift of the plasma into the interstitial fluid occurs, causing dehydration, edema, hypotension, decreased cardiac output, increased pulse, oliguria and anuria, hyperkalemia, hyponatremia, increased hematocrit and a bicarbonate deficit.

2. The second phase is the phase of diuresis that occurs 48 to 72 hours postburn. A tremendous increase in urinary output occurs, as well as pulmonary edema because of circulatory overload, decreased hematocrit, hyponatremia, hypokalemia, and a bicarbonate deficit.

3. The third and final phase is called *recovery* and begins around the fifth day. In this phase the patient has hypocalcemia, hyponatremia, hypokalemia, a negative nitrogen balance, and weight loss. The most serious complication in patients with burns is sepsis, and identifying initial signs in the patient can save his or her life. These signs include changes in sensorium, fever, tachycardia, tachypnea, paralytic ileus, abdominal distention, and oliguria.

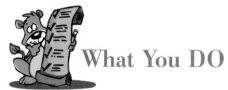 # What You DO

1. Initially, the nurse should try to extinguish and remove the source of the burn. For thermal heat burns the subject should be rolled on the ground and a blanket or shirt should be used to cover the fire. Water should be used on smoldering clothes and chemical burns. The nurse should remember to remove objects that can conduct heat, such as clothing, jewelry, eyeglasses, and false limbs, because ischemia could result from swelling because of a tourniquet-like effect. For radiation seed burns, the nurse should remove the radiation source using special forceps and place the source immediately in a lead-lined box. For chemical burns, the chemical should be removed by copious amounts of irrigation with water or known antidote.

 The web site for care of burns can be found at www.burnsurgery.com.

FIRST-LINE AND INITIAL TREATMENTS FOR BURNS

- **STOP** the burning process. The type or extent of burn will determine whether this may be implemented in the prehospital setting or in the receiving hospital's emergency department.

2. Assess ABCDEF (**A**irway; **B**reathing; **C**irculation, **C**-spine immobilization, Cardiac status; **D**isability, **N**eurologic deficit; **E**xpose body for assessment; **F**luid resuscitation, **F**ahrenheit for assessment of signs of hypothermia).
   - Assess the airway for patency, and note any cyanosis or pharyngeal edema.
   - Assess breathing for shortness of breath, hoarseness, and difficulty swallowing. Be prepared for the possibilities of intubation, suctioning, hemodynamic monitoring, central venous catheter insertion, oxygenation, and mechanical ventilation.
3. Call 911 for emergency assistance.
4. Assess for cervical spine injury; if cervical spine injury is probable, do not move the person.
5. Assess the level of consciousness. Burns will not alter the level of consciousness. Therefore it is important to collect a detailed history from the patient: How did the burn happen? Did it occur in a closed space? Was there a possibility of smoke inhalation? Were chemicals involved? Was there any related trauma? Were any medications used?
6. Initiate body substance isolation to protect from infectious organisms.

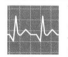 The nurse should assess distal circulation to extremity burns, especially when encircled, because a decreased or absence of a pulse to a given area can result in limited circulation, ischemia, or cell death and ultimately result in amputation of the extremity for the patient.

7. Initiate emergency burn management associated with specific type of burn.
   - **Thermal burns:**
     - Evaluate for smoke inhalation and respiratory burn. Maintain the airway.
     - Cool the burn with water at 2 to 5 minutes.
     - Cover the burn with a dry dressing.
   - **Electrical burns:**
     - Check and monitor vital signs. Anticipate cardiopulmonary arrest. Perform cardiopulmonary resuscitation (CPR) if needed.
     - Look for entrance and exit sites.
     - Cover burns with dry dressings.
   - **Chemical burns:**
     - Remove all contaminated clothes.
     - Flush with water 20 minutes after brushing off powders.
     - Apply a dry dressing.
8. In general, potential problems should be assessed, such as respiratory distress, sepsis, gastrointestinal (GI) bleeding, pain, anxiety, paralytic ileus, and oliguria.
9. Pain should be relieved.
10. Generally, the priority treatment interventions are focused on ventilation and oxygenation, fluid replacement for hypovolemia and electrolytes with Ringer's lactate, humidity regulation, dressing changes, and skin grafting. Closed dressings for superficial to partial thickness usually include Xeroform-Bacitracin, silver sulfadiazine, or biobrane followed by a layer of gauze and Flexnet or ace bandage. Lipidocolloid dressings, such as Urgotul, helps patients heal faster with second-degree burns.
11. Emotional support should be provided. The nurse should be sensitive to the variable emotions that burn patients and their families will experience. Feelings of guilt, fear, anxiety, anger, and depression must be recognized and addressed.
12. Suicide management is important. Self-immolation or other forms of suicide by burning should be considered when a reasonable explanation of the mechanism of the burn is lacking. After an unsuccessful suicide attempt, the patient is usually lucid and talkative, either denying the attempt or voluntarily providing information. Pertinent historical information that may facilitate special case management includes the following:
    - Recent onset of problems involving family, marriage, job, finances, or health
    - Expressions of hopelessness
    - History of alcohol or drug abuse
    - History of emotional problems

Immediate management is directed toward protection of the patient from further attempts at self-destruction by controlling agitation, screening for drug and alcohol overdose, and prescribing a mandatory psychiatric consultation.

After emergency treatment is completed, the interventions for the postemergency phase begin. These interventions include ventilator- and respiratory-dependent management, 12-lead electrocardiogram (ECG) monitoring, hemodynamic monitoring (via central venous pressure [CVP] line, pulmonary artery [PA] catheter, or arterial line), assessment of laboratory and diagnostic tests (complete blood count [CBC]; electrolytes; type and cross match for blood transfusion; serum creatinine for kidney function; albumin and total protein for nutritional status; arterial blood gases [ABGs] for respiratory function; and serum glucose, alkaline phosphatase, calcium, phosphorus, chest radiograph, computed tomographic [CT] scans), nasogastric (NG) tube to low suction for decompression, pain medication as needed, strict intake and output, tetanus toxoid injection to prevent infection from the *Clostridium tetani* organism, antibiotics as prescribed, nutritional management, wound care (including skin grafts with artificial skin such as Integra or with donor skin), and assessment for other injuries (fractures, head injury, chest injuries, and abdominal injury).

Patients with burns have four major systems in which physical complications can occur: (1) the immune system related to infection, (2) GI system related to hemorrhage or paralytic ileus (paralysis of the intestine leading to obstruction), (3) pulmonary system related to respiratory distress syndrome or pneumonia, and (4) the musculoskeletal system associated with contractures. Infections are one of the most serious complications with *Pseudomonas*, most commonly occurring within 36 hours postburn, and hemolytic *Staphylococcus aureus*, occurring up to 1 week postburn. Sepsis is the most serious complication, and patients who are more susceptible have impaired production of macrophage inflammatory protein 1 (MPH-1) alpha. Contractures are a problematic sequelae that can limit mobility and function. The use of devices, such as the Watusi neck collar, can improve function, comfort, and mobility.

A need also exists for house assessment, especially for the elderly. Do they have signs of dementia? Is their tap water temperature regulated so that it is not above 43° C? Do they have ashtrays that are large enough to use? Do they have moderate alcohol consumption?

- Insertion of central venous catheter near or overlapping an open wound should be avoided and not left in place more than 3 days to prevent catheter-related infections.
- The use of intravenous (IV) albumin has been shown to increase the risk of death by 5%, and therefore its use needs to be substantiated.
- Electrical wires should only be removed with wood, rubber, or plastic objects (never with metal objects or bare hands).

TAKE HOME POINTS

Urinary output >70 ml/hr is beneficial to survival.

What IS Inhalation Injury?

Inhalation injury occurs with the aspiration of heated gases or by-products of burned materials. Approximately 20% of patients admitted with burns have some degree of inhalation injuries, which result in impaired gas exchange and altered hemodynamics.

TAKE HOME POINTS

Inhalation injuries have a profound effect on mortality.

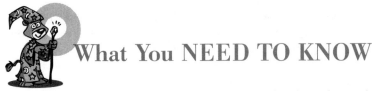

What You NEED TO KNOW

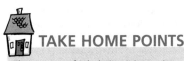

TAKE HOME POINTS

Three types of inhalation injury exist: (1) above the glottis, (2) below the glottis, and (3) carbon monoxide poisoning.

The respiratory system from the upper airway to the alveoli can be involved in inhalation injury. The mucosal barrier can be burned, resulting in edema, tissue sloughing, and airway obstruction. Chemicals and irritating gases can trigger bronchospasm. Inhalation injuries result in mucosal edema and loss of airway patency, bronchospasm, intrapulmonary shunting, decreased lung compliance, pneumonias, bronchiectasis, and respiratory failure.

Inhalation injuries are primarily diagnosed through physical assessment data obtained from the patient. On initial presentation, patients may have little or no pulmonary distress and the initial chest radiograph may appear normal. The most useful adjuncts include history, physical exam, and bronchoscopy. Singed nasal hairs, facial burns, carbonaceous material on teeth, and a history of aspiration of hot steam or liquid may indicate the presence of inhalation injuries.

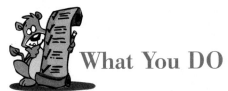

What You DO

Airway patency is essential in the management of patients with inhalation injuries. Change in vocal volume, character of voice, lack of ability to handle secretions, hoarseness, and stridor requires intubation. Laryngoscopy or fiberoptic bronchoscopy can be useful in accomplishing intubation in a timely manner before edema becomes advanced.

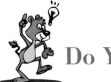

Do You UNDERSTAND?

DIRECTIONS: **Match the types of burn in Column A with the appropriate interventions in Column B.**

Column A	Column B
_____ 1. Chemical	a. Use wood to remove source.
_____ 2. Electrical	b. Remove source with copious amounts of water.
_____ 3. Thermal	c. Use blanket to smother fire.

DIRECTIONS: **Identify the following statements as *True* (T) or *False* (F).**

_____ 4. Partial thickness is a co-morbid condition.

_____ 5. Superficial burns are never painful.

_____ 6. Hypotension is a common physiologic response to an initial burn.

Answers: 1. b; 2. a; 3. c; 4. F; 5. F; 6. T.

DIRECTIONS: Circle all the assessment criteria for assessing breathing in a patient who has been burnt.

7. hoarseness   pharyngeal edema   finger clubbing

   limb flaccidity   difficulty swallowing   color of sclera

DIRECTIONS: Match the laboratory tests in Column A with the associated body systems in the burned patient in Column B.

Column A   Column B

_____   8. Type and cross match   a. Hematologic for blood transfusion
_____   9. Serum creatinine   b. Nutritional status
_____ 10. Albumin and total protein c. Respiratory
_____ 11. ABGs   d. Kidney

DIRECTIONS: Fill in the blanks to complete the following statements.

12. The most serious complication of burns is _____.

13. A CVP line is used for _____ monitoring.

14. A(n) _____ tube is inserted to decompress the stomach.

15. The GI complication of burn patients that includes paralysis of the

    intestines is called _____ _____.

What IS Skin Breakdown?

Skin breakdown may include redness, edema, heat, and broken barriers in the body's largest organ, the skin. Nurses in the critical care environment are constantly challenged by variables that can make patients more susceptible to skin injury. Multiple lines from monitoring devices, feeding tubes and catheters, restraints, and the patient's limited capability to protect himself or herself can lead to skin breakdown.

To prevent damage to a patient's skin, the nurse must be able to identify factors in the management that may result in breakdown. In patients with low tissue tolerance, irreversible damage can occur in as little as 2 hours. The ulcer may not appear for 3 to 5 days after the initial insult occurs. Damages incurred to the

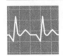

Skin and pressure areas should be monitored daily for any signs of actual or impending breakdown.

TAKE HOME POINTS

Skin breakdown is expensive to manage.

skin may not only be painful and debilitating to the patient but also can be very expensive. Statistics for the cost incurred with a pressure ulcer ranges from $5000 to $40,000 per ulcer. With a larger portion of patients being Medicare eligible, the complete identification of disease-related groups (DRGs) on the admission diagnosis becomes increasingly important. Failure to document actual or impending breakdown on admission can penalize the hospital in terms of reimbursement for services rendered.

In evaluating data regarding skin breakdown, one has to look at the prevalence and incidence of pressure ulcers. **Prevalence** looks at the percentage of patients with breakdown at one point in time. One can also look at admissions to determine the percentage of patients with breakdown on admission versus those who acquired a pressure ulcer or some other form of skin injury after admission (nosocomial breakdown). This is known as **incidence.**

Additionally, the incidence of lawsuits related to skin breakdown are increasing. The public is better informed and realizes that most pressure ulcers are preventable. The liability to the hospital and its personnel increases when protocols and policies are not consistent with national guidelines, or if the guidelines are not being followed. This section looks at the normal physiology of the skin, identifies those variables that cause skin breakdown, the subsequent staging of pressure ulcers, and the nursing management and wound care that can be implemented to promote healing while controlling costs.

What You NEED TO KNOW

The skin is the largest organ in the body. It covers approximately 3000 square inches or an area almost equivalent to 2 m^2. One role of the skin is to protect the individual from factors in the environment that might cause harm, and it also helps to maintain a state of internal homeostasis. The skin consists of several layers including the epidermis, basal membrane zone, dermis, and subcutaneous tissue. The skin lies directly over the fascia and muscle; it normally has a good blood supply and is very sensitive to pressure changes. This sensitivity aids the patient in determining when things may cause harm or injury.

Structure of Skin
and its Relationship to Subcutaneous Tissue

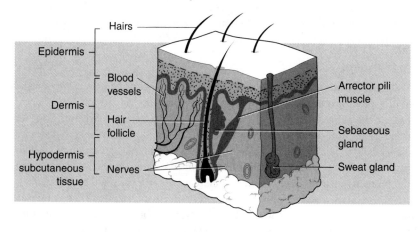

The skin normally has certain neighbors (bacteria) that take up residence on the skin's surface. Other bacteria come and go as the opportunity presents itself. When the outer layer of skin becomes disrupted from maceration, shear, or pressure, this invites certain opportunistic bacteria to establish themselves in a warm, moist environment. This environment is a great soil medium for bacterial and fungal growth. This may result in an infection and further cellular destruction. A young adult can normally replace the epidermis within 21 days. By age 35, this same process can take up to 42 days. This prolonged turnover time leads to a thinner skin covering, wrinkling, increased risk of tears, reduced activity of oil and sweat glands, decreased sensation, loss of thermal insulation, reduced blood flow, and an increased risk for infection. All of these increase the patient's potential for skin breakdown and trauma.

TAKE HOME POINTS

Several functions of the skin are protection, heat regulation, sensory perception, excretion, synthesis of vitamin D, and enhancement of self-image.

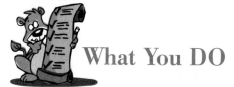
What You DO

Nurses must act as the patient's eyes and ears when it comes to completing a thorough assessment of the many variables that may lead to a disruption of the skin's integrity. The nurse must be skilled in the evaluation of actual or impending breakdown (evidenced by areas of discoloration, warmth, fluctuance, or indurations over a bony prominence) and take measures that will prevent further damage. Numerous risk assessment tools are on the market today that can help the staff nurse to determine if the patient is at risk for breakdown. The Agency for Healthcare Research and Quality (AHRQ) provides guidelines for identifying those individuals that are at risk. The Braden scale for predicting pressure ulcer development identifies six subscales: (1) sensory perception, (2) moisture, (3) activity, (4) mobility, (5) nutrition, and (6) friction and shear that are used to determine the patient's potential for skin breakdown. The nurse's clinical judgment is used to score the patient and intervene with the appropriate measures that will maintain the patient's intact skin. In an acute care setting, the initial assessment should be completed on admission and then reassessed at least every 24 hours or when the patient's condition changes, which could be as often as once a shift.

Assessment

Moisture. Is the patient's skin moist as a result of incontinency or diaphoresis? Will a prescription for an indwelling catheter or fecal incontinence collector benefit the patient? To prevent maceration one can initiate lubricants or other skin barrier protectants to retard water loss from the skin. Commercial pads or a diaper help to wick moisture away from the skin. The nurse should offer a bed-pan or urinal in conjunction with turning. The use of alkaline soaps that remove the protective barrier on the skin and increase water loss should be avoided.

Sensory status, activity, and mobility. The nurse must assess the mental and physical variables of the patient. Is the patient mobile? Can the patient turn himself or herself? Is the patient restrained? Has he or she had a stroke? Does he or she have a complication such as diabetic neuropathy that limits the ability to recognize when the damage from continuous pressure is occurring? Is the patient spending most of the day in bed or in a chair without turning? Will the patient's condition allow turning at 30-degree angles at least every 2 hours with emphasis on pressure-reducing devices being implemented for the heels, as well as pillows between the knees and under bony prominences such as the elbows?

Friction and shear. What is the patient's weight? Is a lift sheet available for repositioning the patient in bed? Is the skin susceptible to shearing? With age, reduced cohesion between the epidermis and dermis increases the risk for shearing. Drugs such as prednisone (Deltasone), a steroid, causes the layers of the skin to become thinner over time.

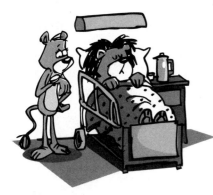

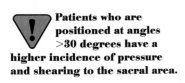 **TAKE HOME POINTS**

- When a patient sits or rests in one position for an extended period of time (more than 2 hours), all layers of the skin become compressed. The layer most affected is the muscle because of the compression of the vital blood supply.
- The nurse should remember that pressure ulcers start deep at the muscle and bone interface.

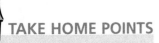 **Patients who are positioned at angles >30 degrees have a higher incidence of pressure and shearing to the sacral area.**

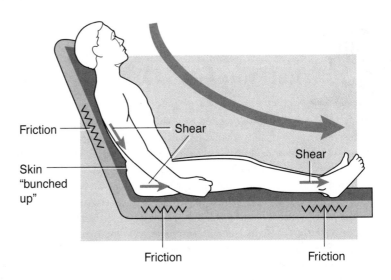

Friction

Shear

Skin "bunched up"

Shear

Friction

Friction

Nutritional status. How much of the patient's meal did he or she eat and drink? Is the patient near ideal body weight? Has there been a 10 lb weight gain or loss over the past week. What is the patient's prealbumin level? What is the 24-hour urine output? What route is the patient presently being fed? Is there any related disease that may affect the patient's nutritional status (i.e., inflammatory bowel disease, Crohn's disease, diabetes)? The nurse should consult a dietitian to determine if a supplement with a multivitamin containing vitamins A, C, and E would be beneficial or a diet high in protein, iron, and vitamin C would help to improve healing.

When All Else Fails

As noted previously, skin damage can occur from a multitude of variables. This section will identify some of the most common types, including partial- and full-thickness skin loss as they relate to pressure ulcer development, shear injuries, and the management of each. Other injuries to the skin that include venous stasis and arterial ulcers are not be covered in this chapter.

PARTIAL-THICKNESS SKIN LOSS

With this injury the epidermis and possibly a portion of the dermis are lost. It is caused by friction, blunt trauma, or sanding away of the surface layer. It is superficial, painful, red, or displays a pale, moist base with visible epidermal islet cells. The injury usually starts with erythema and tenderness. If left untreated, it may extend down through the subcutaneous fat.

NURSING MANAGEMENT

The nurse should try to eliminate the cause (shear, moisture, pressure, irritant) of loss of skin integrity. Shear results from a combination of friction and gravity. If the nurse drags a patient up in bed while allowing the skin to maintain contact with the sheets, he or she is going to promote friction, shear, and probable skin damage. Gentle skin care with moisturizers should be provided if the skin is unbroken.

The nurse should apply heel and elbow protectors and avoid taping over fragile skin as much as possible. A moist wound surface should be maintained while keeping the surrounding surface dry. A transparent dressing may work nicely for minimal exudates and healthy skin, whereas a foam dressing may be a better choice for heavy drainage and fragile skin that would not hold up well under the aggressive adhesiveness of transparent dressings. A sealant (clear liquid plastic polymer usually contained in a cotton swab) can be applied to the skin surrounding the wound. This prevents moisture from coming in contact with the intact skin while preventing stripping from tapes. Considerations for the topical dressing must include the status of the surrounding skin and the amount of moisture that needs to be absorbed. A new linear or flap type of skin tear may need to be cleansed thoroughly with a commercial saline-based skin cleanser, steri-stripped to approximate the wound edges, and then covered with a nonadherent dressing (e.g., Telfa), an oil-coated product such as Adaptic, and 4 × 4 inch gauze or foam. These dressings can be secured with wrap gauze or elastic mesh netting. Other choices may include a thin hydrocolloid or a solid hydrogel wafer.

FIRST-LINE AND INITIAL TREATMENTS FOR SKIN BREAKDOWN

- Eliminate the cause of loss of skin integrity.
- Provide gentle skin care.
- Apply skin protection (i.e., heel and elbow protectors).
- Maintain a moist wound surface.
- Use a sealant.
- Apply dressings.

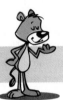

What IS A Pressure Ulcer?

A pressure ulcer (also called a *bed sore*) is an injury caused by constant pressure to the skin and muscle.

What You NEED TO KNOW

Stage I Pressure Ulcer

A Stage I pressure ulcer is an observable pressure-related alteration of skin with indicators (as compared with an adjacent or opposite area on the body) that may include changes in one or more of the following: skin temperature (warmth or coolness), tissue consistency (firmness or boggy feel), and sensation (pain, itching). The ulcer appears as a defined area of persistent redness in lightly pigmented skin, whereas in darker skin tones the ulcer may appear with persistent red, blue, or purple hues (see Color Insert Plate 7a).

Stage II Pressure Ulcer

A Stage II pressure ulcer has a partial-thickness loss of skin involving epidermis, dermis, or both. The ulcer is superficial and presents clinically as an abrasion, blister, or shallow crater (see Color Insert Plate 7b).

Stage III Pressure Ulcer

A Stage III pressure ulcer has a full-thickness loss of skin involving damage or necrosis of subcutaneous tissue that may extend down to, but not through, underlying fascia. The surface of the wound may contain **slough,** which is necrotic or dead tissue and bacteria. It can be white, beige, yellow, or rust colored. Slough consistency can be dry, crusty, slimy, rubbery, or moist. Removal of this devitalized tissue is necessary for wound healing (see Color Insert Plate 7c).

The ulcer presents clinically as a deep crater with or without undermining of adjacent tissue. A Stage III wound may also contain **eschar.** Eschar is the necrotic "leathery" covering on the wound at the skin surface. It can be black-brown-tan and hard-pliable. Eschar is a form of necrotic tissue. Removal of devitalized tissue is necessary for wound healing. The wound can become larger as the débridement progresses. When a wound involves necrotic tissue, staging cannot be confirmed until the wound base is visible.

Stage IV Pressure Ulcer

A Stage IV pressure ulcer has a full-thickness skin loss with extensive destruction, tissue necrosis, or damage to muscle, bone, or supporting structures (i.e., tendon, joint capsule). Undermining and sinus tracts may also be associated with Stage IV pressure ulcers (see Color Insert Plate 7d).

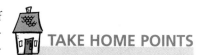

TAKE HOME POINTS

The AHCPR guidelines recommend heel ulcers with dry eschar need not be débrided if they do not develop complications such as edema, erythema, or drainage.

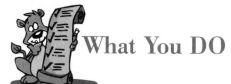

What You DO

Treatment of Stage I Pressure Ulcer

The nurse should do the following:
1. Cleanse the skin area with tap water.
2. Pat it dry.
3. Consider the following options for topical applications:
   - Apply barrier ointment daily as indicated until the ulcer is healed.
   - Apply a transparent dressing sized to at least 2 inches beyond the affected area. Change it every 5 days as needed until it is healed.
   - Apply second-generation barrier cream (about $1/4$ inch depth initially).
   - Reapply barrier ointment and dressing every 12 hours until healed. It is not necessary to remove all layers of the cream with each cleansing. Simply remove fecal- or urine-contaminated layers only. Reapply a thin layer only.
4. Suspend heels off the bed with a pillow or another supportive device.

Treatment of Stage II Pressure Ulcer

The nurse should do the following:
1. Cleanse Stage II pressure ulcer with normal saline (NS) or a commercial wound cleanser.
2. Pat it dry.
3. Consider the following options for topical applications:
   - Apply a hydrocolloid dressing (thin or regular thickness at least 2 inches beyond the affected area). Apply a sacral-shaped dressing if near the anal verge. Change every 3 to 5 days and as needed if loose or soiled until healed. Remove dressing with an adhesive removal wipe.

- Apply a transparent dressing if drainage is minimal and the patient is not elderly with fragile skin.
- Apply a hydrogel sheet approximately 2 inches wider than the wound. Secure with a perforated tape. Change every 3 to 5 days.
- Apply a second-generation barrier cream. Cleanse and reapply three times daily and as needed until healed. It is not necessary to remove the entire old barrier cream with each cleansing.
- Apply foam dressing to the site if the drainage is copious. Apply impermeable secondary dressing and change every 2 to 3 days or as needed if soiled until healed.

Treatment of Stage III Pressure Ulcer

The nurse should do the following:
1. Prepare for surgical debridement.
2. Dressing changes as prescribed.

Treatment of Stage IV Pressure Ulcer

The nurse should do the following:
1. Cleanse Stage IV pressure ulcer with NS or an appropriate commercial wound cleanser.
2. Pat it dry.
3. Consider the following options for topical applications:
   - Apply a barrier ointment or a skin barrier protectant swab to the skin immediately surrounding the wound.
   - Apply hydrogel-impregnated gauze or amorphous hydrogel. Cover it with gauze, bordered gauze, composite dressing, or rolled gauze. Change the dressing daily, every other day, or three times a week until the ulcer is healed.
   - Apply a hydrogel sheet sized approximately 2 inches larger than the actual wound. Secure it with tape, stretch net, or rolled gauze. Change it every 3 to 5 days and as needed if it is loose or soiled until the ulcer is healed.
   - Apply an alginate dressing sheet (allow dressing to overlap slightly onto intact skin). Cover with a gauze, bordered gauze, or composite dressing. Secure it with tape or a stretch net. Change it daily, every other day, or three times a week, depending on the amount of exudates or saturation of secondary dressing until the ulcer is healed.
   - Apply an alginate dressing rope (fill cavity loosely). Cover it with a gauze, bordered gauze, and composite dressing or roll gauze. Secure it with tape or stretch net if needed. Change daily, every other day, or three times a week, depending on the amount of drainage.

- Apply an alginate rope dressing to fill any cavity loosely. Cover it with a foam dressing if drainage is heavy. Secure it with tape or stretch net. Change every other day or three times a week, depending on the amount of exudates until the ulcer is healed.
- Apply a hydrogel pad (polyacrylate) slightly wet, sized to overlap slightly onto the intact skin, impregnated with Ringer's solution (green stripes away from the wound). Cover it with an appropriate gauze dressing and secure it in place with tape or stretch net. Change it daily.

An enzymatic débridement ointment (Collagenase Santyl, Accuzyme, or Panafil) may also be used to chemically remove devitalized tissue. One must determine whether the tissue is dry or moist. This will affect the time required to remove the dead tissue.

A surgeon using a scalpel and suture may perform sharp débridement. A nurse certified in WOCN may perform conservative sharp débridement using forceps and surgical scissors.

Wound Care Dressings

DRESSING	DESCRIPTION	WEAR TIME	CONSIDERATIONS
Transparent film	They are clear dressing sheets that are adhesive, waterproof, and allow for the transmission of oxygen and water vapor. They are impermeable to bacteria and contaminates. They maintain an optimal environment in a dry to slightly moist wound. They will facilitate autolytic débridement and promote growth of living tissue.	7 days	Moisture should stay within the confines of what can be managed within the borders of the dressing.
Hydrocolloid	This is made mostly of hydroactive or absorptive particles that will interact with wound exudates to form a gelatinous material. It is indicated for wounds that have minimal-to-moderate exudates. The dressing maintains an optimal moist environment and will facilitate autolytic débridement.	7 days	They should not be changed more often than every 3 days.

Continued

Wound Care Dressings—cont'd

DRESSING	DESCRIPTION	WEAR TIME	CONSIDERATIONS
Hydrogel	This is a starch- or glycerin-based compound than can insulate the wound and will provide and promote an optimal moist environment. These dressings facilitate cell migration in wounds. They can hydrate necrotic tissue and provide for autolytic débridement. They are ideal for wounds with minimal-to-moderate amounts of exudate.	3 days	They should not be changed more often than every 3 days.
Hydrogel sheet	They are ideal for shallow wounds with zero-to-minimal exudate. The wafer maintains an optimal moist environment. This is an excellent option when the peri-wound integrity is compromised. The glycerin-based hydrogel sheets are bacterio-static and fungistatic and can be used in conjunction with antimicrobial ointments.	5 days (when gentle adhesion is needed)	They are good product for skin tears.
Hydrogel pad	These are polyacrylate pads that contain super-absorbent polymer, activated by saturating with Ringer's solution. They rapidly débride necrotic tissue. As the debris in the wound moves into the pad, the pad releases the Ringer's solution into the wound. This results in a constant washing or rinsing of the wound.	Every 24 hours	
Alginate	This is derived from the calcium salt of sea-weed and is appropriate for moderate-to-heavy exudate. It will autolytically débride by creating an optimal moist wound environment. It promotes growth of living tissue.	2-3 days	They are not appropriate for nondraining wounds.
Foam	This is used for moderate to heavily exu-dating wounds.	2-5 days (depending on amount of drainage)	This should not be used on dry wounds. It may be used on occasion to provide pressure reduction to potential pres-sure ulcers over bony promi-nences. It is less adherent and aggressive to friable skin.

Wound Care Dressings—cont'd

DRESSING	DESCRIPTION	WEAR TIME	CONSIDERATIONS
Composite	This combines physically distinct components into a single dressing to include a bacterial barrier and an absorptive layer.	2-3 days	This should not be used for heavily exudating wounds.
Antimicrobial dressing	This is a nonionic silver-fused transparent film. It is effective against numerous fungi, yeast, and bacteria including MRSA and VRE.	7 days	This is noncytotoxic. The length of the dressing reduces labor requirements of daily dressing changes.
Second-generation barrier plate	This is a starch- or petroleum-based paste used to protect and support denuded areas of the skin.	1-2 days	This is used to protect the skin against urine, stool, fistula, and G-tube drainage.

MRSA, Methicillin-resistant *Staphylococcus aureus; VRE,* vancomycin-resistant enterococci; *G-tube,* gastrostomy tube.

What You NEED TO KNOW

In addition to the dressings described previously, the nurse's institution may have access to a number of therapeutic support surfaces that can be used as an adjunct to the dressing therapy. The information presented is not intended to be an all-inclusive list of products that are on the market. It is intended to give readers an appreciation of the generic products that may be available to their institutions.

Pressure Reduction Mattresses

Pressure reduction mattresses provide a surface that reduces the pressure over a bony area beyond what a standard bed mattress or chair cushion can provide. Examples include the following:

Static air mattress overlays. These are vinyl air mattresses that have interlocking air chambers that permit air to move from chamber to chamber, thus providing very effective pressure reduction. The mattresses could be beneficial to patients who are at high risk for skin breakdown as determined by the appropriate risk assessment tool (i.e., patients who cannot turn themselves, patients in severe pain, and patients who can be turned and have at least two intact turning surfaces). Very little protection exists from shear and moisture, which can be a problem for incontinent patients. The mattress is inflated with a hand held pump, and pressures must be checked daily. Maintenance of these mattresses is high, but individual purchase cost per unit is low. These are normally sold as single patient use, but some hospitals may choose to terminally clean them after the patient's discharge and use them again.

Foam products. These were developed as overlays or mattress replacements. Depending on the design and thickness of the product, it can be therapeutic or nontherapeutic. The egg crate mattress can be purchased at most local discount chain stores and has very limited potential of preventing pressure ulcers. It may provide some temporary relief for those individuals that are mobile in bed, on limited incomes, or both. Foam mattresses should be designed to be 4 inches thick and in such a way that dispersal of the patient's weight is supported (the patient will not bottom out). This can be determined by placing a hand between the foam mattress and the hospital mattress. If the nurse can feel the bony prominence, the patient is bottoming out and not receiving the pressure reduction that he or she needs. Moisture is an issue for all foam products and can be a problem for patients who are incontinent or diaphoretic. If no plastic mattress cover is available, the foam must be disposed of when it becomes soiled. Waste disposal of these products is a primary concern for landfills.

Water fluid medium. It is available in an overlay or mattress replacement. The advantage to this type of mattress is it evenly distributes pressure over bony prominences. It can be used long-term and is cost-effective in long-term settings. It can be used with incontinent patients. Disadvantages include the weight of the mattress, it must use a thermometer to guarantee temperature, and it is easy to puncture.

Gel. It is used as a mattress overlay, in wheel chair cushions, and rental replacement mattresses. It is very effective for heavier patients, is waterproof, and reduces shear. Disadvantages include its weight; in addition, no mechanism is available to promote airflow.

Alternating pressure mattress system. A dynamic air support system designed with multiple air chambers (incorporated into either a mattress overlay or a mattress replacement) that are alternately inflated and deflated by a computerized pump system. The system is designed to provide frequent shifts in pressure points. Depending on the quality of the mattress this can be either pressure reduction or relief. With mattress overlays the nurse has to ensure that the additional height of the overlay does not jeopardize patient safety. When a disoriented patient rolls over, there may not be enough height to the side rail to keep the patient from falling out of bed.

Pressure Relief

The following can also be used to provide pressure relief:

Dynamic air support surfaces: low air loss mattresses and specialty beds. These include zoned air support surfaces with the inflation maintained by a computerized pump. Zoned means that groups of air sacs in the mattress can be calibrated to provide maximum pressure relief. With the provision of constant airflow through the micro pores of the coverlet of the mattress, maceration is prevented. The surface is made out of a material that results in very little friction. Mattress replacement systems, usually rental products, are more financially feasible for the hospital, because many of these systems permit the use of the hospital bed's existing frame. The nurse may also find that a patient will require a specialty bed that cannot mix and match mattresses to the patient's needs. These beds incorporate scales for weighing patients and repositioning aids, such as a chair that the nurse can use to get the patient out of bed after extended periods of being immobile. Bariatric beds incorporate mattresses and frames as a unit that will support the weight and width of patients over 400 pounds. When these patients have surgical procedures that require them to remain intubated overnight, additional modules can be plugged into the computerized mattresses that will support pulmonary toilet and turning.

Air fluidized bead (silicone) beds. These are self-contained specialty beds that are filled with silicone beads that are activated by high volumes of air. Patients who have undergone reconstructive plastic surgery to repair a Stage IV pressure ulcer will require a support surface that will provided the highest level of pressure relief. The consistency of the displacement of the beads by the air allows the patient to lie within a surface that displaces the weight to an extent that the vascular bed to the repaired area can be totally supported. Side effects may include temperature elevation, disorientation, and possible dehydration.

All patients will not respond to nursing measures the same way each time. Variables such as nutritional status, age, medications, and co-morbidities must be taken into account. Nurses in the intensive care environments must have the intuition and assessment skills that alert them to those patients who are at increased risk for skin breakdown. For those patients with some aspect of skin breakdown, the nurse must be able to come up with the best combination of skin protection, dressings, and supportive measures to manage the patient until complete recovery is made.

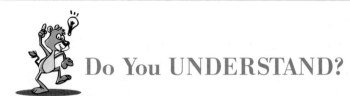

Do You UNDERSTAND?

DIRECTIONS: **Provide a short answer for each of the following questions.**

1. Why is it so important to do skin assessments on patients at regular intervals?

_____

_____

_____

_____

_____

_____

2. When using a risk assessment tool such as the Braden scale, what are some of the variables to consider when evaluating a patient for skin breakdown?

_____

_____

_____

_____

_____

Answers: 1. Skin damage can occur in as little as 2 hours from pressure, moisture, or other skin irritants. Foreign objects left lying near the patient may cause additional pressure. When patients are unable to recognize or respond to pain because of decreased mental status or limitation in mobility, it becomes the nurse's responsibility to protect the patient from injury. 2. Sensory perception, moisture, activity, mobility, nutrition, and friction and shear are all important independent variables that can result in skin breakdown. These criteria can change from the point of admission throughout a patient's stay in the hospital.

3. A patient that was started on vancomycin approximately 24 hours ago now has diarrhea. He is complaining of soreness to the perianal area. What would be an appropriate nursing measure?

_____

_____

_____

_____

_____

4. A patient arrives from the emergency department with a skin tear that apparently resulted from moving the patient. The nurse observes a 3 × 4 cm tear with a large amount of serous exudate coming from the wound. What would be an appropriate dressing to apply to this area once the wound has been cleansed and steri stripped?

_____

_____

_____

5. The nurse is assigned to the night shift of a busy intensive care unit (ICU). One of the patients is ventilated, weights 84 pounds, is incontinent of stool, and his albumin level is 2.5 mg. What would be an appropriate specialty mattress that could be implemented for this patient?

_____

_____

_____

_____

Answers: 3. The nurse should evaluate the skin for breakdown. If none is found, the nurse should apply a second-generation skin barrier petroleum-based ointment or barrier protectant wipe to prevent the enzymatic action of the liquid stool from injuring the skin. One may also decide to remove the diaper and use commercial pads only. This will prevent the drainage from becoming trapped against the skin for any length of time. 4. A nonadherent foam dressing would be minimally aggressive on the skin and provide for exudate control. 5. The best mattress would be a dynamic air support surface that can provide pressure relief. The nurse should also consider a mattress that can rotate the patient from side to side, thus facilitating pulmonary toilet.

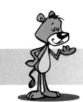

What IS Necrotizing Fasciitis?

- This site provides a nice general overview of the anatomy of the skin:

  http://www.ohsuhealth.com/htaz/derm/anatomy_of_the_skin.cfm.
- This site provides pictures depicting normal skin and the condition of necrotizing fasciitis:

  http://www.emedicine.com/derm/topic743.htm.

Necrotizing (the killing or death of) fasciitis (inflammation of the skin's fascia) is an uncommon, usually acute, severe infection involving the superficial and deep fasciae. Necrotizing fasciitis can affect any part of the body including the abdominal wall, the perianal groin area, face, neck, chest, and most commonly the extremities, particularly the legs.

What You NEED TO KNOW

Infections in general involve three major elements: (1) the abilities of the organism, (2) the point of entry, and (3) the host defense status. More specifically, skin and soft tissue infections can be categorized by the characteristics of the infecting organism, the anatomic location, and the host response or clinical signs and symptoms. Categorizing skin and soft tissue infections can be difficult because different bacterial species may produce similar clinical pictures, but these cutaneous clues can lead to determining the correct diagnosis.

Skin, soft tissue, and muscle conditions that may be difficult to differentiate include cellulitis, necrotizing fasciitis (type I and type II), synergistic necrotizing fasciitis, and clostridial myonecrosis. The term *gangrene* is also associated with these conditions, which means that death of the tissue is usually caused by the lack of blood flow. Gangrene is also associated with inflammation, injury, emboli, and infection. The term *dry gangrene*, particularly, means *an aseptic death to the tissues because of the lack of blood flow.*

CELLULITIS

Cellulitis is defined as an acute spreading infection of the skin that involves the subcutaneous tissues. Generally, cellulitis is caused by a streptococcal or staphylococcal bacteria, and the clinical presentation may be difficult to differentiate. Gangrenous cellulitis can rapidly progress to a crepitant soft tissue wound and cause extensive necrosis of subcutaneous tissues and the overlying skin. Again, depending on the anatomic location, the causative organism, and predisposing condition, a variety of clinical conditions may develop, including necrotizing fasciitis, clostridial myonecrosis (group A streptococcus [GAS] gangrene), and synergistic necrotizing cellulitis.

NECROTIZING FASCIITIS TYPE I

Necrotizing fasciitis type I has nonstreptococcal causes that involve multiple soft tissue layers and is often classified under subcutaneous tissue infections. The

TAKE HOME POINTS

Soft tissues include skin, subcutaneous tissue also known as *superficial fascia,* fascia, and skeletal muscles that are in close proximity. Superficial fascia are subcutaneous loose connective tissues that permit free movement of the skin lying over it. The deeper fascia, are dense, irregular, connective tissues enveloping and binding muscles.

TAKE HOME POINTS

Bacterial infections involving the skin and soft tissues may be a primary infection, a secondary manifestation of infection in some other organ, or even reflect a systemic manifestation of a systemic bacteremia in which timely recognition may be life saving.

cause of type I necrotizing fasciitis includes (1) at least one anaerobic species, commonly *Bacteroides* spp., a gram-negative rod bacteria; (2) *Peptostreptococcus* spp., an anaerobic gram-positive cocci bacteria; (3) one or more facultative (living under certain conditions) anaerobic species such as streptococci (other than group A); and (4) members of the *Enterobacteriaceae* spp., gram-negative rods, such as *Escherichia coli, Enterobacter* spp., *Klebsiella* spp., and *Proteus* spp. An obligate aerobe (one that must have oxygen) such as *P. aeruginosa,* a gram-negative rod, is rarely a component of such a mixed infection. Cases of necrotizing fasciitis in which only anaerobes are present appear to be rare.

Necrotizing Fasciitis Type II

Necrotizing fasciitis type II (also called *hemolytic streptococcal gangrene*) is caused by GAS, which contains pyogenic exotoxin A and is a gram-positive, aerotolerant facultative anaerobe. Streptococcal gangrene is classified with gangrenous cellulitis, because the manifestations are close to cutaneous gangrene. If the GAS infection is profound with a shocklike syndrome, it is called *streptococcal toxic shocklike syndrome* (STSS). STSS is not to be confused with staphylococcal toxic shock syndrome (TSS), caused by the *S. aureus* strains capable of toxin production, acute febrile illness, and often remembered for its relationship to tampon use.

TAKE HOME POINTS

Necrotizing fasciitis is present in about 50% of the STSS cases.

GAS

GAS (*Streptococcus pyogenes)* is often found in the throat and on the skin and is the same bacteria that causes the commonly referred to illness known as *strep throat.* Generally, streptococcal strains from the pharynx and respiratory tract are not the same strains that cause skin infections. As a normal flora, GAS can cause an infection, mainly in the respiratory tract, bloodstream, or the skin, when the host defenses are compromised or normal physiologic defenses penetrated. A small number of people harbor the bacterium, usually in the respiratory tract, without signs of disease. These bacteria are spread via direct contact with drainage from the nose, throat, or wound of a person who is infected, and they may cause mild to severe illness. In addition, an immune-mediated post-streptococcal sequelae may develop such as rheumatic fever and acute glomerulonephritis after acute infections caused by *S. pyogenes.* Typically, antibiotics can kill GAS bacteria; however, the bacteria can become invasive, destroying soft tissue and causing necrotizing fasciitis, myositis, and even TSS. Currently, severe invasive infections caused by GAS have had a puzzling resurgence and are a worldwide health concern. Unfortunately, because of the lack of documentation, the incidence of GAS worldwide is not known.

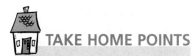

This site provides a nice overview of GAS:

http://www.cdc.gov/ ncidod/dbmd/disease info/groupastreptococcal_g.htm.

   GAS produce a wide array of virulence factors, and many of these factors are related to the cell surface. Six virulence factors of GAS are (1) special proteins for adherence and colonization; (2) the potential for an immunologic disguise along with the ability of antigenic variation and tolerance; (3) the ability to inhibit and kill phagocytes; (4) the ability to produce protein-splitting enzymes, allowing further spread of the bacteria; (5) the ability to release exotoxins; and (6) the ability to induce an exaggerated production of cytokines, contributing to

TAKE HOME POINTS

Streptococcus pyogenes as a pathogen can colonize, rapidly multiply and spread in its host, evade phagocytosis, and confuse the immune system.

the development of systemic toxicity. To add further injury to the host, an immune response and hemolysis can occur because of this bacteria. The host may produce circulating cross-reactive antibodies during a streptococcus infection and indirectly damage tissue. This autoimmune complication can continue even after the GAS organisms have been cleared. Finally, GAS usually are beta-hemolytic and can cause complete lysis of red cells surrounding the colony.

FOURNIER'S GANGRENE

This is a form of necrotizing fasciitis occurring about the male genitals and may extend to the perineum, penis, and abdominal wall. The infection usually starts as a cellulitis and expands with signs symptoms of necrotizing fasciitis. Those that suffer from diabetes mellitus, local trauma, and perirectal or perianal infections are at risk.

CRANIOFACIAL AND CERVICAL NECROTIZING FASCIITIS

Craniofacial necrotizing fasciitis is commonly caused by GAS, and the usual precipitating cause trauma. A polymicrobial process usually causes cervical necrotizing fasciitis, with the usual precipitating cause being dental, oral, or pharyngeal infections (or a combination of these infections). Cervical necrotizing fasciitis is about four times more lethal than craniofacial necrotizing fasciitis.

Necrotizing fasciitis of the face, eyelids, and neck are life threatening but rare.

SYNERGISTIC NECROTIZING CELLULITIS

Synergistic necrotizing cellulitis is very similar to the clinical presentation of type I necrotizing fasciitis but is more extensive and involves the skin, subcutaneous tissue, fascia, and muscle. The usual cause of synergistic necrotizing cellulitis is a mixture of organisms and typically occurs in the lower extremities or perineal area. Therapy includes antibiotics and early surgical radical débridement, even amputation, if the infection is extensive.

TAKE HOME POINTS

Two characteristics of synergistic necrotizing cellulitis are the presence of the following:
- Reddish-brown pus, sometimes called *dishwater pus*
- Crepitus

CLOSTRIDIAL MYONECROSIS

Clostridial myonecrosis (GAS gangrene) is also similar in appearance to necrotizing fasciitis in that it is an acute process with marked pain, swelling, and systemic toxicity. GAS is often present but may be obscured by the swelling of the subcutaneous tissues. Clostridial myonecrosis differs from necrotizing fasciitis in that the process involves muscle, the skin is yellow-bronze, and bullae contain dark-brown fluid. The exudate is serosanguineous versus seropurulent. Clostridial myonecrosis and clostridial cellulitis is differentiated by direct observation in the operating room. The muscle is normal and pink in cellulitis, but with myonecrosis the muscle appears abnormal, fails to contract on stimulation, and does not bleed when cut.

This site provides regularly updated information regarding general microbiology and medical bacteriology (illustrations and pictures are included within the text, including microscopic photographs): www.textbookof bacteriology.net.

Risk Factors and Mortality Rates

Generally those at higher risk for necrotizing fasciitis include patients with chronic illnesses such as diabetes, cirrhosis, alcoholism, peripheral vascular disease, cancer, parenteral IV drug abuse, dependency on renal dialysis, and those with impaired lymphatic drainage, chronic corticosteroid intake, or both.

The mortality rate of necrotizing fasciitis ranges from 20% to 47% and drops to 12% if the diagnosis is made within 4 days of the initial symptoms. In 1999, according to the Center for Disease Control, there were approximately 9400 cases of GAS in the United States, and of those 600 developed necrotizing fasciitis and 300 developed STSS. The mortality of STSS is more than 50%. Of those patients who develop necrotizing fasciitis, about 20% die; of those who develop other forms of GAS, about 10% to 15% die.

Most often the bacteria enter the body through an opening in the skin (quite often a very minor opening such as a laceration, abrasion, or even an insect bite). In some instances, infection occurs after a major trauma or surgery, such as a laparotomy or the repair of an intestinal perforation. In other cases of necrotizing fasciitis an existing wound may be the site of entry such as a perirectal abscess or a decubitus ulcer. Necrotizing fasciitis from intestinal sources may occur in the groin, abdominal wall, or in the lower extremities by following the psoas muscle. In some cases of necrotizing fasciitis, no identifiable point of entry exists.

Signs and Symptoms

Signs and symptoms of both type I and type II necrotizing fasciitis are very similar and can be easily misdiagnosed. The beginning symptoms look like so many other minor afflictions causing many health care workers to not consider necrotizing fasciitis until the patient is critically ill. The initial signs and symptoms include the following:

- Point of entry may be obvious, minor, or none
- Use of nonsteroidal antiinflammatory drugs (NSAIDs) may delay diagnosis by reducing inflammatory features
- Fever
- Severe pain (local or referred)
- Disproportionate pain to the appearing injury or condition
- Ordinary flulike symptoms, nausea, weakness, malaise, diarrhea, dizziness
- Local erythema without sharp margins, hot, shiny, swollen skin
- Complaints of feeling very badly but the inability to explain why

During the next 1 to 3 days, the following signs and symptoms continue:

- The skin begins to become dusky as fibrin thrombi may form in the small arteries and veins of the dermis and subcutaneous fat.
- A purplish rash may appear on the area.
- Pain may decrease before necrosis is seen (a clue that this is not a simple cellulitis but is necrotizing fasciitis).
- Crepitus is seen with type I but not with type II (especially in those with diabetes).

 Young children with varicella can be super-infected with GAS, and this may place them at risk for necrotizing fasciitis.

 TAKE HOME POINTS

Earlier outbreaks of invasive GAS were typically in older individuals with underlying disease; however, more recent outbreaks have involved younger healthy adults after a minor trauma. Bacteria invading the skin will elicit local inflammatory reactions; however, the character of the reaction may be related to the condition of the host.

 http://www.cdc.gov/ncidod/dbmd/diseaseinfo/groupastreptococcal_g.htm. This site provides information regarding GAS vaccine to prevent strep throat and impetigo, as well as more serious invasive disease and postinfectious complications like rheumatic fever. An overview of cellulitis and a fact sheet on streptococcal infections is available (provides references for other sites). http://www.niaid.nih.gov/factsheets/strep.htm.

 Omphalitis in the newborn (an inflammation around the umbilical cord) can lead to swelling and erythema, can progress to periumbilical necrosis, and can advance into the abdominal wall.

The signs and symptoms worsen.

• Large dark marks develop into bullae containing thick, pink to red-black fluid rupturing at about 3 to 4 days.

• Sharply demarcated areas with necrotic eschar develop with a border of erythema resembling thermal burns and anesthesia of the area.

• Extensive necrotic sloughing can result because of deep penetration of the infection along fascial planes.

If the penetration deepens, compartment syndrome may develop (the result of infection and inflammation within a confined muscle compartment space that may result in pressures exceeding arterial pressure). Typical signs and symptoms of compartment syndrome include pain on passive stretching and later pallor, paresthesia, and pulselessness similar to necrotizing fasciitis. Early measurement of compartment pressure using an intracompartmental pressure monitor may identify compartment syndrome early and decisively. The monitor is a definite asset in that the typical signs and symptoms of compartment syndrome are difficult to differentiate from those of necrotizing fasciitis.

With both type I and type II necrotizing fasciitis, systemic toxicity can develop. With type II necrotizing fasciitis, STSS may develop from the toxins given off by the bacteria. The typical signs and symptoms of STSS are chills, fever, a flat red rash over large areas of the body, confusion, vomiting, diarrhea, tachycardia, hypotension, renal impairment, decreasing level of consciousness with overwhelming infection, and multiorgan failure. With systemic involvement, decreased platelets, disseminated intravascular coagulopathy (DIC), acute respiratory distress syndrome (ARDS), and renal impairment may occur. Death may result if treatment is not promptly initiated.

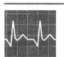

Compartment syndrome is important to identify in that this syndrome necessitates an emergency fasciectomy to prevent further necrosis of the tissues by prompt incision and division of a fascia.

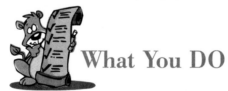

What You DO

If necrotizing fasciitis is clearly suspected on clinical grounds with signs and symptoms such as deep patchy areas of surface hypoesthesia, crepitation, advancing erythema, bullae, and skin necrosis, direct operative intervention is indicated. While probing the area of necrotizing fasciitis an instrument will easily pass along the superficial plane, which would not occur with ordinary cellulitis. Incisions need to go beyond the area of involvement until normal fascia is found, excision of necrotic fat and fascia is accomplished, and the wound is left open.

Laboratory work can also support diagnosis of necrotizing fasciitis. Specimens for cultures and Gram stain smears should be taken from areas of exudate, erosions, ulcerations, abscesses, and or drainage and not from areas of eschar to have the best chance of isolating the infecting organism. Gram-stained smears of exudate usually reveal a mixture of organisms, or with streptococcal gangrene, chains of gram-positive cocci. Cultures from the early bulbous lesions and from blood are frequently positive. The best biopsies are performed during surgical

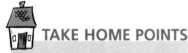

TAKE HOME POINTS

Direct visualization helps confirm the diagnosis of necrotizing fasciitis.

débridement. Leukocytosis, thrombocytopenia, and azotemia are often present. Increased serum levels of creatine phosphokinase reflects progression from cellulitis to fasciitis and myositis.

Imaging studies such as computerized tomography (CT) and magnetic resonance imaging (MRI) can help pinpoint subcutaneous and fascial edema. MRI can reliably detect fascial necrosis in the absence of contrast enhancement. Imaging studies may also show tissue gas and can help distinguish necrotizing fasciitis from cellulitis. However, the presence of tissue gas does not necessarily mean a clostridial infection, because other species can produce gas under certain conditions, and gas can result from surgical débridement.

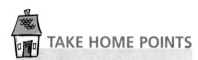

TAKE HOME POINTS

If the specimen is taken from a necrotic area or a granulating area, the bacteria detected may not be the bacteria causing the infection.

Treatment

Cellulitis is treated with a semisynthetic penicillinase-resistant penicillin so that both staphylococcal and streptococcal bacterial cellulitis will be killed. Antibiotics may be prescribed for short or long courses, by oral, IV, or intramuscular (IM) routes depending on the client condition and provider decision. If the cellulitis is known to be just streptococcal, IM, or intravascular, penicillin is the drug of choice. If methicillin-resistant strains of S. *aureus* are suspected, vancomycin is the drug of choice.

Immediate treatment of the more invasive necrotizing fasciitis is critical and requires prompt diagnosis and immediate action. Necrotizing fasciitis must be treated in the hospital with antibiotic IV therapy and aggressive débridement of the affected tissue beyond the involved gangrenous and undermined area (or areas) because of the rapidity with which the process can progress. As noted previously, surgical incisions must go beyond the area of involvement until normal fascia is found, necrotic fat and fascia excised, pus drained, and the wound left open. Reexploration of the wound is often necessary in 24 hours to be sure the initial débridement was adequate.

FIRST-LINE AND INITIAL TREATMENTS FOR NECROTIZING FASCIITIS

- Make prompt diagnosis.
- Provide antibiotic therapy.
- Encourage aggressive débridement.
- Administer ancillary therapies (IV immunoglobulin, hyperbaric oxygen [HBO] chamber therapy).

Powerful broad-spectrum antibiotics must be administered immediately. Initial IV antibiotics are based on the Gram-stained smears and the presumed presence of anaerobic bacteria, *Enterobacteriaceae*, and various streptococci in necrotizing fasciitis. Presumptive antibiotic coverage may include penicillin or ampicillin plus gentamicin, as well as clindamycin or metronidazole to treat anaerobic organisms. Ampicillin-sulbactam and gentamicin, as well as imipenem and metronidazole, are other combination options. Subsequent antimicrobial therapy is based on cultures and antimicrobial susceptibility tests. It is important to identify the causative organism and not be misdirected by coexisting flora.

Surgery is required to open and drain infected areas and débride dead tissue. Initially after surgery, moist dressings are applied; later skin grafting may be required. The nurse should watch for signs and symptoms of expanding infection, including any skin changes, fever, systemic toxicity, and severe pain. Treatment can also depend upon the level of toxicity or organ failure being experienced by the patient. In severe cases of STSS systemic toxicity exists and emergency interventions may be required, including CPR. Prompt diagnosis, IV antibiotics, and aggressive débridement are indicated, as well as the treatment for the systemic shock. Intravascular fluids and vasoactive medications may help support the patient in shock, and a thermodilution catheter may be placed to help guide treatment therapies ultimately affecting tissue oxygenation, including delivery and consumption.

Ancillary therapies, but never a replacement for surgery, include IV immunoglobulin (IVIG) (antibodies) to treat STSS and the HBO chamber therapy for certain cases involving a mixed bacterial infection. HBO therapy uses a special pressure chamber that allows the patient to breathe 100% oxygen while the pressure in the chamber is higher than 1 atmosphere absolute (atm abs), generally 1.4 atm abs. HBO involves the use of oxygen at an increased pressure in a chamber and increases the oxygen saturation in the infected wounds by 1000-fold, leading to a bactericidal effect, improved polymorphonuclear function, and enhanced wound healing.

Nursing Responsibilities

Recognizing the signs and symptoms of necrotizing fasciitis is critical, and prompt diagnosis is paramount. Early recognition and treatment of necrotizing fasciitis may prevent further advancement of the condition and may ultimately be life saving. Nurses caring for patients need to be aware of the signs and symptoms of necrotizing fasciitis when assessing patients, because they may be the first to identify what is developing.

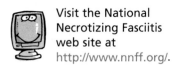
Visit the National Necrotizing Fasciitis web site at http://www.nnff.org/.

The National Necrotizing Fasciitis Foundation is a nonprofit organization founded by survivors of necrotizing fasciitis. The purpose of this foundation is to serve as a resource for the general public regarding necrotizing fasciitis. The mission of this foundation is to educate for public awareness, educate for the recognition of symptoms and preventative measures, advocate research, offer resources and support for those affected by necrotizing fasciitis, and to save lives.

When working with patients with necrotizing fasciitis, the nurse should do the following:

- Obtain an accurate health history and identify those at risk (especially if on corticosteroids).
- Further investigate and report complaints of severe pain that are out of proportion to the condition.
- Assess, treat, and reassess pain, especially for the effectiveness of interventions.
- Report increasing and severe pain.
- Monitor closely those who state they feel extremely ill or unusual and cannot explain why.
- Watch for fever and skin changes, especially quickly moving margins of redness that are not demarcated nor raised.

- Immediately report if a patient that is a few days into the condition has advanced signs and symptoms of deep patchy areas of surface hypoesthesia, crepitation, bullae, and skin necrosis; direct operative intervention may be indicated.
- Remember if the skin is open a physician may examine the patient with a gloved hand, passing the finger easily between the subcutaneous tissue and the deeper fascia. Typically the necrosis is more advanced than it appears.
- Monitor level of consciousness; if it is decreasing, report the finding to the physician.
- Monitor for the patient's ability to protect his or her airway. Intervene and protect the patient's airway as needed. Report findings to the physician immediately.
- Monitor vital signs, intake, and output in proportion to the severity of illness.
- Remember that intravascular volume loss may be detectable and common. Obtain intravascular access, but do not use the affected extremity. Administer intravascular fluids as ordered.
- Insert a Foley catheter if ordered to monitor urine output; however, the risk benefit should be addressed in patients with Fournier gangrene.
- Assess for allergies and start prescribed antibiotics immediately.
- Monitor lab data and report significant information such as new culture results or abnormal reports that may change therapy decisions. Lab studies may include CBC with differential, electrolytes, glucose, BUN, creatinine, blood and tissue cultures, urinalysis, urine electrolytes, and ABG.
- Monitor diagnostic data and report significant information such as new results or abnormal reports that may change therapy decisions. Diagnostic studies can include imaging studies such as local radiographs, CT scanning, and MRI.
- Implement wound care as prescribed. Premedicate the patient for dressing changes; however, if the wound is large, the patient may require visits to the operating room for dressing changes.

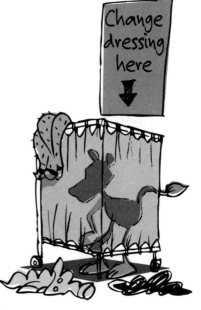

- Accurately assess and measure the wound or wounds and document them in the patient record.
- Monitor for signs and symptoms of compartment syndrome: pain on passive stretching, and later, paresthesia, pallor, and loss of pulse. Early measurement of compartment pressure using an intracompartmental pressure monitor may identify compartment syndrome early and decisively. The intracompartmental pressure monitor is a definite asset in that the signs and symptoms of compartment syndrome are difficult to differentiate from necrotizing fasciitis.
- Ready a patient for surgery if compartment syndrome occurs, because this may necessitate emergency fasciectomy to prevent further necrosis by prompt incision and division of fascia.
- Watch for systemic toxicity that can develop with both types I and II necrotizing fasciitis. With systemic involvement, decreased platelets, DIC, ARDS, and renal impairment may occur. Death may result if treatment is not promptly initiated.
- Watch for STSS with type II GAS infections that may develop from the toxins the bacteria are giving off. The typical signs and symptoms of STSS are chills, fever, a flat red rash over large areas of the body, confusion, vomiting, diarrhea, tachycardia, hypotension, renal impairment, decreasing level of consciousness with overwhelming infection, and multiorgan failure.

- Discuss nutritional needs with the physician, patient, and family. Consult a dietician.
- Educate the patient and family concerning this condition.
- Monitor the patient and family for role conflict and monetary stress; involve case management and psychologic therapy early.
- Address psychologic issues such as anxiety, fear, worry, anger, hopelessness, depression, and concerns regarding disfigurement. Consult clinical psychology as needed.
- As with any patient, provide caring and compassionate emotional support.
- Assist the patient and family to identify goals for the rehabilitation process; include coping skills learned from previous experiences.
- Consult other professional therapies, such as a clinical nurse specialist in psychiatric-mental health; a psychologist; and a speech, physical, or occupational therapist.
- Help the patient and family regain an optimal level of health.

The following are important points for the nurse to remember regarding necrotizing fasciitis:

1. Those at risk should be remembered, especially persons taking corticosteroids.
2. Patients with the condition frequently complain of severe pain out of proportion to the condition.
3. Patients often state that they feel extremely ill or unusual and cannot explain why.
4. Advanced signs and symptoms include deep patchy areas of surface hypoesthesia, crepitation, bullae, and skin necrosis; direct operative intervention may be indicated.

Patient Teaching

When caring for patients the prevention of infection may be encouraged by educating the public to practice frequent good hand washing. Hand washing is an excellent preventive practice regarding many illnesses, especially after coughing, sneezing, and before preparing or eating foods. The nurse should also do the following:

- Avoid contact with persons showing sore throat symptoms. If they have a known exposure to GAS, they should consult a physician.
- Educate patients to clean and care for even the smallest traumas using an antibiotic ointment and a sterile covering with frequent dressing changes. Instruct patients to watch for signs of infection in a wound site and to seek care, especially if fever occurs.
- Educate the public regarding necrotizing fasciitis. Knowledge of this potential condition may result in early treatment and prevention of systemic conditions.
- Educate the public regarding risk factors that may contribute to the possibility of aggressive infections (alcoholism, parenteral drug abuse).
- Provide information regarding appropriate support systems, counseling, social services, and psychosocial support as appropriate.

Necrotizing fasciitis may exist with systemic toxicity and or organ failure. Treatment of systemic shock may include respiratory support with mechanical ventilation and vascular support with intravascular fluids and vasoactive medications. A thermodilution catheter may be placed to guide treatment therapies affecting tissue oxygenation, both delivery and consumption.

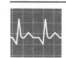

The nurse should always be aware that the patient may progress to this toxic state and may require emergency interventions, including CPR.

Outcomes

Outcomes will vary depending on the type of infecting organism, condition of the host, rate of spread, susceptibility to antibiotics, and how early the condition was diagnosed. Most survivors will have some removal or destruction of tissue and skin, scarring, and later require skin grafting. Negative pressure wound closure is sometimes used to help effectively close open wounds. Amputation may be required if the infection is in a limb and cannot be contained or controlled. Amputation of a limb, aggressive treatment, and powerful antibiotics may save some, but not all patients live.

Do You UNDERSTAND?

DIRECTIONS: **Choose the correct answer to each of the following questions, and place the corresponding letter in the space provided.**

_____ 1. What type of bacteria causes necrotizing fasciitis type II?
  a. *Escherichia coli*
  b. *Enterobacter* spp.
  c. GAS
  d. *Klebsiella* spp.

_____ 2. What two therapies may be chosen but never replace surgical débridement?
  a. HBO chamber therapy and intravenous immunoglobulin (IVIG)
  b. Insulin IV and physical therapy
  c. Acupuncture and physical therapy
  d. HBO therapy and anticoagulants

DIRECTIONS: **Fill in the blanks to complete the following statements.**

3. When caring for any patient, prevention of infections may be encouraged

  by educating the public to practice _____.

4. Necrotizing fasciitis means _____.

CHAPTER

12 Multisystem

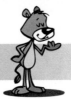

What IS Code Management?

Code management is the organization and direction of resuscitation. The American Heart Association (AHA) is a leader in providing guidance for organizing these efforts. Many things seem to be happening all at once. For resuscitation to be effective, there must be a systematic approach to the delivery of care. The code team must have a captain to lead the efforts, direct, and organize. The team leader should immediately assign one team member to each of the following tasks: managing the airway; providing chest compressions; starting an intravenous (IV) line; administering medications; handling the monitor, code cart, and defibrillator; and recording the events of the code. Personnel not involved directly in the resuscitation effort should provide support for the family and control the number of people observing the resuscitation.

A *code* is the commonly used term in the medical community for a cardiopulmonary arrest. Breathing stops, cardiac contractions are absent or ineffective, and little or no cardiac output (CO) occurs. The heart and brain are deprived of oxygenated blood. Clinical death has occurred, and biological death will quickly follow if appropriate action is not taken.

For the purposes of this text, we will explore adult resuscitation management. Pediatric, infant, and neonatal resuscitation management may vary, because the physiologic cause of the arrest is often different, especially in children.

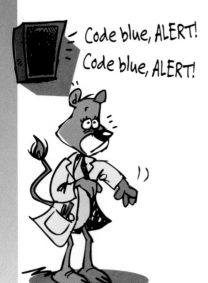

Code blue, ALERT!
Code blue, ALERT!

What IS an Advanced Directive?

Advanced directives are documents that a person writes in anticipation of the fact that at some point they will be unable to make their wishes known to their health care providers. The Patient Self-Determination Act (PSDA) is a law that requires all health care institutions to provide patients with information on advanced directives and to discuss advanced directives with patients. Two types of advanced directives are (1) a *living will* and (2) a *durable power of attorney* for health care. A living will describes what kind of health care a person is to receive in the event of certain medical conditions. A durable power of attorney for health care appoints another person to speak for the patient if he or she is no longer able to do so. For purposes of code management, we are most concerned with the patient's wishes related to the administration of cardiopulmonary resuscitation (CPR) and mechanical ventilation.

TAKE HOME POINTS

Most often a living will addresses the patient's wishes on such issues as CPR, mechanical ventilation, artificial nutrition or hydration, dialysis, surgery, or antibiotic treatment.

What You NEED TO KNOW

The PSDA allows patients to make decisions about their care. Does the patient have an advanced directive? If the patient has a living will, what does it say? If the patient is unable to verbalize his or her wishes, does he or she have a durable power of attorney for health care?

Patients are permitted to refuse care. Some patients do not want CPR or to be placed on a ventilator. These wishes will affect the patient's *code status*. Most health care institutions have polices concerning the limitation of this type of emergency care. The nurse must follow the policies of the institution where he or she works; however, if a patient refuses CPR, mechanical ventilation, or both, his or her wishes must be respected. Resuscitation should not be started. The challenge for a health care provider is to follow the patient's advanced directives, even if they conflict with the health care provider's own ideas and values.

What You DO

All patients must be asked about advanced directives on admission to the hospital. If a patient has a living will, a copy should be placed in the medical record. If a copy is not available, the nurse should ask the family to bring a copy to the hospital. If the document is not readily available, the nurse should ask the patient about his or her wishes. Health care institutions have polices regarding notification of the health care team regarding the contents of the patient's advanced directives. The nurse must know the status of the advanced directives for any patient in his or her care. It is important to be aware before an emergency arises and to follow the institution's policies.

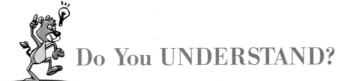

Do You UNDERSTAND?

DIRECTIONS: **Provide short answers to the following questions.**

1. List the two types of advanced directives.

   _____

   _____

2. What is the nurse's responsibility related to advanced directives?

   _____

   _____

   _____

What ARE the Advanced Cardiac Life Support Guidelines?

The AHA's Advanced Cardiac Life Support (ACLS) guidelines organize resuscitation efforts into a primary and a secondary ABCD (**A**irway, **B**reathing, **C**irculation, **D**efibrillation) survey. These eight steps are appropriate for all cardiac emergencies. They are organized in order of priority. Each step involves assessment and management of a problem. By following this approach, the nurse can manage each problem before moving on to the next one.

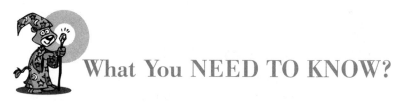

What You NEED TO KNOW?

Before beginning the primary survey, assess for responsiveness. Shake and shout to arouse the patient.

Primary ABCD Survey

ASSESS	MANAGE
Airway: Is the airway open? **Breathing:** Is the patient breathing? **Circulation:** Does the patient have a pulse? **Defibrillation:** Does the rhythm require defibrillation?	**Airway:** Open the airway. **Breathing:** If not breathing, provide ventilation. **Circulation:** If there is no pulse, begin chest compressions. **Defibrillation:** Is the rhythm VF? Is an AED available?

VF, Ventricular fibrillation; *AED,* automatic external defibrillator.

Secondary ABCD Survey

ASSESS	MANAGE
Airway: Provide advanced airway management. **Breathing:** Confirm endotracheal tube placement and adequate oxygenation. **Circulation:** Obtain IV access and determine rhythm. **Differential diagnosis:** Search for and find reversible causes.	**Airway:** Provide intubation with an endotracheal tube if possible. **Breathing:** Confirm tube placement by listening to breath sounds and use of an end-tidal carbon dioxide detector. **Circulation:** Identify the cardiac rhythm. Is IV access available to give medications? **Differential diagnosis:** What is wrong with this patient? Why did they go into cardiac arrest?

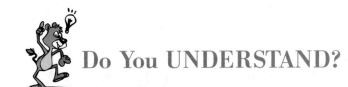

Do You UNDERSTAND?

DIRECTIONS: **List the four steps of the primary and secondary survey.**

PRIMARY SURVEY

1. _____

2. _____

3. _____

4. _____

SECONDARY SURVEY

5. _____

6. _____

7. _____

8. _____

What IS Respiratory Arrest?

A respiratory arrest is defined as *the absence of breathing*. A respiratory arrest is often preceded by progressively worsening respiratory distress or compromise (or both). Patient assessment and intervention is critical to prevent respiratory compromise from becoming arrest. Patients who have a respiratory arrest will have a pulse. If the respiratory arrest is not treated, a cardiac arrest will follow.

Answers: 1. Assess airway; 2. Assess breathing; 3. Assess circulation; 4. Defibrillate; 5. Airway (intubation); 6. Breathing (confirm ventilation) 7. Circulation (IV access); 8. Differential diagnosis.

What You NEED TO KNOW

Many causes for respiratory compromise and arrest exist. Although the underlying causes are important, emergency treatment is the same no matter what the cause. Adequate oxygenation must be maintained. Slow respiratory rates, shallow respirations, or both that do not provide adequate oxygenation may require ventilatory support using a bag-mask. Untreated respiratory compromise may progress to respiratory arrest. Occasional gasping breaths, known as *agonal respiration*, are ineffective. These patients must be treated as if they were in respiratory arrest.

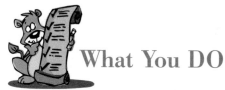

What You DO

If the patient shows any kind of respiratory distress, assessment is critical. The nurse should assess the patient's respiratory rate and quality, assess the work of breathing, and look for use of accessory muscles. Is the patient short of breath? Is the rate too fast or too slow? Does the patient need to sit up or sit in a particular position to breathe? The nurse should auscultate breath sounds. Are they present, absent, abnormal? The patient should be placed on a pulse oximeter if possible. Oxygen saturation below 95% requires attention. The nurse should be prepared to report findings to the physician in charge of the patient's care.

TAKE HOME POINTS
Patients with carbon monoxide poisoning will have a normal pulse oximeter reading, although they require O_2 therapy.

If the patient is not breathing, the nurse must breath for the patient. Initial ventilation may be provided with mouth-to-mouth, mouth-to-mask, or bag-mask breathing. The nurse may give bag-mask ventilation with or without supplemental oxygen; however, 100% oxygen should be delivered as soon as possible. If continued airway support is needed, the patient should be intubated to provide a secure airway.

Do You UNDERSTAND?

DIRECTIONS: **Fill in the blanks to complete the following statements.**

1. Untreated respiratory compromise may lead to _____

_____ .

2. When assessing respirations, the nurse should assess the _____,

_____ , and _____ .

Answers: 1. respiratory arrest; 2. rate, quality, breath sounds.

What IS a Cardiac Arrest?

A cardiac arrest is identified by the absence of a palpable pulse. No blood pressure (BP), CO, or breathing is detected. Clinical death has occurred. With prompt action clinical death is reversible. If pulse and respiration are not promptly restored, biologic death follows.

What You NEED TO KNOW

Three rhythms may be seen in cardiac arrest. The AHA provides algorithms for the treatment of each of the following arrest rhythms:

Ventricular Fibrillation or Pulseless Ventricular Tachycardia

Ventricular fibrillation (VF) or pulseless ventricular tachycardia (PVT) is a chaotic rhythm that does not produce effective contractions. It is by far the most common rhythm in an adult cardiac arrest.

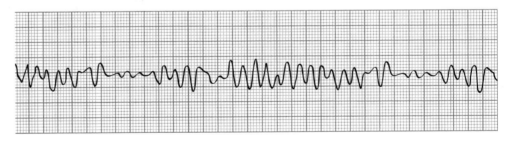

Pulseless Electrical Activity

In pulseless electrical activity (PEA), any organized electrical activity can be visualized on the cardiac monitor. However, no cardiac contractions or CO occur is seen. What defines PEA is the fact that the patient is pulseless.

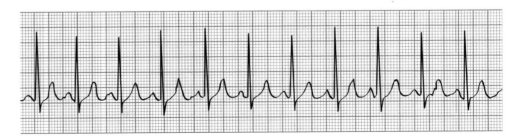

Asystole

Asystole is the absence of electrical activity in the heart. Asystole is generally considered a terminal rhythm. Very few patients will be resuscitated from asystole.

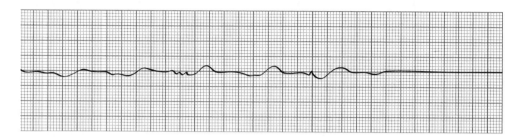

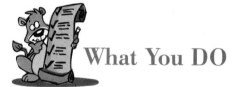

What You DO

The following is a summary of the main treatment points from the AHA Advanced Cardiac Life Support algorithms:

Ventricular Fibrillation or Pulseless Ventricular Tachycardia

When treating patients with VF or PVT heart rhythms, the nurse should do the following:

- Assess the patient. Complete the primary ABCD survey.
- If the patient is not breathing and does not have a pulse, begin CPR.
- If an AED is available, put it on the patient as soon as pulselessness is determined and follow the voice prompts. Electrical defibrillation is the definitive treatment for VF. Do **NOT** delay defibrillation.
- If a monitor defibrillator is available, attach it to the patient and determine the rhythm on the monitor.
- If the patient is in VF or pulseless PVT, prepare to defibrillate. Initially defibrillate at 200 joules (J). If the rhythm does not convert, the energy is increased to 300 J. If the rhythm does not convert, the energy is increased to the maximum dose of 360 J. Deliver these three shocks in rapid succession.
- Resume CPR, intubate the patient, and start an IV if the first three shocks do not convert the rhythm.
- Administer treatment in the following sequence: (1) drug; (2) CPR for 30 to 60 seconds; and (3) defibrillation. Many practitioners remember this as drug, shock, drug, shock with CPR in between.
- Remember that epinephrine (adrenaline) is the first-line drug. Administer epinephrine 1 mg IV every 3 to 5 minutes during the resuscitation. No maximum dose of epinephrine exists.
- Remember that vasopressin (Pitressin) 40 U IV **MAY** be given in place of epinephrine. Vasopressin may only be given once. The nurse should not give vasopressin and epinephrine.

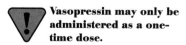

The nurse should always assess and reassess the patient during a code, and he or she should not rely strictly on the monitor.

Vasopressin may only be administered as a one-time dose.

- Remember that antidysrhythmic drugs are the next drugs to be administered. The antidysrhythmic drugs of choice are lidocaine (Xylocaine HCL) 1 mg/kg IV **OR** amiodarone (Coradone) 300 mg IV. The physician should choose one, not both.
- Remember that magnesium sulfate 1 to 2 g IV push is generally indicated in two circumstances: (1) in torsades de pointes (a type of PVT that has both positively and negatively deflected complexes) and (2) in patient's with clinical conditions such as alcoholism or malnutrition that lead to low serum magnesium levels.

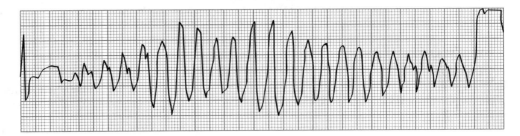

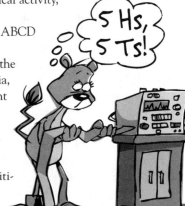

TAKE HOME POINTS

- The nurse should defibrillate VF as soon as possible. He or she should not delay for intubation or obtaining IV access.
- The nurse should remember the sequence of actions is drug, shock, drug, shock.

- Remember that procainamide (Pronestyl) is indicated for recurrent VF and PVT. Procainamide must be administered slowly and has limited usefulness in a cardiac arrest.
- When IV access is not available, remember that certain medications may be given via the endotracheal tube. One aid to help the nurse remember the drugs is the word *LANE*—lidocaine, atropine, naloxone hydrochloride (Narcan), and epinephrine (adrenaline). Tracheal doses of these drugs should be two to four times the IV dose because of the absorption in the lungs. For example, endotracheal epinephrine should be given at 2.0 to 2.5 times the IV dose.

Pulseless Electrical Activity

When treating patients with pulseless electrical activity, the nurse should do the following:

- Assess the patient. Complete the primary ABCD survey.
- Begin CPR. Check the cardiac rhythm on the monitor. Normal sinus rhythm, bradycardia, or tachycardia may be seen, but the patient will be pulseless.
- Complete the secondary survey. Intubate the patient, confirm adequate ventilation, and obtain IV access.
- Remember that differential diagnosis is critical in PEA. One memory aid is to think of the five Hs and the five Ts.

Differential Diagnosis for Pulseless Electrical Activity

FIVE CAUSES THAT START WITH H	TREATMENT
Hypovolemia	Volume infusion
Hypoxia	Oxygenation, ventilation
Hydrogen ion (acidosis)	Sodium bicarbonate, hyperventilation
Hyperkalemia/hypokalemia	Hyperkalemia: sodium bicarbonate, glucose plus insulin, calcium chloride.
	Hypokalemia: rapid but controlled infusion of potassium.
Hypothermia	Warm patient

FIVE CAUSES THAT START WITH T	TREATMENT
Tablets (drug overdose)	Drug screen, lavage, activated charcoal
Tamponade (cardiac)	Pericardiocentesis
Tension pneumothorax	Needle decompression
Thrombosis (coronary)	Thrombolytic agents
Thrombosis (pulmonary)	Thrombolytic agents, surgical embolectomy

- Remember that hypovolemia and hypoxia are the most common causes of PEA.
- Administer epinephrine 1 mg IV every 3 to 5 minutes if ordered to do so by the physician.
- Atropine may be administered if the electrical activity is bradycardia (heart rate [HR] <60).

Asystole

When treating patients in asystole, the nurse should do the following:
- Assess the patient. Complete the primary survey. Begin CPR. Check the monitor in a second lead to confirm asystole.
- Complete the secondary survey. Search for treatable causes—five Hs and five Ts.
- Consider transcutaneous cardiac pacing. This may be effective because no electrical activity occurs with this rhythm.
- Administer epinephrine 1 mg IV every 3 to 5 minutes if ordered by the physician.
- In addition, give atropine 1 mg IV every 3 to 5 minutes (maximum dose of 0.04 mg/kg) if ordered by the physician.
- Because asystole is often a terminal rhythm, consider termination of the code.

 The nurse should not treat the monitor! If a patient has normal electrocardiographic activity and is pulseless, this is PEA.

TAKE HOME POINTS

Remember the five Hs and the five Ts when looking for underlying causes of PEA.

 Cardiac rhythm simulator: www.skill stat.com/home1.htm. ACLS self-testing and assessment tool: www.skillstat.com/ACLS_STAT_demo.html.

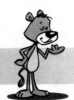

Do You UNDERSTAND?

DIRECTIONS: **Provide short answers to each of the following questions.**

1. What is the most common rhythm seen in adult cardiac arrest?

   _____

2. What is the definitive form of treatment for VF? _____

3. What is the sequence of treatment for VF after the first three shocks?

   _____   _____

   _____   _____

4. What is the first drug of choice in all three cardiac arrest rhythms?

   _____

5. List the five Hs and five Ts to be considered in PEA and asystole.

   _____   _____

   _____   _____

   _____   _____

   _____   _____

   _____   _____

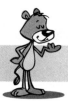

What IS Multiorgan Dysfunction Syndrome?

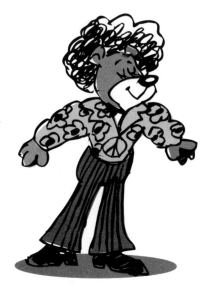

Multiorgan dysfunction syndrome (MODS) is the progressive dysfunction of more than one organ in patients that are critically ill or injured. It is the leading cause of death in intensive care units (ICUs). The initial insult that stimulates MODS may result from a variety of causes including, but not limited to, extensive burns, trauma, cardiorespiratory failure, multiple blood transfusions, and most commonly, systemic infection.

As health care treatments and procedures become increasingly effective, a greater number of patients are surviving traumatic insults. As a result, ICUs are seeing more cases MODS. The term *MODS* has been referred to interchangeably as systemic inflammatory response syndrome (SIRS) and multisystem organ failure (MSOF). In this presentation, we will use the term *MODS*.

What You NEED TO KNOW

Pathogenesis

The body is designed to respond to illness and injury by activating compensatory mechanisms to adjust to the insult. These changes include increased HR, contractility, CO, and oxygen consumption. The neurologic and endocrine systems respond by releasing the following mediators to address this insult: catecholamines, cortisol, antidiuretic hormone (ADH), growth hormone, and glucagons. These changes occur within the first 3 to 5 days after the event and begin to diminish within 7 to 10 days. For some patients the response does not diminish and tachycardia, fever, and a state of hypermetabolism continue.

Whatever the initial illness or injury, the cause of MODS seems to be an uncontrolled systemic inflammatory response and effects of multiple mediator systems. The by-products of these interactive systems cause effects in the vascular system at an intracellular level, and they eventually affect cell function. Vascular occlusive events disrupt blood flow by enhancing release of thromboxane (a potent vasoconstrictor) and by inhibiting synthesis of prostacyclin (a vasodilating substance). The result is an overall vasoconstrictive effect. Intracellular injury and hyperactivity lead to increased intracellular oxygen demand. Leukocyte activation and other effects that amplify a systemic inflammatory response result in organ distress, organ failure, or both.

Systemic Impact of Multiorgan Dysfunction Syndrome

ORGAN SYSTEM	CLINICAL MANIFESTATIONS OF FAILURE
CNS	Altered level of consciousness
Heart	Heart rate (HR) <54 or >100 bpm MAP <49 mm Hg Mean PA < or >15 mm Hg Cardiac output (CO) <4 or >8 LPM CVP <2 or >6 mm Hg Cold, pale skin Weak pulses Urine output <30 ml/hr Irregular rhythm
Pulmonary	Respiratory rate <5 or >49 breaths per minute O_2 saturations <90 mm Hg pH <7.35 or >7.45 $PaCO_2$ <35 or >45 mm Hg HCO_3 <22 or >26 mEq
Kidney	Urine output <30 ml/hr Serum BUN >100 mg/dl Serum creatinine >3.5 mg/dl
GI	Decreased or absent bowel sounds Abdominal distention Diarrhea or constipation Heme-positive stools
Liver	Jaundice Serum bilirubin >6 mg% PTT >4 sec over control in the absence of systemic anticoagulation
Hematologic	WBC count <1000/μl Platelets <20,000/μl Hematocrit <20%
Immune system	Generalized immune depression

CNS, Central nervous system; *MAP*, mean arterial pressure; *PA*, pulmonary artery; *CO*, cardiac output; *LPM*, liters per minute; *CVP*, central venous pressure; O_2, oxygen; CO_2, carbon dioxide; *PaCO$_2$*, arterial platelet level of CO_2; *HCO$_3$*, serum bicarbonate; *BUN*, blood urea nitrogen; *GI*, gastrointestinal; *PTT*, prothrombin time; *WBC*, white blood count.

At-Risk Populations

Patients at greatest risk for developing MODS include the following:

1. Patients with systemic infection (particularly, a gram-negative sepsis)
2. Extensive burns
3. End-organ failure
4. Pancreatitis

5. Hypovolemia
6. Cardiogenic shock
7. Human immunodeficiency virus (HIV)
8. Aspiration
9. Multiple blood transfusions
10. Trauma

Prognosis

Although the mortality is high with MODS, patients can recover, even when multiple organs are involved. Potential for recovery depends upon the severity of illness or injury, underlying organ reserve, the speed of instituting effective treatment, the adequacy of treatment, and the number and severity of subsequent injuries and complications. If treatment is unsuccessful, death usually occurs between 21 and 28 days after the initial insult.

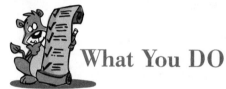 **What You DO**

The treatment of MODS is directed toward the following six goals: (1) identifying the underlying cause, (2) maintaining tissue oxygenation, (3) providing nutritional support, (4) avoiding additional complications, (5) preventing infection, (6) and supporting individual organs by means of mechanical ventilation, dialysis, transfusions of blood products, and pharmacological support as required.

MODS is most commonly associated with systemic infections; therefore aggressive diagnostics to identify the organism will be performed (i.e., blood, tissue, urine, sputum, and invasive line tips are sent for culture and sensitivity). Tissue oxygenation is maintained by providing adequate airway support, by oxygen administration, and by initiating mechanical ventilation assistance as needed. BP, CO, and fluid volume status may be supported with administration of crystalloids, inotropes, such as dobutamine, and vasopressors, such as dopamine. Nutritional supplementation of carbohydrates, proteins, and amino acids is provided with IV or enteral feedings to support metabolic demands. Additional complications from nosocomial infections may be prevented by replacing emergently placed lines as soon as possible and by changing central lines every 72 hours. Patients that are intubated should be weaned and extubated as expeditiously as tolerated to reduce the risk of infection. Dialysis may be used as a supportive measure for renal insufficiency and failure. The administration of blood and blood by-products such as albumin, platelets, and fresh frozen plasma may be required to replace those lost as the result of trauma, infection, disseminated intravascular coagulation (DIC), or thrombocytopenia. Additional pharmacological support may include antibiotics to which the organism is sensitive, antioxidants, antiprostaglandins, antihistamines, and corticosteroids. Xigris is a miscellaneous class drug currently being used for the treatment of sepsis in MODS. The mechanism of action is achieved through complex antithrombotic and antiinflammatory effects.

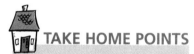 **TAKE HOME POINTS**

Aggressive support in the ICU is usually required for days or weeks.

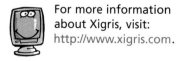 **For more information about Xigris, visit:** http://www.xigris.com.

Nursing Responsibilities

Clinical Manifestations of Multiorgan Dysfunction Syndrome

SYSTEM	NURSING RESPONSIBILITIES
CNS	Assess level of consciousness per Glasgow Coma Scale Observe for respiratory depression Monitor ICP (if indicated)
Pulmonary	Observe for and report: Dyspnea Use of accessory muscles Discolored sputum Wheezes, crackles, rhonchi Poor capillary refill Decreased O$_2$ saturation Abnormal ABG values Provide emergent airway support as needed
Cardiovascular	Observe for and report changes in: • HR) • BP • PAP • CO and cardiac index • CVP • SVR Observe for: • Cold, pale skin • Diminished pulses • Decreased urine output • Dysrhythmias • Myocardial ischemia • Elevated isoenzymes • Elevated troponins
GI	Observe for: • Decreased bowel sounds • Abdominal distention • Diarrhea, constipation, or impaction • Jaundice • Ascites • Guaiac stool if GI bleeding is suspected

CNS, Central nervous system; *ICP*, intracranial pressure; *O$_2$*, oxygen; *ABG*, arterial blood gas; *HR*, heart rate; *BP*, blood pressure; *PAP*, pulmonary artery pressure; *CO*, cardiac output; *CVP*, central venous pressure; *SVR*, systemic vascular resistance; *GI*, gastrointestinal; *GU*, genitourinary; *BUN*, blood urea nitrogen.

Clinical Manifestations of Multiorgan Dysfunction Syndrome—cont'd

SYSTEM	NURSING RESPONSIBILITIES
GI (cont'd)	Observe laboratory results for: • Increased ammonia • Decreased plasma proteins • Decreased clotting factors • Increased liver enzymes
GU	Observe for any changes in urine output, color, odor Observe laboratory results for increased BUN and creatinine levels

CNS, Central nervous system; *ICP,* intracranial pressure; *O₂,* oxygen; *ABG,* arterial blood gas; *HR,* heart rate; *BP,* blood pressure; *PAP,* pulmonary artery pressure; *CO,* cardiac output; *CVP,* central venous pressure; *SVR,* systemic vascular resistance; *GI,* gastrointestinal; *GU,* genitourinary; *BUN,* blood urea nitrogen.

The first line of defense is protection. Proper hand washing and use of aseptic technique should always be used. Early recognition of symptoms by the vigilant nurse is the first step in provision of appropriate treatment. These are most powerful tools in combating MODS in the "at-risk" population.

Do You UNDERSTAND?

DIRECTIONS: **Fill in the blanks to complete each of the following statements.**

1. Name ten at-risk populations for MODS:

_____   _____

_____   _____

_____   _____

_____   _____

_____   _____

2. Tissue oxygenation after an insult is maintained by ensuring adequate

_____, administration of _____, and

initiation of _____ support.

DIRECTIONS: **Identify the following statements as** *true* **(T) or** *false* **(F).**

_____ 3. A common clinical sign of MODS is acute respiratory failure.

_____ 4. Dialysis is a treatment for MODS.

_____ 5. Nutritional support for the patient in MODS is provided by frequent high fat feedings.

_____ 6. Encephalopathy is a clinical manifestation of MODS.

_____ 7. Fluid volume excess is a problem with MODS.

References

Chapter 1 Review of Hemodynamics

Ahrens T, Taylor L: *Hemodynamic waveform analysis*, Philadelphia, 1992, WB Saunders.

Alspach J et al: *AACN core curriculum for critical care nursing*, ed 5, Philadelphia, 1998, WB Saunders.

Chernecky C, Berger B: *Tests and diagnostic procedures*, ed 2, Philadelphia, 1997, WB Saunders.

George-Gay B, Chernecky C: *Clinical medical-surgical nursing: a decision making reference*, Philadelphia, 2002, WB Saunders.

Gutierrez KJ, Peterson PJ: *Real-world nursing survival guide: pathophysiology*, Philadelphia, 2002, WB Saunders.

Parsons PE, Wiener-Kronish JP: *Critical care secrets*, ed 2, Philadelphia, 2001, Hanley & Belfus.

Sole ML, Lamborn ML, Hartshorn JC: *Introduction to critical care nursing*, ed 3, Philadelphia, 2001, WB Saunders.

Chapter 2 Shock Trauma

Barker E: *Neuroscience nursing: a spectrum of care*, ed 2, St Louis, 2002, Mosby.

Collins T: Understanding shock, *Nurs Stand* 14(49):35, 2000.

Deglin J, Vallerand A: *Davis's drug guide for nurses*, ed 7, Philadelphia, 2001, FA Davis.

Dhainaut J, Thijs L, Park G, editors: *Septic shock*, London, 2000, Harcourt.

Garcia J, Rule R: Cardiogenic shock. In George-Gay B, Chernecky C, editors: *Clinical medical-surgical nursing*, Philadelphia, 2002, WB Saunders.

Hall JB, Schmidt GA, Lawrence DH: *Principles of critical care*, ed 2, New York, 1998, McGraw-Hill.

Hand H: Shock, *Nurs Stand* 15(48):45, 2001.

Hollenberg SM, Kavinsky CJ, Parrillo JE: Cardiogenic shock, *Ann Intern Med* 131(1):47, 1999.

Kinney M et al: *AACN: clinical reference for critical care nursing*, ed 4, St Louis, 1998, Mosby.

Morgan G, Mikhail M, Murray M: *Clinical anesthesiology*, ed 3, New York, 2002, McGraw-Hill.

Sole M, Lamborn M, Hartshorn J: *Introduction to critical care nursing*, ed 3, Philadelphia, 2001, WB Saunders.

Stillwell S: *Critical care nursing reference*, ed 3, St Louis, 2002, Mosby.

Urden L, Stacey K, Lough M: *Thelan's critical care nursing: diagnosis and management*, ed 4, St Louis, 2002, Mosby.

Chapter 3 Trauma and Emergency Care

American College of Surgeons: *Advanced trauma life support program for doctors (student course manual)*, ed 6, Chicago, 1997, The College.

American Heart Association: *Advanced cardiac life support provider manual*, Dallas, 2001, AHA.

American Heart Association: *BLS manual*, Dallas, 2001, AHA.

Arahm JL: Management of pain and spinal cord compression in patients with advanced cancer. ACP-ASIM End-of-life Care Consensus Panel. American College of Physicians. American Society of Internal Medicine, *Ann Intern Med* 131(1):37 1999.

Arce D, Sass P, Abul-Khoudoud H: Recognizing spinal cord emergencies, *Am Family Phys* 64(4):631, 2001.

Baines MJ: Spinal cord compression—a personal and palliative care perspective, *Clin Oncol* 14(2):132, 2002.

Barker E: Brain attack/stroke management. In *Neuroscience nursing: a spectrum of care*, ed 2, St Louis, 2002, Mosby.

Barker E: Intracranial pressure and monitoring. In Barker E: *Neuroscience nursing: a spectrum of care*, ed 2, St Louis, 2002, Mosby.

Bennett J, Hoyt K, editors: *Trauma nursing core course (provider manual)*, ed 5, Chicago, 2000, Emergency Nurses Association.

Biglioli P et al: Paraplegia after iatrogenic extrinsic spinal cord compression after descending thoracic aorta repair: case report and literature review, *J Thorac Cardiovasc Surg* 124(2):407, 2002.

Brohi K: *Acute management of traumatic brain injury*, 2000, http://www.trauma.org/neuro/acutemanagement.html. Retrieved February 3, 2003.

Bucholtz JD: Metastatic epidural spinal cord compression, *Semin Oncol Nurs* 15:150, 1999.

Burns M et al: *Advanced trauma care for nurses instructor manual*, Santa Fe, 1998, Society of Trauma Nurses.

Cardona V et al: *Trauma nursing from resuscitation through rehabilitation*, ed 2, 1994, Philadelphia, WB Saunders.

Chen TC: Prostate cancer and spinal cord compression, *Oncology* 15(7):841, 2001.

Chong CC, Kneebone A, Sheridan M: Managing malignant spinal cord compression, *Aust Family Phys* 30(9):859, 2001.

Clochesy JM et al: *Critical care nursing*, Philadelphia, 1996, WB Saunders.

Decker W: *Hypothermia E-Medicine Topic* 279, 2001.

Donato V et al: Radiation therapy for oncological emergencies, *Anticancer Res* 21(3C):2219, 2001.

Feurera et al: *Trauma management: an emergency medicine approach*, St Louis, 2001, Mosby.

Flounders JA, Ott BB: Oncology emergency modules: spinal cord compression, *Oncol Nurs Forum* 30(1):E17, 2003.

Garner C: Cancer-related spinal cord compression, *Am J Nurs* 99(7):34, 1999.

Glaser JA et al: Cervical spinal cord compression and the Hoffmann sign, *Iowa Orthop J* 21:49, 2001.

Grace M, Schumacher L: Increased intracranial pressure. In George-Gay B, Chernecky C: *Medical-surgical nursing: a manual for clinical decision making*, Philadelphia, 2002, WB Saunders.

Guyton A, Hall J: Textbook of medical physiology, ed 10, Philadelphia, 2000, WB Saunders.

Hardman JG et al: *Goodman & Gilman's: the pharmacological basis of therapeutics*, New York, 1996, McGraw-Hill. http://www.chendrick.org/healthy/00045850.html

Hardy J R, Huddart R: Spinal cord compression—what are the treatment standards? *Clin Oncol* 14(2):132, 2002.

Harrison S, editor: *Textbook of internal medicine on-line*, New York, 2001, McGraw-Hill.

Hashimoto S et al: Clinical efficacy of telemedicine in emergency radiotherapy for malignant spinal cord compression, *J Digit Imaging* 14(3):124, 2001.

Hock NH: Brain attack: the stroke continuum, *Nurs Clin North Am* 34(3):689, 1999.

Hoit BD: Diseases of the pericardium. In Fuster VF, Alexander RW, O'Rourke RA, editors: *Hurst's: the heart*, ed 10, vol 2, New York, 2001, McGraw-Hill.

Husband DJ, Grant KA, Romaniuk CS: MRI in the diagnosis and treatment of suspected malignant spinal cord compression, *Br J Radiol* 74:15, 2001.

Janjan N: Bone metastases: approaches to management, *Semin Oncol* 28(4 suppl 11):28, 2001.

Kienstra GE et al: Prediction of spinal epidural metastases, *Arch Neurol* 57(5):690, 2000.

King BS, Gupta R, Narayan RK: The early assessment and intensive care unit management of patients with severe traumatic brain and spinal cord injuries, *Surg Clin North Am* 80(3):855, 2000.

Ma O: Head injury. In Cline D et al, editors: *Emergency medicine: a comprehensive study guide, companion handbook,* ed 5, New York, 2000, McGraw-Hill.

Malcolm GP: Surgical disorders of the cervical spine: presentation and management of common disorders, *J Neurol Neurosurg Psychiatry* 73(suppl 1):i34, 2002.

Manglani HH et al: Orthopedic emergencies in cancer patients, *Semin Oncol* 27(3):299, 2000.

McCall WG: Airway management. In Waugamann W, Foster S, Rigor B, editors: *Principles and practice of nurse anesthesia,* ed 3, Stamford, Conn, 1999, Appleton & Lange.

McCance K, Huether S: *Pathophysiology: the biologic basis for disease in adults & children,* ed 4, St Louis, 2002, Mosby.

McLain RF: Spinal cord decompression: an endoscopically assisted approach for metastatic tumors, *Spinal Cord* 39:482, 2001.

McNeill MM: Pericardial, myocardial, and endocardial disease. In Woods SL, Froelicher E, Adams S, editors: *Cardiac nursing,* 4 ed, Philadelphia, 2000, Lippincott.

Mendez KA: Neurologic therapeutic management. In Urden LD, Stacy KM, Lough ME: *Thelan's critical care nursing: diagnosis and management,* ed 4, St Louis, 2002, Mosby.

Metules TJ: Cardiac tamponade, *RN* 62(12):26, 1999.

Morris J, Cook TM: Rapid sequence induction: a national survey of practice, *Anaesthesia* 56(11):1090, 2001.

Naco GJ, von Gunten C: Refractory neuropathic pain from chronic cord compression, *J Palliat Med* 5(3):433, 2002.

Newberry L: *Sheehy's emergency nursing: principles and practice,* ed 5, St Louis, 2003, Mosby.

Quinn JA, DeAngelis LM: Neurologic emergencies in the cancer patient, *Semin Oncol* 27(3):311, 2000.

Rades D, Heidenreich F, Karstens JH: Final results of a prospective study of the prognostic value of the time to develop motor deficits before irradiation in metastatic spinal cord compression, *Int J Radiat Oncol Biol Phys* 53(4):975, 2002.

Rades D, Karstens JH, Alberti W: Role of radiotherapy in the treatment of motor dysfunction due to metastatic spinal cord compression: comparison of three different fractionation schedules, *Int J Radiat Oncol Biol Phys* 54(4):1160, 2002.

Rogers CL et al: Surgery and permanent 125I seed paraspinal brachytherapy for malignant tumors with spinal cord compression, *Int J Radiat Oncol Biol Phys* 54(2):505, 2002.

Rude M: Selected neurologic complications in the patient with cancer. Brain metastases and spinal cord compression, *Crit Care Nurs Clin North Am* 12(3):269, 2000.

Schlesinger S, Blanchfield D: Modified rapid sequence induction of anesthesia: a survey of current clinical practice, *AANA J* 69(4):291, 2001.

Schoeggl A, Reddy M, Matula C: Neurological outcome following laminectomy in spinal metastases, *Spinal Cord* 40:363, 2002.

Schumacher L: Cerebrovascular accident. In George-Gay B, Chernecky C: *Medical-surgical nursing: a manual for clinical decision making,* Philadelphia, 2002, WB Saunders.

Seol HJ, Chung CK, Kim HJ: Surgical approach to anterior compression in the upper thoracic spine, *J Neurosurg Spine* 97(3 suppl):337, 2002.

Spivak JM: Vertebroplasty: weighing the benefits and the risks, *Am Fam Physician* 66(4):565, 2002.

Spodick DH: Pathophysiology of cardiac tamponade, *Chest* 113:1372, 1998.

Thwaites A J, Rice CP, Smith I: Rapid sequence induction: a questionnaire survey of its routine conduct and continued management during a failed intubation, *Anaesthesia* 54(4):376, 1999.

Vance DL: Treating acute ischemic stroke with intravenous alteplase, *Crit Care Nurse* 21(4):25, 2001.

Walker J: Caring for patients with a diagnosis of cancer and spinal metastatic disease, *Nurs Stand* 16(42):41, 2002.

Weinberg A: Hypothermia, *Ann Emerg Med* 22:370, 1993.

Chapter 4 Cardiovascular System

Abraham WT et al: *MIRACLE trial results presented at ACC clinical trials II session,* Orlando, Fla, March 20, 2001.

American Heart Association web site. Retrieved January 6, 2003 http://www.americanheart.org.

Albert N: Heart failure: the physiologic basis for current therapeutic concepts, *Crit Care Nurse* 19(3 Suppl):2, 1999.

Bowman MA: *Current concepts in the management of heart failure: maximizing medical therapy.* Presentation at St. Joseph Hospital, Augusta, Ga, January 2002.

Carroll DL et al: Activities of the APN to enhance unpartnered elders self-efficacy after myocardial infarction, *Clin Nurse Spec* 15(2):60, 2001.

Consensus recommendations for the management of chronic heart failure. On behalf of the membership of the advisory council to improve outcomes nationwide in heart failure, *Am J Cardiol* 83(2A):1A, 1999.

Corrigan M, Cupples ME, Stevenson M: Quitting and restarting smoking: cohort study of patients with angina in primary care, *BMJ* 324(7344):1016, 2002.

Dib N: *Muscle cell transplants repair damaged heart tissue.* Presented at the American Heart Associations' Scientific Sessions 2002, November 2002, Chicago.

Fallon E, Roques J: Acute chest pain, *AACN Clin Issues* 8(3):383, 1997.

Fife A, Farr E: Acute myocardial infarction, *Nurs Stand* 12(26):49, 1998.

Garrett K: Heart failure. In George-Gay B, Chernecky C, editors: *Clinical medical-surgical nursing: a decision-making reference,* Philadelphia, 2002, WB Saunders.

Hand H: Myocardial infarction: part 1, *Nurs Stand* 15(36):45, 2001.

Hand H: Myocardial infarction: part 2, *Nurs Stand* 15(37):45, 2001.

Hunt SA et al: ACC/AHA guidelines for the evaluation and management of chronic heart failure in the adult: executive summary. A report of the American College of Cardiology/American Heart Association Task Force on Practice Guidelines (committee to revise the 1995 Guidelines for the Evaluation and Management of Heart Failure), *J Am Coll Cardiol* 38(7):2101, 2001.

InSync Cardiac Resynchronization Therapy, Medtronic, 2002.

Kucia AM, Taylor KTN, Horowitz JD: Can a nurse trained in coronary care expedite emergency department management of patients with acute coronary syndromes? *Heart Lung* 30(3):186, 2001.

Scios: *Natrecor (nesiritide): questions and answers about Natrecor,* Fremont, Calif, 2001, Scios.

Patton JA, Funk M: Survey of use of ST-segment monitoring in patients with acute coronary syndrome, *Am J Crit Care* 10(1):23, 2001.

Pelter MM, Adams MG, Drew BJ: Association of transient myocardial ischemia with adverse in-hospital outcomes for angina patients treated in a telemetry unit or a coronary care unit, *Am J Crit Care* 11(4):318, 2002.

Pitt B et al: The effect of spironolactone on morbidity and mortality in patients with severe heart failure, *New Engl J Med* 341(10):709, 1999.

Publication Committee for the VMAC (Vasodilation in the Management of Acute CHF) Investigators: Intravenous nesiritide vs nitroglycerin for treatment of decompensative congestive heart failure: a randomized controlled trial, *JAMA* 287(12):1531, 2002.

Roberts A, Johnstone J, Miles M: An evaluation of nurse-led thrombolysis in the management of patients with acute myocardial infarction, *Nurs Crit Care* 6(6):267, 2001.

Roettig ML, Tanabe P: Emergency management of acute coronary syndromes, *J Emerg Nurs* 26(6 Pt 2):S1, 2000.

Smith M, Irving JB: Managing heart failure in the community: role of the nurse specialist, *Health Bull* 59(5):340, 2001.

Yeghiazarians Y et al: Medical progress: unstable angina pectoris, *New Engl J Med* 342:101, 2000.

Chapter 5 Respiratory System

Ball C et al: Clinical guidelines for the use of the prone position in acute respiratory distress syndrome, *Intensive Crit Care Nurs* 17(2):94, 2001.

Brower RG et al: Treatment of ARDS, *Chest* 120(4):1347, 2001.

Goll CA: Respiratory dysfunctions: acute respiratory distress syndrome. In Swearingen PL, Keen JH, editors: *Manual of critical care nursing,* ed 4, St Louis, 2001, Mosby.

Hynes-Gay P, MacDonald R: Using high-frequency oscillatory ventilation to treat adults with acute respiratory distress syndrome, *Crit Care Nurs* 21(5):38, 2001.

Lee LC, Shah K: Clinical manifestation of pulmonary embolism, *Emerg Med Clin North Am* 19(4):925, 2001.

Marion BS: A turn for the better: prone positioning of patients with ARDS: a guide to the physiology and management of this effective, underused intervention, *Am J Nurs* 101(5):26, 2001.

Moccia JM: Using the ECG to identify pulmonary embolism, *Dimens Crit Care Nurs* 19(5):27, 2000.

Mortelliti MP, Manning HL: Radiologic decision-making: acute respiratory distress syndrome, *Am Fam Physician* 65(9):1823, 2002.

Rosenberg SG: Modes of mechanical ventilation. In Duke J, editor: *Anesthesia secrets,* ed 2, Philadelphia, 2000, Hanley & Belfus.

Spritzer CJ: Unraveling the mysteries of mechanical ventilation: a helpful step-by-step guide, *J Emerg Nurs* 29(1):29, 87, 2003.

Stacy KM: Pulmonary disorders: pulmonary embolus. In Urden LD, Stacy KM, editors: *Priorities in critical care nursing,* ed 3, St Louis, 2000, Mosby.

Stacy KM: Pulmonary therapeutic management. In Urden LD, Stacy KM, editors: *Priorities in critical care nursing,* ed 3, St Louis, 2000, Mosby.

Welsh CH: Mechanical ventilation. In Parsons PE, Wiener-Kronish JP, editors: *Critical care secrets,* ed 2, Philadelphia, 1998, Hanley & Belfus.

Wood KE: Major pulmonary embolism: review of a pathophysiologic approach to the golden hour of hemodynamically significant pulmonary embolism, *Chest* 121(3):877, 2002.

Chapter 6 Nervous System

Alspach JG, editor: *Core curriculum for critical care nursing,* Philadelphia, 1998, WB Saunders.

Barker E: *Neuroscience nursing: a spectrum of care,* ed 2, St Louis, 2002, Mosby.

Best J: Action stat: cauda equina syndrome, *Nursing* 31(4):43, 2001.

Ignatavicius DD, Workman ML: *Medical-surgical nursing: critical thinking for collaborative care,* ed 4, Philadelphia, 2002, WB Saunders.

Kammerman S, Wasserman L: Seizure disorders: part 1. Classification and diagnosis, *West J Med* 175(2):99, 2001.

Kammerman S, Wasserman L: Seizure disorders: part 2. Treatment, *West J Med* 175(3):184, 2001.

McDonald JW, Sadowsky C: Spinal-cord injury, *Lancet* 359(9304):417, 2002.

Munden J, McCleery JG, editors: *Springhouse review for critical care nursing certification,* ed 3, Philadelphia, 2002, Lippincott, Williams & Wilkins.

Parini SM: The meningitis mind-bender, *Nurs Manag* 33(8):21, 2002.

Tipton KD: Action stat: autonomic dysreflexia, *Nursing* 28(11):33, 1998.

Chapter 7 Gastrointestinal System

Alspach JG, editor: *Core curriculum for critical care nursing,* ed 5, Philadelphia, 1998, WB Saunders.

Bucher L, Melander S: *Critical care nursing,* Philadelphia, 1999, WB Saunders.

Burke M: Acute intestinal obstruction: diagnosis and management, *Hosp Med* 63(2):104, 2002.

Burkill G, Bell J, Healy J: Small bowel obstruction: the role of computed tomography in its diagnosis and management with reference to other imaging modalities, *Eur Radiol* 11(8):1405, 2001.

Casey P: Assessment and management of patients with endocrine disorders. In Smeltzer S, Bare B, editors: *Brunner and Suddarth's textbook of medical-surgical nursing,* ed 9, Philadelphia, 2000, Lippincott, Williams & Wilkins

Chambers J: Gastrointestinal alterations. In Sole ML, Lamhorn ML, Hartshorn JC: *Introduction to critical care nursing,* ed 3, Philadelphia, 2001, WB Saunders.

Chernecky C, Macklin D, Murphy-Ende K: *Real-world nursing survival guide: fluids & electrolytes,* Philadelphia, 2002, WB Saunders

Cohen A: Liver diseases. In Copstead LC, Banasik JL, editors: *Pathophysiology: biological and behavioral perspectives,* ed 2, Philadelphia, 2000, WB Saunders.

Crist D, Cameron J: The current management of acute pancreatitis, *Adv Surg* 20:69, 1987.

Dauphne CE et al: Placement of self-expanding metal stents for acute malignant large-bowel obstruction: a collective review, *Ann Surg Oncol* 9(6):74, 2002.

Davis MP, Nouneh C: Modern management of cancer-related intestinal obstruction, *Curr Pain Headache Rep* 5(3):257, 2001.

De Giorgio R et al: Review article: the pharmacologic treatment of acute colonic pseudo-obstruction, *Aliment Pharmacol Ther* 15(11):1717, 2001.

Edlich RF, Woods JA: Wangensteen's transformation of the treatment of intestinal obstruction from empiric craft to scientific discipline, *J Emerg Med* 15(2):235, 1997.

Fischer CP, Doherty D: Laparoscopic approach to small bowel obstruction, *Semin Laparosc Surg* 9(1):40, 2002.

Fleshner PR et al: A prospective, randomized trial of short versus long tubes in adhesive small-bowel obstruction, *Am J Surg* 170(4):366, 1995.

Frager D: Intestinal obstruction role of CT, *Gastroenterol Clin North Am* 31(3):777, 2002.

Furukawa A et al: Helical CT in the diagnosis of small bowel obstruction, *Radiographics* 21(2):341, 2001.

Gavaghan M: The pancreas-hermit of the abdomen, *AORN J* 75(6):1110, 2002.

Ignatavicius DD, Workman ML: *Medical-surgical nursing: critical thinking for collaborative care,* ed 4, Philadelphia, 2002, WB Saunders.

Kavic SM, Kavic SM: Adhesions and adhesiolysis: the role of laparoscopy, *JSLS* 6(2):99, 2002.

Khot UP et al: Systematic review of the efficacy and safety of colorectal stents, *Br J Surg* 89(9):1096, 2002.

Kinney MR et al: *AACN clinical reference for critical care nursing,* ed 4, St Louis, 1998, Mosby.

Lehne RA: *Pharmacology for nursing care,* ed 4, Philadelphia, 2001, WB Saunders.

Liakakos T et al: Peritoneal adhesions: etiology, pathophysiology, and clinical significance. Recent advances in prevention and management, *Dig Surg* 18(4):260, 2001.

Matter I et al: Does the index operation influence the course and outcome of adhesive intestinal obstruction? *Eur J Surg* 163(10):767, 1997.

Miettinen P et al: The outcome of elderly patients after operation for acute abdomen, *Ann Chir Gynaecol* 85(1):11 1996.

Munoz A, Katerndahl DA: Diagnosis and management of acute pancreatitis, *Am Fam Physician* 62(1):164, 2000.

Odom B: Intestinal obstruction. In George-Gay B, Chernecky C, editors: *Clinical medical-surgical nursing: a decision making reference,* St Louis, 2002, Mosby.

Onoue S et al: The value of contrast radiology for postoperative adhesive bowel obstruction, *Hepatogastroenterology* 49(48):1576, 2002.

Phipps W et al: *Medical-surgical nursing: health and illness perspectives,* ed 7, St Louis, 2003, Mosby.

Platt V: Malignant bowel obstruction: so much more than symptom control, *Int J Palliat Nurs* 7(11):547, 2001.

Ripamonti C, Bruera E: Palliative management of malignant bowel obstruction, *Int J Gynecol Cancer* 12:135, 2002.

Sagar PM et al: Intestinal obstruction promotes gut translocation of bacteria, *Dis Colon Rectum* 38(6):640, 1995.

Shelton BK: Intestinal obstruction, *AACN Clin Issues Crit Care* 10(4):478, 1999.

Singh S, Gagneja HK: Stents in the small intestine, *Curr Gastroenterol Rep* 4(5):383, 2002.

Sole ML, Lamborn ML, Hartshorn JC: *Introduction to critical care nursing,* ed 3, Philadelphia, 2001, WB Saunders.

Taourel P et al: Non-traumatic abdominal emergencies: imaging of acute intestinal obstruction, *Eur Radiol* 12(9):2151, 2002.

Urden L, Stacy KM, Lough M: *Thelan's critical care nursing: diagnosis and management,* ed 4, St Louis, 2002, Mosby.

Wilson MS, Hawkswell J, McCloy RF: Natural history of adhesional small bowel obstruction: counting the cost, *Br J Surg* 85(9):1294, 1998.

Chapter 8 Renal System

Ahmed S: *Manual of clinical dialysis,* London, 1999, Science Press.

Black J, Hawks J, Keene A: *Medical-surgical nursing: a clinical management for positive outcomes,* ed 6, Philadelphia, 2001, WB Saunders.

Bullock BA, Henze RL: *Focus on pathophysiology,* Philadelphia, 2000, Lippincott.

Buttaro T et al: *Primary care: a collaborative practice,* St Louis, 1999, Mosby.

Campbell D: How acute renal failure puts the brakes on kidney function, *Nursing* 33(1):59, 2003.

Cotran RS, Kumar V, Collins J: *Robbin's pathological basis of disease,* ed 6, Philadelphia, 1999, WB Saunders.

Hudak CM, Gallo BM, Morton PG: *Critical care nursing: a holistic approach,* ed 7, Philadelphia, 1998, Lippincott.

Huether SE, McCance KL: *Understanding pathophysiology,* ed 2, St Louis, 2000, Mosby.

Petroni K, Cohen N: Continuous renal replacement therapy: anesthetic implications, *Anesth Analges* 94(5):1288, 2002.

Ross C: Dialysis disequilibrium syndrome, *Am J Nurs* 100(2):53, 2000.

Schrier R, Gottschalk C: Acute renal failure. In *Diseases of the kidney,* ed 6, Philadelphia, 1997, Lippincott, Williams & Wilkins.

Sole ML, Lamborn ML, Hartshorn JC: *Introduction to critical care nursing,* ed 3, Philadelphia, 2001, WB Saunders.

Chapter 9 Endocrine System

Alspach J et al: *Core curriculum for critical care nursing,* ed 5, Philadelphia, 1998, WB Saunders.

Barker E: Metabolic disorders. In Barker E: *Neuroscience nursing: a spectrum of care,* ed 2, St Louis, 2002, Mosby.

Chernecky C, Berger B: *Laboratory tests and diagnostic procedures,* ed 3, Philadelphia, 2001, WB Saunders.

Clark JM: Endocrine disorders and therapeutic management. In Urden LD, Stacy KM, Lough ME: *Thelan's critical care nursing: diagnosis and management,* ed 4, St Louis, 2002, Mosby.

George-Gay B, Chernecky C: *Clinical medical-surgical nursing: a decision making reference*, Philadelphia, 2002, WB Saunders.

Gutierrez KJ, Peterson PJ: *Real-world nursing survival guide: pathophysiology*, Philadelphia, 2002, WB Saunders.

Guyton AC, Hall JE: *Textbook of medical physiology*, ed 10, Philadelphia, 2000, WB Saunders.

Harrigan MR: Cerebral salt wasting syndrome: a review, *Neurosurgery* 38(1):152, 1996.

Jones RE, Huether SE: Alterations of hormonal regulations. In McCance KL, Huether SE, editors: *Pathophysiology: the biological basis for disease in adults and children*, ed 4, St Louis, 2002, Mosby.

McEldowney DK: Endocrine alterations. In Sole ML, Lamborn ML, Hartshorn JC: *Introduction to critical care nursing*, ed 3, Philadelphia, 2001, WB Saunders.

Milionis HJ, Liamis GL, Elisaf MS: The hyponatremic patient: a systemic approach to laboratory diagnosis, *CMAJ* 166:1056, 2002.

Ousman Y et al: A standardized nurse-adjusted insulin infusion algorithm (SIIA) is safe and effective, *Diabetes* 51(suppl 2):A110, 2002.

Parobek V, Alaimo I: Fluid and electrolyte management in the neurologically impaired patient, *J Neurosci Nurs* 28(5):322, 1996.

Parsons PE, Wiener-Kronish JP: *Critical care secrets*, ed 2, Philadelphia, 2001, Hanley & Belfus.

Schafer SL: Oncologic complications. In Otto SE, editor: *Oncology nursing*, ed 4, St Louis, 2001, Mosby.

Sole ML, Lamborn ML, Hartshorn JC: *Introduction to critical care nursing*, ed 4, Philadelphia, 2001, WB Saunders.

Chapter 10 Hematologic System

Anastasia PJ: Nursing considerations for managing topotecan-related hematologic side effects, *Clin J Oncol Nurs* 5(1):27, 2001

Barel C et al: Treatment of hepatitis C virus associated thrombocytopenic purpura with a combination of interferon alfa-2b and ribavirin, *J Clin Gastroenterol* 35(2):200, 2002.

Chan G, DiVenuti G, Miller K: Danazol for the treatment of thrombocytopenia is patient with myelodysplastic syndrome, *Am J Hematol* 71(3):166, 2002.

Chemnitz J et al: Successful treatment of severe thrombotic thrombocytopenia purpura with the monoclonal antibody rituximab, *Am J Hematol* 71(2):105, 2002.

Chernecky C, Berger B: *Laboratory tests and diagnostic procedures*, ed 4, Philadelphia, 2003, WB Saunders.

Deitcher SR et al: Lepirudin anticoagulation for hepatin-induced thrombocytopenia, *J Pediatr* 140(2):264, 2002.

Dhainaut JF, Thijs LG, Park G, editors: *Septic shock: critical care management series*, London, 1999, Bailliere Tindall.

Fishbein TM et al: Recurrent portal hypertension after composite liver/small bowel transplantation, *Liver Trans* 8(7):639, 2002.

Friedman AM et al: Do basic laboratory tests or clinical observations predict bleeding in thrombocytopenic oncology patients? A reevaluation of prophylactic platelet transfusions, *Transfusion Med Rev* 16(1):34, 2002.

George-Gay B, Chernecky C: *Clinical medical-surgical nursing: a decision-making reference*, Philadelphia, 2002, WB Saunders.

Gesundheit B et al: Thrombocytopenia and megakaryocyte dysplasia: an adverse effect of valproic acid treatment, *J Pediatr Hematol Oncol* 24(7):589, 2002.

Harkness M: Neonatal issues. Neonatal alloimmune thrombocytopenia, *Br J Midwif* 10(2):99, 2002.

Hashimoto H et al: Hematologic findings associated with thrombocytopenia during the acute phase of exanthem subitum confirmed by primary human herpesvirus-6 infection, *J Pediatr Hematol Oncol* 24(3):211, 2002.

McCance KL, Huether SE: *Pathophysiology: the biologic basis for disease in adults and children*, ed 4, St Louis, 2002, Mosby.

Ruutu T et al: Thrombic thrombocytopenic purpura after allogeneic stem cell transplantation: a survey of the European group for blood and marrow transplantation (EBMT), *Br J Haematol* 118(4):1112, 2002.

Stillwell S: *Critical care nursing reference*, ed 3, St Louis, 2002, Mosby.

Theilen HJ et al: Fatal intracerebral hemorrhage due to leptospirosis, *Infection* 30(2):109, 2002.

Tierney L, McPhee S, Papadakis M, editors: *Current medical diagnosis & treatment*, New York, 2003, Lange Medical Books/McGraw-Hill.

Urden LD, Stacy KM, Lough ME: *Thelan's critical care nursing: diagnosis and management*, ed 4, St Louis, 2002, Mosby.

Uygun A et al: Interferon treatment of thrombocytopenia associated with chronic HCV infection, *Int J Clin Practice* 54(10):683, 2000.

Chapter 11 Integumentary System

Biddle EA, Hartley D: Fire and flame related events with multiple occupational injury fatalities in the United States, 1980-1995, *Inj Control Saf Promot* 9(1):9, 2002.

Hill AJ, Germa F, Boyle JC: Burns in older people—outcomes and risk factors, *J Am Geriatr Soc* 50(11):1912, 2002.

Hurlin Foley K et al: Use of an improved Watusi collar to manage pediatric neck burn contractures, *J Burn Care Rehabil* 23(3):221, 2002.

Kobayashi M et al: An increase in the susceptibility of burned patients to infectious complications due to impaired production of macrophage inflammatory protein 1 alpha, *J Immunology* 169(8):4460, 2002.

Meaume S et al: Urgotul: a novel non-adherent lipidocolloid dressing, *Br J Nurs* 11(16 suppl):S42, S46, 2002.

Medeiros R, Putnam S: First aid for injuries. In George-Gay B, Chernecky C: *Clinical medical-surgical nursing: a decision making reference*, Philadelphia, 2002, WB Saunders.

Monstrey S et al: A conservative approach for deep dermal burn wounds using polarized-light therapy, *Br J Plast Surg* 55(5):420, 2002.

Palmieri TL, Greenhalgh DG: Topical treatment of pediatric patients with burns: a practical guide, *Am J Clin Dermatol* 3(8):529, 2002.

Ramos GE et al: Catheter infection risk related to the distance between insertion site and burned area, *J Burn Care Rehabil* 23(4):266, 2002.

Ryan CM et al: Use of Integra artificial skin is associated with decreased length of stay for severely injured adult burn survivors, *J Burn Care Rehabil* 23(5):311, 2002.

Saraiya M, Hall HI, Uhler RJ: Sunburn prevalence among adults in the United States, 1999, *Am J Prev Med* 23(2):91, 2002.

Zhou YP et al: (2002). Experience in the treatment of patients with burns covering more than 90% TBSA and full-thickness burns exceeding 70% TBSA, *Asian J Surg* 25(2):154, 2002.

Bergstrom N, Braden BJ: Predictive validity of the Braden scale among black and white subjects, *Nurs Res* 51(6):398, 2002.

Bryant RA: *Acute and chronic wounds: nursing management*, ed 2, St Louis, 2001, Mosby.

Emory University: *WOCNEC syllabus: skin and wound module*, February 1, 1997.

Harada C, Shigematsu T, Hagisawa S: The effect of 10-degree leg elevation and 30-degree head elevation on body displacement and sacral interface pressure over a 2-hour period, *J Wound Ostomy Continence Nurs* 29(3):43, 2002.

Lindgren M, Unosson M, Krantz AM: A risk scale for the prediction of pressure sore development: reliability and validity, *J Adv Nurs* 38(2):190, 2002.

Lyder CH: Pressure ulcer prevention and management, *Ann Rev Nurs Res* 20:35, 2002.

Ackley BJ, Ladwig GB: *Nursing diagnosis handbook, a guide for planning care*, ed 5, St Louis, 2002, Mosby.

Centers for Disease Control and Prevention: *Group A streptococcal disease (on-line)*, 2002. Available: http://www.cdc.gov/ncidod/dbmd/diseaseinfo/groupastreptococcal_g.htm

Grindel CG, Crowley LV, Johnston CA: *Anatomy and physiology*, Springhouse, Penn, 2002, Springhouse.

Swartz MN: Cellulitis and subcutaneous tissue infections. In Mandell GL, Bennett JE, Dolin R, editors: *Mandell, Douglas, and Bennett's principles and practice of infectious diseases*, vol 1, Philadelphia, 2000, Churchill Livingstone.

Toder K: *On-line textbook of bacteriology*, 2002. Available: www.textbookofbacteriology.net: University of Wisconsin-Madison–Department of Bacteriology.

Chapter 12 Multisystem

American Heart Association: *Advanced cardiac life support*, Dallas, 2001, AHA.

American Heart Association: *Guideline 2000 for cardiopulmonary resuscitation and emergency cardiovascular care*, Dallas, 2001, AHA.

Autonomy and the Patient Self-Determination Act. http://www.med.upenn.edu/bioethic/Museum/Felder/Ethics.html

Black JM, Matassarin-Jacobs E: Multiple-organ system failure: systemic inflammatory response syndrome. In Framboise LN, editor: *Medical-surgical nursing*, Philadelphia, 1997, WB Saunders.

Chernecky C et al: *Real-world survival guide: ECGs & the heart*, Philadelphia, 2002, WB Saunders.

Dennison RD: Systemic inflammatory response syndrome and multiple organ dysfunction, *Pass CCRN*, ed 2, St Louis, 2000, Mosby.

Xigris: *Welcome to Xigris.com*. Retrieved November 21, 2002 from http://xigris.com.

Illustration Credits

Page 4, 6, 9, 230. From Sole ML, Lamborn ML, Hartshorn JC: *Introduction to critical care nursing*, ed 3, Philadelphia, 2001, WB Saunders.

Page 11, 37, 54, 224. From Bucher L, Melander S: *Critical care nursing*, Philadelphia, 1999, WB Saunders.

Page 19, 20, 27, 86, 117, 121, 130, 191, 295, 296. Phipps et al: *Medical-surgical nursing: health and illness perspectives*, ed 7, St Louis, 2003, Mosby.

Page 21, 332-334. Chernecky et al: *Real-world nursing series: ECGs & the heart*, Philadelphia, 2002, WB Saunders.

Page 23, 83, 119, 162, 166. Lewis SM, Heitkemper MM, Dirksen SR: *Medical-surgical nursing: assessment and management of clinical problems*, ed 5, St Louis, 2000, Mosby.

Page 35, 59, 123, 205, 206. Urden L, Stacy K, Lough M: *Thelan's critical care nursing: diagnosis and management*, ed 4, St Louis, 2002, Mosby.

Page 43, 46. Courtesy of Matthew W. Kervin, RN, BS, BSN, CRNA, Medical College of Georgia, Augusta, Georgia.

Page 82, 94, 134. Conover M: *Understanding electrocardiography*, ed 8, St Louis, 2003, Mosby.

Page 103. Feurera et al: *Trauma management: an emergency medicine approach*, St Louis, 2001, Mosby.

Page 133. Aehlert B: *ECGs made easy*, ed 2, St Louis, 2002, Mosby.

Page 155. From Pierce LNB: *Guide to mechanical ventilation and intensive respiratory care*, Philadelphia, 1995, WB Saunders.

Page 183. Barker E: *Neuroscience nursing: a spectrum of care*, ed 2, St Louis, 2002, Mosby.

Page 193, 194, 197, 231, 248, 249, 304. Ignatavicus DD, Workman ML: *Medical-surgical nursing: critical thinking for collaborative care*, ed 4, Philadelphia, 2002, WB Saunders.

Page 295. Newberry L: *Sheehy's emergency nursing: principles and practice*, ed 5, St Louis, 2003, Mosby.

Page 303. Morison et al: *Nursing management of chronic wounds*, ed 2, St Louis, 1999, Mosby.

NCLEX® Examination Review Questions

CHAPTER *1*

Review of Hemodynamics

1. At the end of diastole, the degree of ventricular stretch is referred to as:
   1 Preload.
   2 Afterload.
   3 Contractility.
   4 Cardiac output (CO).

2. The cardiac conduction system is the stimulus for:
   1 Atrial filling.
   2 Ventricular contraction.
   3 Systemic vascular resistance (SVR).
   4 Afterload.

3. The formula for CO equals:
   1 Stroke volume × heart rate (HR).
   2 Patient weight × HR.
   3 Contractility × HR.
   4 Stroke volume × contractility.

4. Which of the following is *not* a determinant of stroke volume?
   1 Contractility
   2 Preload
   3 HR
   4 Afterload

5. Preload is:
   1 A measurement of SVR.
   2 A measurement reflecting contractility.
   3 Reflective of left ventricular end–diastolic volume.
   4 Reflective of CO.

6. Afterload is reflective of:
   1 Pulmonary capillary wedge pressure (PCWP).
   2 CO.
   3 Contractility.
   4 SVR.

7. A substance that affects contractility is referred to as:
   1 Chronotropic.
   2 Inotropic.
   3 Vasoactive.
   4 Vasodilatory.

8. Preload can be measured with a pulmonary artery catheter by obtaining:
   1 SVR.
   2 PCWP.
   3 Left ventricular stroke work index (LVSWI).
   4 Pulmonary artery systolic pressure.

9. The sum of resistance in peripheral arterioles reflected in mean aortic pressure is:
   1 Pulmonary vascular resistance (PVR).
   2 SVR.
   3 Mean arterial pressure (MAP).
   4 PCWP.

10. Miscellaneous influences that *decrease* contractility include:
    1 Hypoxia, hyperkalemia, sympathetic stimulation.
    2 Hypercarbia, hyponatremia, sympathetic stimulation.
    3 Hypoxia, myocardial scar tissue, parasympathetic stimulation.
    4 Hypokalemia, hypernatremia, parasympathetic stimulation.

349

CHAPTER 2

Shock Trauma

1. You are the nurse for a 56-year-old woman who has been admitted for a gastrointestinal (GI) bleed. On the second day of hospitalization, the physician orders two units of packed red blood cells (RBCs) to be given over 4 hours each. You hang the first unit of blood at 9 AM. At 9:25 the patient calls the nurses' station for her nurse. The patient states that her hands are itching and she cannot get her wedding ring off. You should first:
   1 Remind the patient that she should not be wearing her wedding ring in the hospital and that if it should get lost or stolen, the hospital would not be responsible.
   2 Run and get a syringe of epinephrine to administer it subcutaneously because the patient is having an anaphylactic reaction.
   3 Stop the blood transfusion immediately because you suspect that it may be the cause of the patient's itching and swollen hands.
   4 Call the physician to let him or her know about the patient's complaints and request an order for Benadryl to help with the itching.

2. You are working as a nurse in the radiology department of your hospital. Your patient is a 34-year-old man needing a diagnostic computed axial tomographic (CAT) scan of the abdomen. He states that he has never had such a test before. You start a 20-gauge peripheral intravenous (IV) line in his left hand because the patient will receive iodinated radiocontrast media for the procedure. Once the patient's procedure has started, and the IV injection of the contrast has started, the patient complains of "feeling funny" and of not being able to swallow. Knowing that the patient may be experiencing an allergic reaction, your next step is to:
   1 Call the physician because you believe the patient is having an allergic reaction to the contrast media, and you will need some help taking care of the patient.
   2 Assess the patient's airway, administer 100% oxygen, and determine whether intervention such as intubation needs to take place immediately.
   3 Assure the patient that he is experiencing a normal reaction to the contrast media and that people often feel that way.
   4 Immediately start a large bore peripheral IV in the opposite arm as the existing IV because you need to administer large amounts of IV fluids to treat the allergic reaction.

3. In the situation in Question 2, you suspect that the patient is having a _____ reaction to the contrast media.
   1 Anaphylactic
   2 Acidotic
   3 Basophilic
   4 Anaphylactoid

4. You are the nurse taking care of a 55-year-old man who has been hospitalized for cellulitis of the left calf. You are about to go to lunch but decide to hang the patient's newly ordered antibiotic early so it will be finished when you return. You hang 1 piperacillin (PCN) 1 g in the IV piggyback and start the infusion to go over 1 hour. You tell the patient that you will return when it is finished to flush his IV. On your way to lunch you hear another nurse yell, "He's not breathing" from your patient's room. You then recall that your patient stated that he was allergic to PCN on his admission assessment. You immediately:
   1 Go to the room to see what the commotion is all about.
   2 Bring a syringe of epinephrine into the room and administer 0.3 to 0.5 ml of a 1:1000 solution subcutaneously (SC).
   3 Go to lunch because if you do not go now, you will probably not be able to eat later.
   4 Call the physician and tell him what has happened and that he ordered the wrong antibiotic for your patient.

5. You are a critical care nurse in the intensive care unit (ICU). You have just admitted a 44-year-old woman from the surgical floor who is having an anaphylactic reaction from eating a peanut butter cookie. The patient is deathly allergic to peanuts. So far the patient has been given oxygen and two doses of epinephrine SC. You apply the ICU monitors to the patient; the SaO_2 is 82%, and the patient is experiencing supraventricular tachycardia (SVT). The patient is looking lethargic and difficult to arouse. Your next step is to:
   1 Assist the patient's ventilation with an ambubag and 100% oxygen, and call for an emergent intubation.
   2 Establish two large-bore peripheral IV lines, and start normal saline (NS) wide open.
   3 Start cardiopulmonary resuscitation (CPR) because the patient is not responsive.
   4 Give the patient a beta blocker medication to slow the HR, which will decrease the oxygen consumption of the heart.

6. Continue with situation in Question 5. The anesthesia personnel are at the bedside to intubate the patient. You notice that they are having difficulty with the oral intubation; the patient's oxygen saturation is 50% and the HR is 60 beats per minute (bpm). If the team cannot get the patient orally intubated, the next step should be to:
   1 Continue to try to intubate the patient orally because the patient needs to be ventilated.
   2 Page the head of the anesthesia department to try to intubate the patient.
   3 Perform an immediate cricothyrotomy or tracheotomy to establish an airway because the anesthesia provider believes that orally intubating the patient is impossible.
   4 Stop all efforts because if the patient cannot be intubated, then nothing else can be done.

7. Continue the situation in Questions 5 and 6. The anesthesia provider successfully intubates the patient orally on the final attempt. A 6.0-oral endotracheal (ET) tube is placed, and the patient is given 100% oxygen via an ambubag. The oxygen saturation in now 98%, but the HR is decreasing rapidly and the patient has no pulse. The next step is to:
   1 Follow the airway, breathing, circulation (ABCs) of patient care, and initiate CPR.
   2 Adjust the IV fluids wide open, and give a bolus of NS 500 ml.
   3 Call the physician taking care of the patient to ask him or her what he or she wants you to do.
   4 Keep administering oxygen because the patient is experiencing hypoxia, which leads to the low HR.

8. Continue the situation in Questions 5, 6, and 7. CPR has been started. The respiratory therapist is controlling the patient's respirations, your colleague is performing CPR, and you are administering medications per the physician's orders. The physician orders epinephrine 0.5 mg IV now. Before you can administer the medication, your colleague inadvertently pulls out the only IV the patient has. Your next step is to:
   1 Scream at your colleague because he or she has lost the only IV access you have for the patient.
   2 Immediately try to start a new peripheral IV because you must give the epinephrine along with the required IV fluids.
   3 Administer the epinephrine via the ET tube while trying to establish another IV line.
   4 Stop CPR, and have the physician place a central line preferably in the right internal jugular vein.

9. The major, immediate risk associated with the use of a left ventricular assist device (LVAD) is:
   1 Infection.
   2 Embolus.
   3 Pump failure.
   4 Immobility.

10. Patients with cardiogenic shock often require vasopressor therapy. Select the most potent vasoconstrictor from the following list:
    1 Nitroprusside
    2 Dopamine
    3 Dobutamine
    4 Epinephrine

11. A person who develops ____% damage to the heart will likely develop cardiogenic shock.
    1 10%
    2 25%
    3 30%
    4 50%

12. During deflation, the intraaorta balloon pump (IABP) assists the heart by:
    1 Increasing preload.
    2 Decreasing afterload.
    3 Increasing cardiac oxygen demand.
    4 Decreasing preload.

13. How is cardiogenic shock different from hypovolemic shock?
    1 No difference exists between cardiogenic shock and hypovolemic shock.
    2 The BP is increased in cardiogenic shock and lowered in hypovolemic shock.
    3 An increase of fluid exists in the heart during cardiogenic shock but not during hypovolemic shock.
    4 The pulse rate is decreased in cardiogenic shock and increased in hypovolemic shock.

14. What is the ultimate goal of initial treatment of cardiogenic shock?
    1 To prevent further heart muscle damage
    2 To decrease HR
    3 To decrease core temperature
    4 To increase vascular volume

15. What patient sign or symptom will assist in determining cardiogenic shock versus another shock state?
    1 Blood loss
    2 Temperature 104° F
    3 Hives with breathing difficulty
    4 Angina with electrocardiographic (ECG) changes

16. Dobutamine works by stimulating which of the following receptors?
    1 Alpha-1
    2 Alpha-2
    3 Beta-1
    4 Beta-2

17. What is the underlying pathophysiology of all forms of shock?
    1 Inadequate tissue perfusion
    2 Respiratory alkalosis
    3 Decreased SVR
    4 Increased basal metabolic rate

18. Causes of hypovolemic shock include which absolute or direct loses?
    1 Diabetes insipidus (DI) and hyperglycemic osmotic diuresis
    2 Hypotension
    3 Sepsis and thermal injuries
    4 Protein albumin and magnesium

19. Hypovolemic shock causes:
    1 A decrease in CO and pulmonary capillary wedge pressure.
    2 Alkalosis.
    3 The release of nosocomial infection mediators.
    4 The release of antiplatelet factor (APF).

20. A patient in hypovolemic shock experiences hypotension and a narrow pulse pressure. The patient is in what stage of shock?
    1 Compensatory
    2 Progressive
    3 Refractory or irreversible
    4 Multiple-organ failure

21. The most sensitive indicator for evaluating a patient's fluid status is:
    1 Urine output.
    2 BP.
    3 Central venous pressure.
    4 pH of the skin.

22. First-line treatment of hypovolemia is:
    1 Dopamine.
    2 IV crystalloids.
    3 Whole blood transfusions.
    4 Platelet transfusions.

23. A patient arrives at the ED with the chief complaint of fever of 102° F, as well as nausea and vomiting for 3 days. The patient is experiencing tachycardia with a sustained HR of 120 bpm, BP of 95/60 mm Hg, tachypneic at 26 bpm. The nurse starts an IV knowing that the patient has deficient volume and is going to need a bolus of IV fluids. The initial treatment is with:
    1 NS 4 to 5 L.
    2 Colloids such as Hetastarch.
    3 Ringer's lactate (RL) 1 to 2 L.
    4 Mannitol 10%.

24. A contributing factor that can lead to the deterioration of a patient in hypovolemic shock is:
    1 Colloid administration.
    2 Hypothermia.
    3 Head of bed elevated 30 degrees.
    4 Urticaria.

25. The cause of neurogenic shock is anything that disrupts which nervous system?
    1 Reticuloendothelial
    2 Autonomic
    3 Sympathetic
    4 Central third ventricular

26. Which of the following is a common cause of neurogenic shock?
    1 Head trauma
    2 Diabetes mellitus
    3 Hypertension
    4 Spinal cord injury

27. Which vital sign would indicate neurogenic shock?
    1 BP 160/100 mm Hg
    2 Temperature 38.1° C
    3 Pulse 50 bpm
    4 Respiration rate (RR) 16 bpm

28. In neurogenic shock a decrease in CO occurs. How does this decrease affect tissue perfusion?
    1 Tissue perfusion is increased.
    2 Tissue perfusion is decreased.
    3 Tissue perfusion is without change.
    4 Tissue perfusion increases and decreases hourly.

29. The primary cause of hypothermia in patients with neurogenic shock is:
    1 Hypertension.
    2 Tachycardia.
    3 Vasoconstriction.
    4 Vasodilation.

30. The management goal of the patient in neurogenic shock is to improve:
    1 Pain control.
    2 Tidal volume with the use of metered dose inhalers.
    3 Tissue perfusion.
    4 Urinary output with the use of angiotensin-converting enzyme (ACE) inhibitor medications.

31. Which of the following is an appropriate way to monitor hypoxia in the patient who has neurogenic shock?
    1 Serum glucose levels
    2 Pulse oximeter
    3 Electrocardiogram
    4 Tidal volume caliper

32. Treatment of neurogenic shock with the use of IV fluids assists in managing the problem of:
    1 Tissue perfusion.
    2 Hypertension.
    3 Diabetes insipidus.
    4 Increased intracranial pressure (ICP).

Questions 33 and 34 relate to the following situation: A 76-year-old woman is admitted with a temperature of 102° F, mental confusion, HR of 117 bpm, respiratory rate (RR) of 32, BP of 64/40 mm Hg, oxygen saturation of 85%, and a scant amount of dark amber urine with sediment from her suprapubic catheter.

33. What is your initial intervention?
    1 Establish IV access.
    2 Obtain cultures.
    3 Supplement oxygen.
    4 Provide patient comfort.

34. Appropriate therapies at this time would probably include:
    1 Crystalloids and inotropes.
    2 Crystalloids and beta blockers.
    3 Colloids and beta blockers.
    4 Colloids and inotropes.

35. A patient arrives at the ED and is diagnosed with septic shock. He is confused and agitated. What initial intervention would best address one of the possible reasons for the confusion?
    1 Obtain consent from the closest relative for a lumbar puncture.
    2 Medicate the patient for fever reduction per department protocol.
    3 Replace fluids.
    4 Deliver oxygen.

36. What would be an appropriate intervention for a patient in septic shock who has the following?
    pH: 7.29
    pCO_2: 69
    pO_2: 60
    HCO_3: 32
    SaO_2: 83
    RR: 36 breaths/min, obviously labored
    Diaphoretic and complains of being tired
    1 Deliver oxygen by 100% nonrebreather.
    2 Place patient in upright position, and give supplemental oxygen and the prescribed anxiolytic.
    3 Provide intubation and mechanical ventilation.
    4 Consult respiratory therapy for a breathing treatment, and give supplemental oxygen.

37. Which of the following patients is at greatest risk for septic shock?
    1 A 45-year-old man who has had coronary artery bypass surgery with a sternal infection 2 weeks earlier
    2 An 86-year-old insulin-dependent, diabetic woman with stage 4 sacral decubitus who is incontinent and has an indwelling Foley catheter
    3 A 60-year-old man with pneumonia
    4 A 35-year-old man who has tested positive for human immunodeficiency virus (HIV) and is being treated for cellulitis of his hand on an outpatient basis

38. What causes the decreased SVR in septic shock?
    1 Fever
    2 Decreased CO
    3 Respiratory acidosis
    4 Cellular mediators from the infectious organisms

39. What is the terminal result of septic shock?
    1 Multiple-organ failure
    2 Hypotension
    3 Acidosis
    4 Coma

40. Positive inotropic agents are given during septic shock to:
    1 Decrease anxiety.
    2 Decrease BP.
    3 Increase contractility of the heart.
    4 Increase the calcium pump of the heart

CHAPTER 3

Trauma and Emergency Care

1. Rapid sequence intubation (RSI) is used most often in:
   1 Routine elective intubations.
   2 Any case involving airway trauma.
   3 Any case in which a potential for aspiration exists.
   4 Any case in which the patient cannot extend or flex his or her neck.

2. Preoxygenation:
   1 Should be used only on patients who are unconscious.
   2 Is limited to 2 minutes of 100% forced inspiratory oxygen (FIO_2) in emergencies.
   3 Can be accomplished via nasal canula over 5 minutes.
   4 Can consist of 4 vital capacity breaths of 100% FIO_2.

3. Application of pressure to the cricoid cartilage:
   1 May interfere with tracheal intubation.
   2 Is a benign procedure.
   3 Requires a minimum of 10 pounds per foot.
   4 Is performed at the cricothyroid membrane.

4. The use of succinylcholine (Anectine) during RSI:
   1 Is contraindicated.
   2 Allows for rapid return of spontaneous ventilation in patients with failed intubation.
   3 Has no contraindications.
   4 May cause serious precipitation in the IV line.

5. By not performing a "test breath" ventilation during RSI:
   1 Less time is taken.
   2 The patient is allowed to ventilate spontaneously.
   3 Laryngeal distention is prevented.
   4 The risk of aspiration is decreased.

6. When performing cricoid pressure, the following should be performed:
   1 Remove pressure while an ET tube is being inserted.
   2 Apply backward and downward pressure.
   3 Apply enough pressure for left displacement.
   4 Apply pressure so that the ET tube is backward, upward, and to the right.

7. Mr. Jones, an 84-year-old quadriplegic patient with significant history of gastroesophageal reflux disease (GERD) and chronic renal failure (CRF), is exhibiting signs of respiratory distress. The decision has been made to provide intubation and mechanical ventilation. As the ICU house staff enters the patient's room they ask for your assistance. You recognize that:
   1 Some of the medications used to intubate Mr. Jones will have a delayed onset because of the CRF.
   2 Mr. Jones will require a fiberoptic intubation because of his history of quadriplegia.
   3 Succinylcholine (Anectine) may induce a hyperkalemic response in Mr. Jones.
   4 Mr. Jones will need more induction medication because of upregulation of central nervous system (CNS) receptors secondary to quadriplegia.

8. You are assisting a certified registered nurse anesthetist (CRNA) who is performing an RSI on your patient in the ICU. The CRNA asks you to apply cricoid pressure. You know that:
   1 The cricoid cartilage is the first cartilage ring caudal to the thyroid cartilage and that it lies directly below the cricothyroid membrane.
   2 The cricoid cartilage lies above the larynx and requires 5 pounds per foot of pressure.
   3 Cricoid pressure is used to occlude the trachea.
   4 Cricoid pressure should be held until a chest x-ray confirms the ET tube placement.

9. In the time between administering medications and laryngoscopy:
   1. Two to three ventilations of 100% oxygen are delivered.
   2. An oxygen mask should remain on the patient's face.
   3. The patient's eyelids should be taped shut to prevent corneal abrasions.
   4. One "test breath" should be attempted in conscious patients.

10. The ability of the brain to tolerate increases in intracranial volume is called compliance. Compliance is based on which two concepts?
    1. RR and BP
    2. Temperature and CO
    3. Volume and pressure
    4. Temperature and volume

11. Which of the following would result in a significant increase in ICP?
    1. Normal compliance
    2. High compliance
    3. Low elastance
    4. High elastance

12. According to the Monroe-Kellie hypothesis, if a patient has an increase in cerebrospinal fluid (CSF), then he or she should compensate by having a(n):
    1. Increase in blood viscosity.
    2. Decrease in blood volume.
    3. Increase in brain volume.
    4. Increase in BP.

13. A pressure gradient across the brain defined as mean arterial pressure (MAP)–ICP is the definition of:
    1. Cerebral blood flow.
    2. CO.
    3. Brain volume.
    4. Cerebral perfusion pressure.

14. Mr. Kwon is in good health except he has hay fever and is sneezing, which causes fluctuations in ICP. By what process is Mr. Kwon's ICP regulated?
    1. Autoregulation
    2. Perfusion
    3. Hypoxia
    4. Thermal dilation

15. Which of the following patients is at increased risk for increased ICP?
    1. Left leg compound fracture
    2. Postcraniotomy as a result of partial tumor removal
    3. Diabetic patient with 138 mg/dl blood sugar
    4. Bradycardic patient with a sinus infection

16. Sustained increased ICP can lead to brainstem herniation. The outcome of brainstem herniation is:
    1. Cerebral stroke.
    2. Seizure.
    3. Death.
    4. Migraine headache.

17. Which of the following body positions is best for a patient with increased ICP?
    1. Prone
    2. Trendelenberg
    3. Head of bed (HOB) elevated 90 degrees and hips flexed
    4. HOB elevated 20 degrees

18. The ABCs of trauma resuscitation are the primary life saving measures used in stabilization. The letter D represents:
    1. Decision time.
    2. Disability.
    3. Dextrose.
    4. Deep tendon reflexes.

19. A patient during examination opens his eyes in response to pain, makes no verbal response, but withdraws from pain. What is the Glasgow Coma Score (GCS) for this patient?
    1. 3
    2. 5
    3. 7
    4. 11

20. Cushing response is associated with:
    1. Cardiac tamponade.
    2. Tension pneumothorax.
    3. Cervical spine fracture in response to traumatic brain injury (TBI).
    4. Increased ICP.

21. A 26-year-old man is the victim of a motor vehicle crash (MVC) and is brought to the ED by a friend. Examination of the patient reveals an abrasion on the forehead. The patient is able to state his name but does not know what time it is and has no recall of the events involving the MVC. Based on your understanding of the types of TBI, you suspect this patient *most* likely sustained a(an):
    1 Open skull fracture to the occiput of cranium.
    2 Concussion.
    3 Diffuse axonal injury.
    4 Subdural hematoma.

22. A child is admitted to the ICU with a head injury after being in an MVC. The nurse notes a small amount of bloody drainage in the left ear with mild ecchymosis around the eyes. The nurse suspects:
    1 Linear skull fracture.
    2 Subdural hematoma.
    3 Basilar skull fracture.
    4 Increased ICP.

23. The appropriate drug for reducing ICP, which helps reduce fluid on the brain is:
    1 Mannitol (Osmitrol).
    2 Morphine.
    3 Midazolam (Versed).
    4 Epinephrine (Adrenaline).

24. A 21-year-old man was struck on the right side of the head. This injury may cause a compression of the third (III) cranial nerve, resulting in:
    1 Dilation of the contralateral pupil.
    2 Constriction of the ipsilateral pupil.
    3 Dilation of the ipsilateral pupil.
    4 Constriction of the contralateral pupil.

25. A 40-year-old man was transported to the ED via emergency medical service (EMS), after suffering a severe TBI in an MVC. The health care team's attempt at stabilizing the patient is futile. He is pronounced dead after 20 minutes. The family is directly notified by the attending physician. Soon after, the nurse observes the patient's wife consoling other family members. Which of the following interpretations of this behavior *best* explains her response?
    1 She has already moved through the stages of the grieving process.
    2 She is repressing anger related to her husband's death.
    3 She is experiencing shock and disbelief related to her husband's death.
    4 She is demonstrating resolution of her husband's death.

26. The cause of symptoms of a brain attack that resolves quickly is known as:
    1 Cerebrovascular accident (CVA).
    2 Transient ischemic attack TIA).
    3 Brain herniation.
    4 Peripheral neuropathy.

27. Which of the following patients is at the greatest risk for a brain attack?
    1 A 33-year-old diabetic
    2 A 45-year-old obese, drug addict
    3 A 48-year-old patient who has had a myocardial infarction (MI) has hyperlipidemia and a previous stroke, and is a smoker
    4 A 74-year-old with hypotension and migraine headaches

28. In assessing for signs of acute ischemic stroke, you ask the patient to smile or show his or her teeth. This tests for what physical finding?
    1 Hearing loss
    2 Speech difficulties
    3 Facial droop
    4 Motor arm drift

29. Which of the following indicates a positive motor arm drift?
    1 Both arms are equal in height.
    2 The left arm is lower in height.
    3 The left leg and left arm pronate.
    4 Both pupils are dilated.

30. What is the window of time for instituting thrombolytic therapy in a brain attack?
    1 30 minutes
    2 1 hour
    3 3 hours
    4 24 hours

31. Dosing of recombinant tissue plasminogen activator (rt-PA) is dependent on the patient's:
    1 Age.
    2 Height.
    3 Weight.
    4 Temperature.

32. Which of the following patients would *not* be a candidate for rt-PA?
    1 Patient with lupus erythematosus
    2 Patient younger than 18 years of age
    3 MI within the past 3 years
    4 GI bleed within 1 week

33. Which of the following areas is the first priority for assessing the patient who is dysphagic as a result of a brain attack?
    1 Circulation
    2 Airway
    3 Incontinence
    4 Methods of communication

34. Which statement best characterizes Class III hemorrhage?
    1 Up to 750 ml blood loss
    2 1200 ml blood loss
    3 2000 ml blood loss
    4 3500 ml blood loss

35. Blood is replaced at what rate with crystalloid in the hemorrhaging patient?
    1 1:1
    2 2:1
    3 3:1
    4 5:1

36. What percentage of loss of blood volume describes Class II hemorrhage?
    1 10%
    2 45%
    3 20%
    4 35%

37. Urinary output is sometimes used to monitor renal perfusion. How much urine output would indicate adequate intravascular volume?
    1 0.1 ml/kg/hr
    2 0.2 ml/kg/hr
    3 0.3 ml/kg/hr
    4 0.5 ml/kg/hr

38. Which of the following is a contraindication for the use of Medical Antishock Trousers (MAST) or Pneumatic Antishock Garment (PASG)?
    1 Hypovolemic shock
    2 Pelvic or lower extremity fractures
    3 Septic shock
    4 Left ventricular dysfunction

39. Mr. JW, an 18-year-old man, is brought to your level 1 ED by car. His friends state he has been shot. You note multiple gunshot wounds. He is tachycardic, tachypneic, and lethargic. Vital signs are HR of 146 bpm, RR of 40 breaths/min, and BP at 60/40 mm Hg. He is bleeding profusely from a gaping abdominal wound. When considering care for this patient, what would you presume to be the most likely sequence of events?
    1 Start an IV, and administer vasopressors and IV fluids. Monitor vital signs in the ED until bleeding is controlled.
    2 Secure airway and cervical spine, administer oxygen, support respirations, start two large-bore peripheral IVs, and administer crystalloids and blood while assessing and preparing the patient for immediate transport to the surgical department.
    3 Transport the patient to an ED that is better equipped to manage a patient like this.
    4 Stabilize the patient, and immediately transport to CAT scan for evaluation.

40. What type blood can be given to the hemorrhaging trauma patient who has not been typed and crossed?
    1 AB
    2 A+
    3 O−
    4 AB−

41. The main goal for transfusion in the patient with hemorrhage is to:
    1 Increase oxygenation and tissue perfusion.
    2 Attain a hemoglobin of 36.
    3 Obtain an oxygen saturation of 100%.
    4 Equalize blood in to blood lost.

42. A 65-year-old man has recently had a balloon angio-plasty. Which of the following signs could be indicative of cardiac tamponade?
    1 Crackles in both lung fields
    2 Bradycardia
    3 Muffled heart tones
    4 Hypertension

43. A premature infant with a newly placed central line catheter develops hypotension. What other sign is associated with cardiac tamponade in premature infants?
    1 Increased urine output
    2 Fever
    3 Bradycardia
    4 Decreased CVP

44. Which of the following patients are at greatest risk for developing cardiac tamponade?
    1 Middle-aged man who has had a cardiac catheteri-zation 1 week earlier
    2 Older woman who has had a balloon angioplasty 2 hours earlier
    3 Premature infant who has had a central line removed 3 days earlier
    4 Male adolescent with a history of acute pericarditis 1 year ago

45. Which of the following classes of medications predis-poses a patient to cardiac tamponade?
    1 Anticoagulants
    2 Antidepressants
    3 Antihypertensives
    4 Antibiotics

46. Cardiac tamponade is caused by:
    1 Excess fluid or clots collecting in the ventricles of the heart.
    2 Decreased venous return.
    3 Excess fluid accumulation of fluid in pericardial sac.
    4 Increased CO.

47. The nurse suspects that a patient may be developing cardiac tamponade and has notified the physician. What will be the next most likely intervention?
    1 Prepare the patient for heart catheterization.
    2 Prepare the patient for surgery.
    3 Administer oxygen.
    4 Administer nitroglycerin sublingually.

48. The physician requests a STAT potassium level before performing a pericardiocentesis. The rationale for this order is:
    1 Potassium is lost in the fluid removed during the procedure.
    2 Hyperkalemia causes cardiac tamponade.
    3 Potassium is injected into the pericardial space.
    4 Hypokalemia can result in arrhythmias during the procedure.

49. The nurse is assessing the patient for cardiac tamponade. Which of the following is the *least* reliable indicator?
    1 ECG tracing
    2 Alterations in BP
    3 Jugular venous distention
    4 Muffled heart tones

50. Which type of disease *best* describes the patient at greatest risk for developing spinal cord compression?
    1 Onycholysis
    2 Osteoporosis
    3 Melanoma
    4 Meningitis

51. A spinal cord compression in the lumbar spine region may result in which of the following physical symptoms?
    1 Loss of buttock sensation
    2 Quadriplegia
    3 Paralysis of the diaphragm
    4 Constipation

52. The earliest and most common symptom of spinal cord compression is identified as:
    1 Weakness.
    2 Paresthesias.
    3 Pain.
    4 Ataxia.

53. Which of the following is a risk factor for the develop-ment of a cervical spinal cord compression?
    1 Rheumatoid arthritis
    2 Prostate cancer
    3 Breast cancer
    4 Systemic lupus erythematosus (SLE)

54. Autonomic dysfunction (AD) may occur as a result of spinal cord compression. Which of the following assessment findings would alert you to the possibility of a related AD occurring in your patient?
    1 Hypertension
    2 Tachycardia
    3 Confusion
    4 Bradycardia

55. In patients with spinal cord compression and AD, treatment and management strategies may need to be modified for bowel and bladder dysfunction. Which of the following strategies would you expect to be taught to the patient and family?
    1 Correct technique to transfer from the wheelchair
    2 Correct technique to apply a brace or splint
    3 Correct administration of an antidepressant medication
    4 Correct technique for self-catheterization

56. A patient has a spinal cord compression in the cervical spine. The patient is complaining of radiating pain across the shoulders and down to his or her right elbow. The patient is also complaining of numbness and weakness of both arms (right greater than left) and difficulty catching his or her breath. Which of the following interventions would be the priority?
    1 Reassess the patient in 30 minutes.
    2 Instruct to perform arm exercises twice daily.
    3 Perform a complete respiratory assessment.
    4 Administer pain medication as ordered.

57. Magnetic resonance imaging (MRI) is typically used to diagnose spinal cord compression. Which of the following is correct regarding the diagnostic use of MRI in a patient with suspected spinal cord compression?
    1 Is able to obtain a CSF specimen
    2 Is able to distinguish the type of tissue and lesion
    3 Allows for dye to be injected into the epidural space
    4 Permits visualization of the compressed area

58. The diagnosis of hypothermia is made by:
    1 Twelve-lead ECG.
    2 Axillary temperature when shivering is observed
    3 Core temperature below 35° C, measured at two sites.
    4 Presence of bradycardia.

59. Factors that may increase the risk of hypothermia include:
    1 Paraplegia or quadriplegia.
    2 Obesity.
    3 Hyperthyroidism.
    4 Respiratory failure.

60. Mechanisms of heat loss in the human body are:
    1 Conviction.
    2 Elevation.
    3 Convection.
    4 Reaction.

61. A nurse is asked to care for a hypothermic patient with a core temperature of 27° C. Rewarming methods suitable for this patient include:
    1 Immersing patient in a room-temperature Hubbard tank.
    2 Providing warmed blankets.
    3 Providing warm oral fluids.
    4 Providing hemodialysis.

62. When considering what laboratory tests are appropriate for the severely hypothermic patient:
    1 Coagulopathies do not occur because coagulation enzymes are not sensitive to temperatures.
    2 Hemoglobin is not needed. No blood loss occurs during treatment of hypothermia.
    3 Potassium must be checked because both hypokalemia and hyperkalemia are possible.
    4 Changes in blood sugar are minimal because of the greatly reduced metabolic rate during hypothermia.

63. When the nurse must perform CPR in the hypothermic patient:
    1 Between 30 and 45 seconds may be necessary to detect a pulse before initiating CPR.
    2 Defibrillation should be continued if not initially successful per basic life support (BLS) protocol.
    3 Defibrillation is difficult because of chest wall stiffness.
    4 A chance of full neurologic recovery is always possible when CPR is initiated.

64. A patient intoxicated with alcohol may arrive hypothermic in the ED. Which of the following is *true* concerning the influence of alcohol on body temperature regulation?
    1 The patient who has had alcohol exhibits peripheral vasoconstriction.
    2 The intoxicated patient shivers excessively, increasing body oxygen consumption.
    3 Alcohol inhibits the cerebellar thermoregulatory center.
    4 Alcohol impairs the patient's ability to recognize and respond correctly to a hypothermic environment.

65. The body has two thermal compartments. The interactions between the two thermal compartments include:
    1 Metabolic heat production from the peripheral compartment is transferred to the core.
    2 Heat generated in the periphery is eliminated from the body through respiration.
    3 Vasoconstriction in the periphery helps prevent heat loss from the core.
    4 The peripheral temperature is kept tightly controlled within a narrow range.

66. Which of the following is *true* of dry drowning?
    1 It occurs in the absence of aspiration.
    2 It is precipitated by laryngospasm.
    3 Prolonged respiratory obstruction is secondary to laryngospasm.
    4 With increased loss of consciousness (LOC), glottic closure occurs, causing asphyxia.

67. Which is *not* true of wet drowning?
    1 It involves aspiration of fluid.
    2 It is precipitated by laryngospasm, which causes LOC.
    3 It occurs in the absence of aspiration.
    4 Glottic relaxation results in aspiration and suffocation.

68. The underlying pathophysiology of drowning is:
    1 Hypoxia, hypercarbia, metabolic acidosis, respiratory acidosis.
    2 Metabolic acidosis, respiratory alkalosis, hypoxia, hyporcarbia.
    3 Hypoxia, metabolic acidosis, hyporcarbia, respiratory alkalosis.
    4 Hypercarbia, metabolic alkalosis, hypoxia, respiratory alkalosis.

69. The most frequent physical respiratory finding in the near-drowning patient is:
    1 Tachypnea.
    2 Apnea.
    3 Cheyne Stokes.
    4 Kushmal breathing.

70. Which of the following factors increases the chance of survival of a near-drowning victim?
    1 Warm water
    2 Suspected spinal injury
    3 Muddy water
    4 Rapid recovery and CPR

71. Cardiac arrhythmias in a near-drowning patient occur from:
    1 Hyperthermia.
    2 Hypoxemia.
    3 Alkalosis.
    4 Renal failure.

72. Rewarming the patient is essential to prevent which of the following?
    1 Anoxic encephalopathy
    2 Acute respiratory distress syndrome
    3 Ventricular fibrillation
    4 Disseminated intravascular coagulation

73. A patient is brought to the ED by ambulance. The patient is alone, confused, and has no form of identification. Who is most likely to become the primary source of information?
    1 ED nurse
    2 Emergency medical technician
    3 ED physician
    4 Patient

74. For the patient in Question 73, what will be the focus of treatment?
    1 Research
    2 Ongoing medical management
    3 Stabilization
    4 Rehabilitation

75. An ED patient has been reported taking an overdose of pills. After stabilizing the patient the focus of further treatment will be to do which of the following?
    1 Eliminate the pills from the body.
    2 Locate the patient's family.
    3 Call the police.
    4 Send the patient for a computed tomographic (CT) scan.

76. What safety measures should be instituted when there is cause to believe the patient attempted to take his or her life with a drug overdose?
    1 Suicide precautions
    2 Fall precautions
    3 Infection control precautions
    4 Delirium tremens precautions

77. A 34-year-old man is brought to the ED for the ingestion of 15 to 20 phenobarbital tablets 45 minutes earlier. What is the first-line treatment choice to eliminate the pills from the GI tract?
    1 Supportive care
    2 Gastric lavage
    3 Antidote
    4 Activated charcoal

78. A cathartic medication has been ordered for the patient with a drug overdose. This patient has a history of congestive heart failure. Which of the following would be safe to administer?
    1 Sorbitol
    2 Magnesium citrate
    3 Ipecac
    4 Nalmefene

79. A patient who has overdosed, been treated, and stabilized reports having suicidal ideations. His history notes an inpatient admission 1 year ago for attempting suicide. What is the best choice for continued care?
    1 Discharge home with instructions to contact his or her private physician.
    2 Contact the patient's family.
    3 Call for a psychiatric consultation.
    4 Discharge with instructions to contact the mental health clinic.

80. A patient in the ED has been ordered to receive gastric lavage for an overdose. The patient has loss of the gag reflex. What is the most effective procedure to carry out the gastric lavage?
    1 Hemodialysis
    2 Intubation with cuffed ET tube
    3 Force diuresis
    4 Trendelenburg positioning

CHAPTER *4*

Cardiovascular System

1. The nurse understands that the most common cause of angina is:
    1 Coronary artery vasospasm.
    2 Atherosclerosis.
    3 Congenital heart defect.
    4 Mitral valve stenosis.

2. According to the American Heart Association, which of the following is an unmodifiable risk factor for angina?
    1 Smoking
    2 Diabetes
    3 Age
    4 Malnutrition

3. The basic underlying pathophysiologic cause of angina is:
    1 Coronary vasodilation.
    2 Myocardial oxygen supply that exceeds demand during periods of increased work.
    3 Impaired myocardial contractility.
    4 Myocardial oxygen demand that exceeds supply during periods of increased work.

4. A patient with stable angina will exhibit which of the following clinical manifestations?
    1 Chest pain that occurs predominantly at rest
    2 Chest pain that is predictable in onset, intensity, and duration
    3 Chest pain that is unrelieved with nitroglycerin
    4 Chest pain that is unpredictable in onset, duration, and intensity

5. During an attack of Prinzmetal's angina the nurse expects an ECG to show:
    1 ST-segment elevation.
    2 Inverted T waves.
    3 Q waves.
    4 ST-segment depression.

6. Which of the following therapeutic action makes nitroglycerin the drug of choice in the pharmacologic management of an anginal attack?
   1 Coronary artery dilation and peripheral venous constriction
   2 Coronary artery constriction and peripheral venous constriction
   3 Coronary artery constriction and peripheral venous dilation
   4 Coronary artery dilation and peripheral venous dilation

7. Which of the following factors worsens the imbalance between myocardial oxygen supply and demand?
   1 Hemoglobin (HGB): 14 g/dl
   2 HR: 98 bpm
   3 HR: 58 bpm
   4 RR: 14 breaths/minute

8. During an attack of new onset chest pain, the ED nurse anticipates which of the following medications will be prescribed?
   1 Meperidine hydrochloride (Demerol)
   2 Furosemide (Lasix)
   3 Cefazolin sodium (Ancef)
   4 Morphine sulfate

9. The predominant cause of an acute MI (AMI) is:
   1 Coronary vasospasm.
   2 Electrocution.
   3 Thromboembolism.
   4 Blunt trauma.

10. A patient who experienced an AMI 24 hours earlier has an elevated leukocyte level. The nurse understands that this is most likely due to:
    1 An inflammatory response.
    2 An infection.
    3 Circulating catecholamines.
    4 Glycogenolysis.

11. The most common complication after an AMI is:
    1 Cardiogenic shock.
    2 Dysrhythmias.
    3 Congestive heart failure.
    4 Myocardial wall rupture.

12. Which subset of the population will have an atypical clinical presentation of AMI?
    1 Patients with renal dysfunction
    2 African Americans
    3 Alcoholics
    4 Women

13. An AMI causes conduction abnormalities because the:
    1 Myocardial cells are forced to engage in aerobic metabolism.
    2 Myocardial cells are over excited.
    3 Myocardial membrane potential is altered.
    4 Myocardial cells contain too much potassium.

14. A patient is complaining of unrelenting, crushing chest pain, nausea, dyspnea, and appears cold and clammy. The nurse suspects the patient is experiencing an AMI and expects to see which of the following changes on the ECG?
    1 T-wave depression
    2 ST-segment elevation
    3 T-wave inversion
    4 P-wave inversion

15. The nurse notices indicative ECG changes in leads II, III, and aVF that are strongly suggestive of an AMI. What area of the myocardium is affected?
    1 Inferior
    2 Anterior
    3 Posterior
    4 Lateral

16. Which of the following cardiac markers is very effective in determining an AMI because it is sensitive, specific, begins rising within 3 to 9 hours, and remains elevated for 10 to 14 days?
    1 Myoglobin
    2 Creatinine kinase (CK)
    3 Lactic dehydrogenase (LDH)
    4 Troponin

17. The term *systolic dysfunction* is best defined as:
    1 A reduction in pumping power of the left ventricle to the point where the left ventricular (LV) ejection fraction (EF) is less than 40%.
    2 An inability of the ventricle to relax during filling, causing increased BP and bradycardia.
    3 Atrial fibrillation.
    4 Increase in ventricular filling pressure with normal EF.

18. The most common cause of right heart failure is:
    1 Adult respiratory distress syndrome (ARDS).
    2 Jugular venous distention.
    3 Left heart failure.
    4 Systemic hypertension.

19. The most important diagnostic test in the initial diagnosis of systolic heart failure is:
    1 Two-dimensional echocardiography with Doppler flow.
    2 A chest x-ray.
    3 An ECG.
    4 A brain natriuretic peptide (BNP) test.

20. Two classes of drugs that have been shown to decrease ventricular remodeling in chronic heart failure are:
    1 Digitalis and diuretics.
    2 ACE inhibitors and beta blockers.
    3 Natriuretic peptides and phosphodiesterase inhibitors.
    4 Nonsteroidal antiinflammatory drugs (NSAIDs) and cathartic blockers.

Questions 21 through 24 relate to the following case study:
Mr. Jacobs, a 63-year-old man, has been treated since 1992 when he suffered an anterior MI. He has been hospitalized several times in the past few years with congestive heart failure and hypertension. He has done reasonably well (New York Heart Association [NYHA] Class III) on digitalis, captopril, and large doses of diuretics. He was discharged from the hospital 2 weeks earlier when he had diuresed 13 pounds. His chief complaint today is increasing shortness of breath, even at rest, and weight gain. His abdomen is swollen. Over the last 3 days, his weight has increased from 166 to between 170 and 176 pounds. His wife gave him an extra dose of furosemide yesterday, but this didn't relieve his symptoms.
Vital signs:
  HR: 132
  BP: 150/90 mm Hg
  RR: 24 breaths/minute and labored
  EF: 35% (confirmed by echocardiogram) (cardiac catheterization last admission)
  Chest x-ray: Increased pulmonary vascular markings, enlarged heart
  Lungs: Coarse crackles bilaterally
  Heart: Third heart sound
  Neck Veins: Distended at 90 degree
  Ascites in abdomen
  Peripheral edema in legs

Mr. Jacobs is placed on oxygen per nasal cannula at 4 L/min. He is given furosemide and potassium IV supplementation. He is placed on Natrecor and Primacor drips, and his shortness of breath begins to resolve within 20 minutes. After one night in the hospital, he is discharged on the following medications:
  Lasix 40 mg twice daily
  Potassium 20 mEq twice daily
  Lanoxin 0.25 mg once daily
  Capoten 25 mg three times daily
  Coreg 3.125 mg twice daily

21. Which of these is *not* the rationale for the Natrecor infusion?
    1 To decrease preload to the heart
    2 To decrease BP by vasodilating the arteriolar beds
    3 To diurese the excess intravascular fluid
    4 To increase the preload of the heart

22. Rationale for the Primacor infusion is to:
    1 Decrease venous return.
    2 Dilate arteriolar beds.
    3 Increase contractility.
    4 Prevent remodeling.

23. With such high doses of diuretics, which electrolyte deficiency is likely to require supplementation?
    1 Hypokalemia
    2 Hyponatremia
    3 Hypocalcemia
    4 Hypophosphatemia

24. After 1 month at home, Mr. Jacobs develops an irregular pulse that is determined to be atrial fibrillation. On a routine home visit, you notice that he has gained 6 pounds since your last visit 1 week earlier. He has no shortness of breath but complains of nausea and decreased appetite. He also states that he has not been awakened with nocturia the last 2 nights, which is unusual for him. His total daily urinary output is diminished. He has an irregular pulse with occasional palpitations noted. His current medications include digoxin (Lanoxin) 0.25 mg once daily, furosemide (Lasix) 40 mg twice daily, potassium chloride (KCl) 20 mEq/L twice daily, Coumadin 5 mg once daily, Capoten 25 mg three times daily, and Coreg 3.125 mg twice daily. You notify Mr. Smith's physician and anticipate which of the following orders?
    1 Increase dose of Lanoxin
    2 Decrease dose of Coumadin; assess serum prothrombin time/international normalized ratio (PT/INR)
    3 Increase dose of furosemide; assess serum digitalis level
    4 Admit to telemetry unit of local hospital

CHAPTER 5

Respiratory System

1. A patient on mechanical ventilation has a tidal volume that is showing 500 to 600 ml, and each breath ends when the pressure reaches 18 mm Hg. What type of mechanical ventilator is the patient connected to?
   1 Volume cycled
   2 Pressure cycled
   3 Flow cycled
   4 Time cycled

2. A patient on mechanical ventilation has a tidal volume of 700 ml, and a breath is given 12 times a minute. The patient is also breathing four spontaneous breaths per minute. What mode of ventilation is the ventilator set on?
   1 Controlled
   2 Assist controlled
   3 Synchronized intermittent mandatory
   4 Pressure controlled

3. The use of positive end-expiratory pressure (PEEP) may cause which of the following to occur?
   1 Decreased intrathoracic pressure
   2 Increased venous return
   3 Increased CO
   4 Decreased BP

4. Normal inspiratory-expiratory (I/E) ratio is which of the following?
   1 1:1
   2 1:2
   3 1:3
   4 2:1

5. Barotrauma is a complication that is associated with mechanical ventilation. Which of the following plays a major role in the development of barotrauma?
   1 High airway pressures
   2 Leakage of fluid into alveoli
   3 Pneumothorax
   4 Air leak into the mediastinum

6. When weaning a patient from mechanical ventilation, which of the following occurs?
   1 Tidal volume is gradually decreased
   2 Ventilation rate is gradually decreased
   3 Tidal volume is gradually increased
   4 Ventilation rate is gradually increased

7. Your patient is on mechanical ventilation and you notice water in the ventilator tubing. You should empty the tubing for which of the following reasons?
   1 Moisture accumulation inhibits bacterial growth.
   2 Moisture accumulation improves the air flow.
   3 Moisture accumulation impedes the flow of oxygen.
   4 Moisture accumulation impedes the removal of carbon dioxide.

8. Which of the following determines how fast the tidal volume will be delivered with each ventilated breath?
   1 Flow rate
   2 RR
   3 I/E ratio
   4 Tidal volume

9. A patient is at risk for development of a pulmonary embolus. Which of the following risk factors would the patient have?
   1 Anticoagulated blood
   2 Early ambulation
   3 Use of pneumatic stockings
   4 Atrial fibrillation

10. Ventilation-perfusion (V/Q) mismatch is frequently seen with pulmonary embolus. Which of the following is caused by the decrease in carbon dioxide associated with V/Q mismatch?
   1 Bronchoconstriction
   2 Decrease in pulmonary resistance
   3 Increase in oxygenation
   4 Shunting of blood to affected area of lungs

11. Which of the following clinical manifestations would lead you to suspect that your patient has developed a pulmonary embolism (PE) if the patient had risk factors?
   1 Chest pain on expiration
   2 Hypertension
   3 Wheezing on exertion
   4 Acute onset of shortness of breath

12. Your patient has developed a PE and is placed on heparin therapy, and serial activated partial thromboplastin time (aPTT) levels are drawn. What is the therapeutic level of aPTT that is used for maintenance of heparin therapy?
   1 1.0 to 1.5 times normal
   2 2.0 to 2.5 times normal
   3 1.5 to 2.0 times normal
   4 0.5 to 1.5 times normal

13. Your patient has suddenly developed shortness of breath and restlessness. An arterial blood gas (ABG) is drawn. Which of the following results may indicate that your patient has developed a PE?
   1 Respiratory acidosis
   2 Respiratory alkalosis
   3 Normal pO_2 levels
   4 Normal pCO_2 levels

14. Which of the following differential diagnostic studies is the most definitive test for the diagnosis of PE?
   1 V/Q scan
   2 ECC
   3 Pulmonary angiography
   4 Spiral CT scan

15. Which of the following medications may be given to a patient who arrives in the ED with a major PE (greater than 50% of lung occluded) and who has no contraindications to the therapy?
   1 Heparin
   2 Urokinase
   3 Coumadin
   4 Protamine

16. Your patient has had a recurrent PE and is scheduled for placement of an umbrella-type filter (Greenfield). Where is the placement of this filter located?
   1 Inferior vena cava
   2 Iliac artery
   3 Superior vena cava
   4 Pulmonary artery

17. The onset of acute respiratory distress syndrome (ARDS) causes the patient to have which of the following?
   1 Alkalosis
   2 Hyperventilation
   3 Hypoventilation
   4 Vasodilatation

18. Refractory hypoxemia is described by which of the following?
   1 Low PaO_2 with increased oxygen concentration
   2 Low $PaCO_2$ with increased oxygen concentration
   3 Low PaO_2 with decreased oxygen concentration
   4 Low $PaCO_2$ with decreased oxygen concentration

19. Which mode of ventilation used in ARDS treatment allows for alveoli to open and lowers airway pressures?
   1 Continuous positive airway pressure (CPAP)
   2 Pressure support ventilation (PSV)
   3 Inverse ratio ventilation (IRV)
   4 Assist-controlled ventilation (ACV)

20. Which of the following medications may be used to maintain tissue perfusion during periods of low CO and hypotension?
   1 Dobutamine (Dobutrex)
   2 Neosynephrine
   3 Nitroglycerine
   4 Sodium Nitroprusside (Nipride)

21. Which of the following is *true* about the use of cortico-
    steroids in the treatment of ARDS?
    1 Increases fluid leakage into alveoli
    2 Provides most benefits if given early after onset
    3 Decreases the risk of nosocomial infections
    4 Decreases the permeability of the respiratory
      membrane

22. Which of the following is a sign of increasing respirato-
    ry distress?
    1 Hypoventilation
    2 Bradycardia
    3 Confusion
    4 Pink mucous membranes

23. Your patient has an arterial line and a pulmonary artery
    catheter in place. While observing hemodynamic
    trends, which of the following should alert you to the
    need to notify a physician?
    1 Decreasing central venous pressure (CVP)
    2 Increasing pulmonary capillary wedge pressure
      (PCWP)
    3 Increasing CO
    4 Decreasing PCWP

24. Symptoms of respiratory distress associated with ARDS
    usually begin within how many hours after insult or
    injury to lungs?
    1 2 to 6
    2 6 to 12
    3 12 to 24
    4 24 to 48

CHAPTER 6

Nervous System

1. Your patient suddenly becomes unresponsive as you are
   speaking to him, and he develops trembling of all
   extremities. Your priority is to:
   1 Notify the physician immediately.
   2 Administer diazepam IV.
   3 Perform a rapid neurologic examination.
   4 Establish an airway.

2. A 49-year-old man is brought to the unit with a diagnosis of status epilepticus. He is having generalized tonic-
   clonic seizures every 5 minutes. Each seizure lasts 30 to
   90 seconds. He is receiving a total of 50 mg diazepam
   before arriving at the ICU. In accordance with accepted
   safety precautions, which of the following drugs does
   the nurse ensure is available at the patient's bedside?
   1 Flumazenil (Mazicon)
   2 Phenobarbital
   3 Naloxone (Narcan)
   4 Phenytoin (Dilantin)

3. Ms. Coletta has suffered a closed head injury secondary
   to an MVC. She has begun to experience tonic-clonic
   (grand mal) seizures. Which of the following nursing
   actions is *most* appropriate for Ms. Coletta?
   1 Pad the bedside rails.
   2 Ensure that someone is with the patient at all times.
   3 Place a padded tongue blade at the patient's bedside.
   4 Place oxygen and suction equipment in the patient's
     room.

4. In preparing a patient for an EEG, before the test the
   nurse should:
   1 Sedate the patient.
   2 Wash the patient's hair.
   3 Keep the patient awake for 48 hours.
   4 Administer phenytoin (Dilantin) as prescribed.

5. If you come upon a patient having a seizure, you
   should:
   1 Protect his or her head from injury and turn him or
     her to the side if possible.
   2 Place an object between the teeth, and move the
     patient to an upright position.
   3 Restrain the patient to prevent injury.
   4 Move the patient to the floor and hold the patient
     down.

6. Which of the following interventions would be effective in minimizing the risk of seizure activity in a
   patient with tonic-clonic seizures?
   1 Maintain the patient on bed rest.
   2 Close the door to the room to minimize stimulation.
   3 Administer sedatives as prescribed.
   4 Administer anticonvulsant medications on schedule.

7. Which of the following observations would the nurse expect in the patient after a tonic-clonic (grand mal) seizure? The patient:
   1 May be drowsy after the seizure.
   2 May be unable to move after the seizure.
   3 Will be hypotensive.
   4 Will remember what triggered the seizure.

8. Tom is a young man who is being placed on long-term seizure treatment with phenytoin (Dilantin). The importance of regular medical follow-up is emphasized. Which instruction is critical to include in the teaching for this patient?
   1 The drug should always be taken on an empty stomach.
   2 Diarrhea is a common side effect, so he should increase his intake of fiber and fluids.
   3 Good oral hygiene and gum massage should be incorporated into his daily routine.
   4 Hyperactivity and insomnia are common early effects, but these should gradually decrease with time.

9. A patient who has meningitis often exhibits photosensitivity and extreme irritability, making it important that the nurse:
   1 Provide a quiet, dimly lit environment for the patient.
   2 Allow frequent visits from family to prevent depression from isolation.
   3 Ventilate the room properly and provide sufficient sunlight.
   4 Eliminate strong odors and unpleasant sights to prevent vomiting.

10. A high fever often accompanies meningitis. A nursing intervention most helpful in relieving febrile delirium would be to:
    1 Apply a warm water bottle to the posterior neck.
    2 Restrain the patient to prevent self-injury.
    3 Apply cool compresses or an ice bag to the forehead.
    4 Increase fluid intake to prevent dehydration.

11. With a diagnosis of acute bacterial meningitis, it is likely that the laboratory data of the CSF will reveal:
    1 Glucose 70 mg/dl.
    2 Protein 450 mg/dl.
    3 White blood cells (WBCs) 4 cells/mm^3.
    4 Specific gravity 1.007.

12. Which of the following is not a likely complication associated with fulminating meningococcal meningitis?
    1 Waterhouse-Friderichsen syndrome
    2 Disseminated intravascular coagulation (DIC)
    3 Encephalitis
    4 Pulmonary embolus

13. All of the following findings are consistent with meningeal irritation *except:*
    1 Nuchal rigidity.
    2 Headache.
    3 Presence of Trousseau's sign.
    4 Presence of Kernig's sign.

14. When caring for a person with meningitis, the critical care nurse should be alert for the development of which complication?
    1 Cerebral dehydration
    2 Deafness
    3 Hypothermia
    4 Hypervigilance

15. A physician performs a lumbar puncture on a 4-year-old with suspected meningitis. The CSF is then sent to the laboratory for testing. The nurse should then:
    1 Assess the child for discomfort at the insertion site and administer narcotics as ordered.
    2 Make sure the child lies flat for at least 8 hours.
    3 Encourage the parents to hold the child.
    4 Place a sandbag over the puncture site for 3 hours.

16. Mr. Schussler is admitted to the hospital with viral meningitis. Which of the following would the nurse *not* expect to find on physical examination?
    1 Positive Kernig sign
    2 Muscle pains
    3 Severe headache
    4 Abdominal pain

17. A 23-year-old man is admitted to the ICU after suffering a traumatic injury to the left side of his neck. The patient has flaccid paralysis of the upper and lower extremities on the left side but retains the sensations of pain and temperature on the left side. He has some movement of his upper and lower extremities on the right side but no sensations of pain or temperature on the right side. What type of spinal cord injury should the nurse suspect when doing an assessment?
    1. Posterior spinal cord injury associated with hyperextension
    2. Central spinal cord compression
    3. Anterior spinal cord syndrome associated with dislocation
    4. Brown-Sequard syndrome associated with intervertebral disk rupture

18. Which of the following is *not* a vital assessment to make on the patient with a spinal cord injury?
    1. Loss of perspiration below level of injury
    2. Ability to speak
    3. Level of loss of sensation
    4. Presence of spontaneous respiration

19. Your patient has had a spinal cord injury and is suffering from autonomic dysreflexia. Which of the following would *not* be a symptom of dysreflexia?
    1. Severe headache
    2. Tachycardia
    3. Rapidly increasing BP
    4. Profuse sweating

20. Which of the following is *not* an effective measure to prevent the occurrence of autonomic dysreflexia?
    1. Maintain the patient in a prone position.
    2. Prevent bladder distention.
    3. Maintain a bowel regime.
    4. Prevent pressure sores.

21. When log-rolling a patient to the side, it is important for the nurse to:
    1. Remove the pillow from under the patient's head and place it under the shoulders.
    2. Elevate the head of the bed slightly to avoid pressure on the back.
    3. Raise the knee gatch slightly to avoid pressure on the hips.
    4. Support the back with pillows and place a pillow between the legs to avoid straining the back.

22. Sam Johnson is admitted to the hospital after falling off his motorcycle. A fracture in the cervical area of the spine is suspected. What is the first priority of nursing care?
    1. Restrict movement of his extremities.
    2. Perform neurologic examinations every 5 minutes.
    3. Keep him on a nothing-by-mouth regimen.
    4. Immobilize his cervical spine.

23. Jack, a 20-year-old college student, suffered a complete C3 transverse cord injury after an MVC involving a drunk driver. Which nursing diagnosis is the highest priority for Jack?
    1. Risk for impaired skin integrity related to paralysis
    2. Impaired urinary elimination related to paralysis and immobility
    3. Impaired physical mobility related to paralysis
    4. Ineffective airway clearance related to high cervical spinal cord injury

24. Mr. Brown has fallen from a ladder and experienced an axial loading injury to L4-L5. After surgery to remove the fragments of bone, which of the following assessments are vital for you to include in your nursing care?
    1. Assess arm strength and arm sensation; assess dressing.
    2. Assess pupils, and check for bladder distention; assess dressing.
    3. Assess leg strength, motion, position sense and sensation, and check dressing.
    4. Assess cranial nerves II, III, IV, and VI, and check dressing.

CHAPTER 7

Gastrointestinal System

1. A patient is admitted to the hospital with the diagnosis of peptic ulcer disease. The patient develops a sudden, sharp pain in the midepigastric region of the abdomen. The abdomen is rigid and boardlike. The clinical manifestations most likely indicate which of the following?
    1. The ulcer has perforated.
    2. Additional ulcers have formed.
    3. The patient has hemorrhagic shock.
    4. An intestinal obstruction has developed.

2. A patient has been diagnosed with chronic gastritis caused by *Heliobacter pylori*. The nurse anticipates that the patient will be administered which of the following categories of medications?
   1 Antacids
   2 Mucosal protectant agents
   3 Histamine 2–receptor antagonists
   4 Antibiotic combinations

3. Which diagnostic tool is used in patients with peptic ulcer disease and provides direct visualization of the GI tract and the bleeding site?
   1 Endoscopy
   2 Angiography
   3 Radionuclide scanning
   4 Barium enema

4. The patient arrives at the ED with nausea and bloody vomitus that has occurred for the past 48 hours. Which of the following acid-base imbalances would you expect to find when laboratory results return?
   1 Respiratory acidosis
   2 Respiratory alkalosis
   3 Metabolic acidosis
   4 Metabolic alkalosis

5. Which of the following statements describes hematemesis?
   1 Bright red or maroon blood passed via the rectum
   2 Blood that cannot be identified on visual examination
   3 Bright red bloody vomitus or vomitus with a coffee-ground appearance
   4 Black, tarry stool passed via the rectum

6. The nurse is completing dietary teaching for the patient recovering from an episode of GI bleeding. The nurse explains that diet will consist of which of the following?
   1 High protein, low-fat foods
   2 Any foods that are tolerated
   3 Low calorie, low-fat foods
   4 High-fiber foods

7. The nurse is caring for a patient who was admitted with massive GI bleeding. The nurse assesses the patient and notes the following: tachycardia, decrease in urine output to less than 30 ml/hr, skin cool to the touch, and pallor. The nurse believes these symptoms are associated with:
   1 Cardiogenic shock.
   2 Neurogenic shock.
   3 Distributive shock.
   4 Hemorrhagic shock.

8. Which of the following cells are responsible for the production of hydrochloric acid?
   1 Chief cells
   2 G cells
   3 Parietal cells
   4 Mucosal cells

9. In small bowel obstruction, absent bowel sounds are found where?
   1 Proximal to the obstruction
   2 Over the obstruction
   3 At a 45-degree angle, 2 inches from the mid-clavicular line
   4 Over the inguinal lymph nodes

10. A patient with intestinal obstruction can often be dehydrated. Which laboratory test best signifies dehydration?
    1 Increased serum magnesium
    2 Decreased blood urea nitrogen (BUN)
    3 Decreased total platelets
    4 Elevated hematocrit

11. Which diagnostic test differentiates the specific cause and location of mechanical bowel obstruction?
    1 Flat-plate x-ray of the abdomen
    2 Handheld Doppler of the abdomen
    3 CT of the abdomen
    4 Gastroscopy

12. A rectal tube is used to reduce dangerous dilation of what bowel in intestinal obstruction?
    1 Small bowel
    2 Large bowel
    3 Appendix
    4 Stomach

13. Which nursing intervention is the key to assessing and evaluating hypovolemia in bowel obstruction?
    1 Serum calcium assessment
    2 Intake and output measurement
    3 Serum WBC count assessment
    4 Bowel sound auscultation

14. Which one of the following patients is a candidate for surgical treatment of bowel obstruction? A patient with:
    1 Hemoptysis.
    2 Bradycardia and low-grade temperature.
    3 Abdominal pain that comes and goes every 4 to 6 hours.
    4 A large immovable tumor of the bowel.

15. A physical assessment of an abdomen in a patient with potential bowel obstruction should be implemented in what order?
    1 Percussion then auscultation
    2 Palpation then auscultation
    3 Auscultation then palpation
    4 Digital rectal examination then flat plate of the abdomen

16. Which nursing intervention is best for a patient with a dry mouth resulting from complete bowel obstruction?
    1 Ice chips as needed
    2 Hard candy as needed
    3 Liquid diet
    4 Oral care as needed

17. The endocrine cells reside in the:
    1 Acini cells.
    2 Islets of Langherhan.
    3 Duodenum.
    4 Liver.

18. The first drug of choice in the treatment of pancreatic pain is:
    1 Hydromorphone (Dilaudid).
    2 Meperidine (Demerol).
    3 Fentanyl citrate (Sublimaze).
    4 Morphine.

19. The main symptom of acute pancreatitis is:
    1 Nausea and vomiting.
    2 Severe pain.
    3 Elevated lipase and amylase serum levels.
    4 Hypocalcemia or hypercalcemia.

20. Tetany should be treated with:
    1 Calcium gluconate.
    2 Atropine.
    3 Pancrelipase (Cotazym).
    4 Cimetidine (Tagamet).

21. Loss of pancreatic function occurs in:
    1 Acute pancreatitis.
    2 Chronic pancreatitis.
    3 Pseudocyst formation.
    4 Pancreatic insufficiency.

22. The best diagnostic procedure available to the physician in determining pancreatitis is:
    1 Plain radiographic films.
    2 Endoscopic retrograde cholangiopancreatography (ERCP).
    3 Contrast enhanced CT.
    4 Ultrasound studies.

23. Which of the following is a nursing diagnosis for the patient with pancreatitis?
    1 Imbalanced Nutrition: More than Body Requirements
    2 Excess Fluid Volume
    3 Ineffective Tissue Perfusion: Peripheral
    4 Potential for Hemorrhage

24. In chronic pancreatitis, diabetes may develop as a result of:
    1 Shock.
    2 Effects of the disease on the islets of Langerhans.
    3 Secondary infection.
    4 The formation of fibrous tissue that replaces healthy acini tissue.

25. Which of the following clinical signs suggest hepatic encephalopathy?
    1 Decrease in urine output
    2 Upper GI bleeding
    3 Decrease in level of consciousness
    4 Shortness of breath

26. Hepatorenal syndrome is caused by:
    1 Decreased renal blood flow and increased levels of aldosterone.
    2 Accumulation of unmetabolized wastes in the renal tubules.
    3 Pressure exerted on the kidneys by ascitic fluids.
    4 Obstruction of the ureters as they exit the renal pelvis.

27. Which of the following diagnoses can lead to liver failure?
    1 Glomerulonephritis, renal carcinoma
    2 Abdominal aortic aneurysm, arteriosclerosis
    3 Gastrointestinal bleeding, bowel obstruction
    4 Hepatitis, biliary atresia

28. The purpose of administering nitrates in a patient who has portal hypertension is to:
    1 Promote the excretion of ascitic fluid.
    2 Reduce portal pressure.
    3 Improve arterial renal blood flow.
    4 Prevent the development of hepatic encephalopathy.

29. Which of the following laboratory tests would be monitored in a patient who is receiving lactulose for hepatic encephalopathy?
    1 Creatinine
    2 Bilirubin
    3 Ammonia
    4 Albumin

30. Which of the following symptoms is associated with liver failure?
    1 Hypoalbuminemia, malnutrition, jaundice, coagulopathies
    2 Hyperalbuminemia, jaundice, weight gain, coagulopathies
    3 Ascites, hypobilirubinemia, weight loss, cyanosis
    4 Asterixis, palmar erythema, hypobilirubinemia, vomiting

31. The nurse is caring for a patient with severe ascites. Which of the following positions is appropriate for the patient?
    1 Fowler's
    2 Trendelenburg
    3 Supine
    4 Prone

32. Which of the following interventions would be the *most* appropriate for the patient who has developed a coagulopathy associated with liver failure?
    1 Monitor urine output.
    2 Observe stool and gastric contents for evidence of bleeding.
    3 Assess for changes in level of consciousness.
    4 Eliminate hepatotoxins.

CHAPTER *8*

Renal System

1. The earliest sign of acute tubular necrosis (ATN) is:
    1 Decreased urinary output.
    2 Uremic frost.
    3 Chills and fever.
    4 Cardiac friction rub.

2. Which of the following is a cause of prerenal failure related to decrease renal perfusion?
    1 Aminoglycosides
    2 Heart failure
    3 Benign prostatic hyperplasia (BPH)
    4 Iodinated contrast dyes

3. The patient asks the nurse what azotemia is. The nurses best response should be increased:
    1 Blood and protein in your urine.
    2 KCl in your blood.
    3 Blood levels of nitrogenous waste products.
    4 Kidney function.

4. Which of the following urine patterns is seen in the maintenance phase of ATN?
    1 Anuria
    2 Polyuria
    3 Oliguria
    4 Hypovolemia

5. Which patient is at the highest risk for the development of postrenal failure?
    1 29-year-old woman who smokes
    2 15-year-old adolescent with diabetes
    3 10-year-old hospitalized child
    4 75-year-old man

6. When the nurse calculates the fluid allotment for a patient in acute renal failure, the nurse adds the previous day's urinary output to the patient's insensible losses. Insensible daily losses allotted are:
    1 250 ml.
    2 500 ml.
    3 400 ml.
    4 1000 ml.

7. As a nurse caring for a patient in acute renal failure, you are observing your patient's HR. Which electrolyte would you be concerned about?
   1 Sodium
   2 Potassium
   3 Chloride
   4 Phosphorous

8. All of the following physical examination findings are consistent with fluid volume excess *except:*
   1 Increased BP.
   2 Increased HR.
   3 Audible basilar crackles.
   4 Negative jugular venous distention.

9. Which of the following should the nurse expect to find when assessing an arteriovenous fistula?
   1 Redness
   2 Pulselessness
   3 Presence of thrill and bruit
   4 Mottled skin distal to site

10. An appropriate short-term goal for a patient preparing to begin dialysis would be to have the patient:
    1 Verbalize understanding of the treatment and its implications.
    2 Demonstrate proper technique for vascular access.
    3 Discuss rationale for administration of Epogen.
    4 Verbalize importance of weighing self on a weekly basis.

11. The nurse knows the patient understands his discharge instructions regarding his arteriovenous fistula when he states:
    1 "I will feel the site each day for a bruit."
    2 "I will listen each day for a thrill."
    3 "I will place my arm under my body at night to keep the site warm."
    4 "I will avoid wearing any tight fitting clothing around my fistula."

12. The nurse understands the term *azotemia* is used to describe:
    1 An elevation in serum BUN and creatinine.
    2 Itching as a result of uremic frost.
    3 An increase in creatinine clearance levels.
    4 A decrease in erythropoietin secretion.

13. A patient newly diagnosed with renal insufficiency asks, "When will I need to start dialysis?" The nurse responds best by saying:
    1 "You will need to start dialysis as soon as possible to prevent further kidney damage."
    2 "It is hard to say, but with proper diet and fluid restrictions you can slow the progress of the disease."
    3 "You will need a kidney transplant, not dialysis."
    4 "Don't worry about dialysis; you'll probably never need it!"

14. The nurse is teaching a patient about the classic signs and symptoms of renal failure. The nurse realizes the patient needs additional instruction when he includes which of the following?
    1 Loss of appetite
    2 Fatigue
    3 Increase in urinary frequency
    4 Fluid retention

15. Which of the following patients does the nurse recognize as being at greatest risk for the development of renal disease?
    1 A 72-year-old African-American woman with osteoporosis
    2 A 55-year-old African-American man with hypertension
    3 A 32-year-old obese white woman
    4 A 15-year-old white adolescent with cerebral palsy

16. Which of the following medications would the nurse most likely question its use when caring for a patient with a diagnosis of end-stage renal disease (ESRD)?
    1 Acetaminophen
    2 Epogen
    3 Calcium carbonate
    4 Phos-Lo

17. For continuous renal replacement therapy (CRRT) to be effective when using continuous arteriovenous hemofiltration (CAVH), mean arterial pressure must be at least:
    1 40 mm Hg.
    2 60 mm Hg.
    3 80 mm Hg.
    4 120 mm Hg.

18. Which of the following medications may be prescribed to prevent clot formation in the extracorporeal circuit?
    1 Vitamin K
    2 Warfarin (Coumadin)
    3 Trisodium citrate
    4 Protamine sulfate

19. When caring for the patient receiving CRRT, the nurse knows an important aspect of her role is:
    1 Selecting the composition of dialysate solution to be used.
    2 Setting the fluid balance goal.
    3 Monitoring electrolyte levels daily.
    4 Calculating amount of fluid replacement.

20. The nurse recognizes one of the benefits of CRRT over intermittent hemodialysis (IHD) is that CRRT:
    1 Can only be used in hemodynamically stable patients.
    2 Enhances fluid volume overload.
    3 Increases electrolyte imbalances.
    4 Provides better azotemic and uremic control.

21. Transient hypotension may occur just after beginning CRRT. The nurse knows this condition is initially best treated by:
    1 Decreasing the rate of blood flow from the patient to the machine.
    2 Aggressively replacing fluids.
    3 Administering vasopressors as prescribed.
    4 Discontinuing CRRT.

22. The patient receiving CRRT has a temperature of 96.2° F. The nurse knows this is best treated by:
    1 Using an in-line fluid warmer to warm the blood returning to the patient.
    2 Ensuring that the patient is fully covered with a warming blanket.
    3 Applying warm compresses to the vascular access site.
    4 Encouraging a family member to bring a pair of warm flannel pajamas for the patient.

23. When setting up the CRRT machine, the nurse knows that the filtered blood will be returning to the body through the:
    1 Red line.
    2 Yellow line.
    3 Green line.
    4 Blue line.

24. The wife of a patient receiving CRRT asks "Can my husband receive this treatment at home?" The nurse responds best by saying:
    1 "Yes, but only after you are trained to perform CRRT."
    2 "Yes, we can arrange for a home health nurse to visit and perform CRRT once a day."
    3 "No, this is a complex procedure that should only be performed by skilled nurses in a critical care setting."
    4 "No, CRRT isn't done at home, but I'll ask the physician if it is possible to do it on an outpatient basis."

CHAPTER 9

Endocrine System

1. Which of the following is caused by a total lack of endogenous insulin?
   1 Metabolic alkalosis
   2 Hypotension
   3 Hyperosmolar hyperglycemic nonketotic (HHNK) coma
   4 Diabetic ketoacidosis

2. Severe hyperosmolarity, dehydration, and blood glucose levels above 1000 mg/dl is most likely associated with:
   1 Metabolic alkalosis.
   2 HHNK coma.
   3 Diabetic ketoacidosis.
   4 Adrenal insufficiency.

3. The most important way to prevent diabetic ketoacidosis (DKA) in a hyperglycemic patient is to:
   1 Monitor blood glucose levels frequently.
   2 Administer insulin and rehydrate the patient.
   3 Administer glucose and fluids.
   4 Replace electrolytes and fluids.

4. A patient is admitted to the ICU with a decreased level of consciousness. She has a 4-year history of type I diabetes. Her skin is dry with poor turgor. A physical examination reveals the following:

RR: 40, deep and rapid
HR: 118 bpm, weak pulse
PB: 100/58 mm Hg
Temperature: 101.8° F, rectally
Serum glucose level: 510 mg/dl
Serum osmolarity: 315 mOsm/L
HGB: 14 g/dl
Hemocrit (HCT): 48%
Na^+: 130 mEq/L
K^+: 5 mEq/L
pH: 7.23

Which of the following is the *main* cause of the patient's dehydration and increased serum osmolarity?

1 Hyponatremia
2 Hyperthermia
3 Ketosis
4 Osmotic diuresis

5. The primary goal during initial treatment of a patient who has HHNK syndrome is to:
1 Lower serum glucose levels as quickly as possible.
2 Correct the patient's dehydrated state.
3 Restore normal serum potassium levels.
4 Identify the precipitating problem.

6. A primary danger of insulin shock is:
1 Increased uptake of glucose.
2 Severe dehydration and hypovolemia.
3 Increased alertness.
4 Irreversible brain damage.

7. Which regulates uptake of glucose into the cell?
1 Somatostatin
2 Glucagons
3 Gastrin
4 Insulin

8. Early signs of hypoglycemia include:
1 Irritability.
2 Seizures.
3 Pain.
4 Hyponatremia..

9. Insulin is released from the pancreas by:
1 Alpha cells.
2 Beta cells.
3 Delta cells.
4 Other pancreatic cells.

10. In critically ill patients, serum glucose levels can be increased by:
   I. Administration of hyperalimentation fluids.
   II. Administration of corticosteroid therapy.
   III. Stress.
   IV. Administration of enteral feedings.
1 I, II, III
2 III only
3 III, IV
4 I, II, III, IV

11. The primary intervention in the treatment of HHNK is:
1 Administration of hypertonic dextrose solutions.
2 Administration of hypotonic solutions.
3 Administration of isotonic fluids.
4 Administration of hypertonic fluids.

12. Which of the following is *true* concerning inappropriate antidiuretic hormone secretion (SIADH)?
1 Antidiuretic hormone (ADH) levels are increased, serum sodium levels are increased, urine specific gravity is increased.
2 ADH levels are increased, serum sodium levels are decreased, urine-specific gravity is increased.
3 ADH levels are decreased, serum sodium levels are decreased, urine-specific gravity is decreased.
4 ADH levels are decreased, serum sodium increased, urine-specific gravity is unchanged.

13. ADH hormone:
1 Is secreted in response to decreased osmolarity.
2 Increases the permeability of distal tubules of the kidney to water.
3 Increases urine volume.
4 Increases the permeability of distal tubules of the kidney to sodium.

14. Clinical manifestations of SIADH include:
1 Serum hyponatremia.
2 Serum hyperosmolality.
3 Urine hypoosmolality.
4 Excess water loss.

15. A patient with SIADH rings the nurse's station and asks to go to the bathroom. You tell him that you will come to assist him based on the fact that:
    1 Patients with SIADH may have symptoms of hypokalemia including muscle cramping.
    2 Fluid intake and output is monitored in patients with SIADH.
    3 Patients with SIADH may have symptoms of hyponatremia including confusion.
    4 Patients with SIADH may have symptoms of hypernatremia including confusion.

16. SIADH is suspected in which of the following patients?
    1 An older patient with a recent stroke who is confused and on diuretics
    2 A patient recovering from surgery with a serum sodium level of 150 mEq/L and increased urine sodium level
    3 A pregnant woman with serum sodium level of 130 mEq/L
    4 A patient with small-cell carcinoma of the lung whose urine-specific gravity is 1.030 and serum sodium is 120 mEq/L. The patient is complaining of muscle cramps

17. A family member of a patient with SIADH asks why the patient is confused. The appropriate response is:
    1 His sodium level is low.
    2 His potassium level is low.
    3 He is dehydrated.
    4 His pH is low.

18. A patient with SIADH asks why he is on water restrictions. The appropriate response is:
    1 The physician has prescribed it.
    2 You are not on fluid restriction. Your sodium level is restricted.
    3 Water restrictions will bring your potassium level back to normal.
    4 Your body is producing too much ADH, causing you to reabsorb water. Limiting your water will help bring your water level down and your sodium level up.

19. A diagnosis of hyponatremia is made in a patient with:
    1 Serum sodium level greater than 134 mEq/L.
    2 Serum sodium level less than 280 mOsm/kg.
    3 Confusion, lethargy, muscle twitching, and convulsions.
    4 Serum sodium level less than 160 mEq/L.

20. Which of the following hormones is deficient in the patient with diabetes insipidus?
    1 Testosterone
    2 Estrogen
    3 Insulin
    4 ADH

21. The clinical symptoms of DI in which the renal tubules are not able to conserve free-water results in:
    1 Bradycardia.
    2 Polyuria.
    3 Sweating.
    4 Polyphagia.

22. Which of the following is a common cause of DI?
    1 Pyelonephritis
    2 Syphilis
    3 Hypotension
    4 Carotid stenosis

23. Which of the following vital signs would indicate DI?
    1 BP 210/140 mm Hg, temperature 97.8° F
    2 HR 66 bpm, temperature 102° F
    3 RR 28 breaths/minute, HR 40
    4 BP 70/40 mm Hg, HR 124

24. What clinical manifestation results in the GI tract as a result of polyuria associated with DI?
    1 Diarrhea
    2 Constipation
    3 Hemorrhage
    4 Ulcerative colitis

25. Which urinary laboratory test is diagnostic for DI?
    1 Sodium
    2 Casts
    3 Osmolity
    4 Potassium

26. The medication of choice in replacing ADH in the person with DI is:
    1 Furosemide (Lasix).
    2 Sodium nitroprusside (Nipride).
    3 Mannitol.
    4 Vasopressin (Pitressin).

27. What two main areas of nursing assessment are crucial in monitoring the patient with DI?
    1 Cardiac rate and psychologic status
    2 Airway and GI loss
    3 Fluid volume and neurologic status
    4 Pain and pulmonary status

28. Cerebral salt wasting (CSW) is characterized by what serum electrolyte abnormally?
    1 Low potassium
    2 High potassium
    3 Low sodium
    4 High sodium

29. In cerebral salt wasting, what happens to the total fluid volume?
    1 It increases.
    2 It decreases.
    3 It remains normal.
    4 It only increases during late-stage disease.

30. In which of the following conditions does weight increase?
    1 CSW
    2 DI
    3 SIADH
    4 Increased ICP

31. Which of the following conditions is attributed to the failure to regulate sodium absorption by the CNS?
    1 Hypotension
    2 DI
    3 SIADH
    4 CSW

32. In CSW, fluid replacement is usually done through:
    1 Nasogastric (NG) tube replacement.
    2 IV replacement.
    3 Percutaneous endoscopic gastrostomy (PEG) tube in stomach.
    4 An enema.

33. Which of the following IV solutions is used for fluid replacement in a patient who has CSW?
    1 NS
    2 $D_{10}W$
    3 LR
    4 $D5_{1/2}NS$ with 40 mg KCl

34. Your patient has CSW. She has a urinary output of 150 ml/hr. What should your rate of IV replacement be?
    1 150 ml/hr
    2 75 ml/hr
    3 300 ml/hr
    4 125 ml/hr

35. Rapid correction of hyponatremia in CSW can cause what side effect?
    1 Blindness
    2 Pontine myelinolysis
    3 Hypotension with bradycardia
    4 Erythroblastosis fetalis

CHAPTER *10*

Hematologic System

1. Which of the following patients is most at risk for developing sepsis?
    1 46-year-old man who is 2 days postoperative for an appendectomy
    2 76-year-old woman with diabetes who is admitted with pneumonia
    3 66-year-old woman hospitalized for 2 days for a dislocated hip
    4 5-year-old girl admitted with a urinary tract infection

2. In which of the following patients would you suspect sepsis?
    1 45-year-old man with abdominal pain and rigidity, temperature of 102.2° F, BP of 100/56 mm Hg, HR of 110 bpm, and RR of 28 breaths/min
    2 35-year-old woman with a productive cough, fever of 101.2° F, BP of 120/76 mm Hg, HR of 84 bpm, and RR of 20 breaths/min
    3 4-month-old infant with one episode of vomiting; vital signs within normal limits
    4 16-year-old woman with hematuria, back pain, temperature of 98.6° F, BP of 110/68 mm Hg, HR of 66 bpm, and RR of 16 breaths/min

3. A nurse is suspicious that a patient with chronic pneumonia is developing sepsis. What would be the first symptom to be observed?
    1 Decreased BP with narrow pulse pressure
    2 Rales upon auscultation to lung fields
    3 Mental confusion
    4 Respiratory acidosis

4. In treating a patient with probable sepsis, the highest priority after establishing patient safety and stability would be to:
   1 Anticipate treating the patient with broad spectrum antibiotics.
   2 Obtain cultures: blood, sputum, urine.
   3 Initiate fluid resuscitation.
   4 Initiate ventilatory management and inotropic therapy.

5. Which of the following is *not* a major component of sepsis?
   1 Inflammation
   2 Coagulation
   3 Suppressed fibrinolysis
   4 Diuresis

6. Which of the following may cause an increase in the incidence of sepsis?
   1 Increased use of invasive hemodynamic monitoring
   2 Increased elective outpatient procedures
   3 Increased awareness of hand washing
   4 Use of appropriate antibiotics after cultures are obtained

7. Which would be considered a treatment for sepsis?
   1 Blood transfusion
   2 Vasopressors
   3 Antibiotics
   4 Possible intubation

8. Diagnosis of sepsis can be made by:
   1 Presence of fever, tachycardia, tachypnea, and an overwhelming infection.
   2 Hypotension and respiratory acidosis.
   3 Possible identification of the infective microorganism through blood cultures.
   4 Chest x-ray and complete blood count (CBC).

9. Which of the following conditions is related to a low production of platelets in the body as a cause of thrombocytopenia?
   1 Vitamin B12 deficiency
   2 Hyperspleenism
   3 Hypothyroidism
   4 Hydrocephalus

10. The average lifespan of a platelet is:
    1 1 to 2 days.
    2 3 to 5 days.
    3 9 to 12 days.
    4 120 days.

11. The risk of hemorrhage is greater than 50% if the total platelet count in an adult is less than:
    1 500,000 cells/mm^3.
    2 250,000 cells/mm^3.
    3 100,000 cells/mm^3.
    4 20,000 cells/mm^3.

12. Vital signs for a patient with thrombocytopenia may include:
    1 Hypertension and a low-grade fever.
    2 Pain of 9 on a 1-to-10 scale and fever greater than 102° F.
    3 Hypotension and tachycardia.
    4 RR less than 5 breaths/min and bradycardia.

13. Which of the following findings would be a sign of thrombocytopenia when implementing an eye assessment?
    1 Sclera yellow in color
    2 Retinal hemorrhage
    3 Encrusted eyelashes
    4 Pupils react to light

14. What is the rationale for trying to avoid vomiting from occurring in patients with thrombocytopenia?
    1 Vomiting leads to constipation.
    2 Vomiting can rupture the liver that can cause the release of large amounts of platelets into the bloodstream.
    3 Vomitus can cause aspiration that causes hypoventilation.
    4 Vomiting raises ICP.

15. Your patient's postplatelet transfusion count raises 200 cells/mm^3 per unit of platelet transfused. The advanced practice nurse states the patient has developed antibodies against human leukocyte antigens (HLA). This is called:
    1 Leukocytosis.
    2 Alloimmunization.
    3 Autoregulation.
    4 Red cell lysis syndrome.

16. Which of the following outcomes can be a complication from a platelet transfusion?
    1 Hemolytic transfusion reaction
    2 Amnesia
    3 Pneumonectomy
    4 Sickle cell disease

17. Your patient's platelet count continues to drip 24 hours and again at 36 hours after platelet transfusion. What could be the cause of this?
    1 Sleep apnea
    2 Hepatosplenomegaly
    3 Anxiety
    4 Chronic scoliosis

18. When describing the first stages of DIC, one would recall the following:
    1 DIC is always precipitated by an infectious pathogen.
    2 Profuse bleeding can be immediately expected.
    3 Microthrombi production can be expected.
    4 Heparin and antifibrinolytic therapy should be started without delay.

19. What organ or organs are especially at risk from microemboli during DIC?
    1 Gastrointestinal
    2 Liver
    3 Kidneys, skin, and lungs
    4 CNS

20. When choosing a nursing diagnosis to best describe the events of DIC, one would likely state which of the following?
    1 Ineffective tissue perfusion
    2 Interrupted family processes
    3 Activity intolerance
    4 Decreased CO

21. Using the best word or words to describe the second phase of DIC, one might use which of the following term or terms?
    1 Fever and dehydration
    2 Microthrombi
    3 Hemorrhaging
    4 Necrosis and gangrene

22. The main reason or reasons for the development of hemorrhage late in DIC includes:
    1 Pathogen-releasing endotoxins.
    2 A further spread of microthrombi.
    3 Activation of the fibrinolytic system and consumption of coagulation factors.
    4 A lack of initiation of heparin and antifibrinolytics.

23. The primary approach to consider when treating a patient with DIC is:
    1 Correct the condition, and treat the underlying precipitating mechanism.
    2 Start heparin therapy.
    3 Begin blood products.
    4 Administer excessive IV fluids.

24. When planning a treatment plan to deal with the symptoms of DIC, one would include which of the following?
    1 Limit intravascular fluids.
    2 Administer antibiotic therapy.
    3 Increase activity.
    4 Prepare possible transfusion of blood products.

25. Which of the following laboratory tests is BEST for diagnosing DIC?
    1 D-dimer
    2 HGB and HCT
    3 WBC count
    4 ABG

CHAPTER *11*

Integumentary System

1. What type of burn occurs when a person's clothes catch on fire as a result of playing with matches?
    1 Chemical
    2 Electrical
    3 Ileal
    4 Thermal

2. The extent of a burn is based on:
    1 Depth.
    2 Percent of body area burned.
    3 Amount of pain experienced.
    4 Patient's gender.

3. Which type of severity of burn can be painless as a result of nerves being burnt?
   1 Superficial
   2 Full thickness
   3 Partial thickness
   4 Epidermal thickness

4. A burned patient of what age is most vulnerable based on co-morbidity status.
   1 62 years old
   2 45 years old
   3 30 years old
   4 12 years old

5. Within 48 hours of a burn, what physiologic responses usually occur?
   1 Hypernatremia, pulmonary edema, paralytic ileus
   2 Dehydration, edema, oliguria
   3 Negative nitrogen balance and weight loss
   4 Tremendous increase in urinary output, hypokalemia, and decreased hematocrit

6. Which of the following patients has the highest co-morbidity risk for burns?
   1 25 year old with ingrown toenail and fractured wrist
   2 8 year old with burns to both great toes and history of suicide
   3 70 year old with chronic obstructive pulmonary disease (COPD) and leukemia with burns to the face and hands
   4 50 year old with schizophrenia and burns to the left calf

7. To prevent a burned patient from being infected by the *Clostridium tetani* organism, what injection may be given?
   1 Vitamin K
   2 Vitamin B12
   3 Mantoux injection
   4 Tetanus toxoid

8. What is the major physical complication associated with the musculoskeletal system that is related to patients who have severe burns?
   1 Loss of pain tolerance
   2 Contractures
   3 Fractures
   4 Muscle spasms

9. Which of the following is *not* a function of the skin?
   1 Protection
   2 Aids in maintenance of homeostasis
   3 Sensory perception
   4 Absorption of nutrients

10. Which of the following is *not* an appropriate nursing measure for preventing skin breakdown?
    1 Eliminating the cause of the skin irritation
    2 Applying adhesive tape to the gauze cover dressing to prevent it from wadding up
    3 Applying a transparent dressing over reddened, bony prominences to prevent shear and friction
    4 Applying heel or elbow protectors

11. A stage II pressure ulcer is defined as:
    1 An observable pressure-related alteration of the intact skin, including temperature, tissue consistency, or changes in color.
    2 Full-thickness loss of skin involving damage or necrosis of subcutaneous tissue that many extend down to but not through the underlying fascia.
    3 Partial-thickness loss of the skin involving the epidermis or dermis.
    4 Full-thickness skin loss with extensive destruction, tissue necrosis, or damage to muscle, bone, or supporting structures (tendon or joint capsule).

12. A transparent dressing is best described as:
    1 A dressing made of hydroactive and absorptive particles that will interact with wound exudates to form a gelatinous material.
    2 A clear, dressing sheet that is adhesive and waterproof. It allows for the transmission of oxygen and water vapor.
    3 A starch or glycerin-based compound that can insulate the wound and provide a moist, wound environment.
    4 A dressing derived from the calcium salt of seaweed.

13. Which of the following best describes a nonionic, silver-fused transparent film that is effective against numerous fungi, yeast, and bacteria?
    1 Transparent film
    2 Hydrogel
    3 Composite dressing
    4 Antimicrobial dressing

14. Specialty mattresses that provide incorporate-zoned air support surfaces that offer constant airflow to maximize the prevention of pressure over a bony prominence is classified as:
    1 Foam.
    2 Pressure relief.
    3 Static-air mattress overlay.
    4 Pressure reduction.

15. What type of specialty bed is best used for the patient weighing more than 400 pounds?
    1 Bariatric
    2 Waterbed
    3 Static air
    4 Air-fluidized bed (silicone bed)

16. The air-fluidized bed is best used for what type of skin management?
    1 Skin tears
    2 Stage II pressure ulcers
    3 Stage III pressure ulcers requiring conservative management
    4 Stage IV pressure ulcers requiring flap surgery

17. The most common location of necrotizing fasciitis is the:
    1 Lower extremities.
    2 Abdomen.
    3 Face.
    4 Neck.

18. Which of the following is a key symptom of necrotizing fasciitis?
    1 Exquisite pain out of proportion to the condition
    2 Cough
    3 Headaches
    4 Incontinence

19. What is one important factor with regards to the treatment of necrotizing fasciitis?
    1 Treatment can be performed at home for 1 week before seeking medical help.
    2 Left-over antibiotics from the patient's last sore throat can be taken before calling his or her physician.
    3 Rest, if fatigued, can help delay the progression of necrotizing fasciitis.
    4 Prompt diagnosis

20. Which group is most likely to develop necrotizing fasciitis?
    1 Those who have received no immunizations
    2 Diabetic patients, parenteral drug users, and alcoholics
    3 Those who live in the Southwest
    4 Those of European descent

21. While monitoring the patient, the nurse notes that the erythema of the skin seems to be increasing, bullae is developing, and the patient complains of surface hypoesthesia. What should the nurse do?
    1 Wait and check the patient in 1 hour.
    2 Immediately report the findings to the physician.
    3 Remove the dressing, redress the wound, and check in 4 hours.
    4 Report the findings to the family.

22. A change in the level of consciousness or mentation may be the first signs of:
    1 Systemic toxicity or sepsis.
    2 Tension pneumothorax.
    3 Fractured femur.
    4 Incomplete lower spinal cord injury.

23. Which of the following are the most likely potential complications of necrotizing fasciitis?
    1 Infertility
    2 Loss of hearing
    3 Scarring and amputation
    4 Anaphylaxis

24. Virulence factors associated with group A streptococci include:
    1 Immunologic disguise, the ability to inhibit and kill phagocytes, the ability to release exotoxins, and the ability to induce an exaggerated production of cytokines.
    2 The inability to cause hemolysis.
    3 The inability to develop an immunologic disguise.
    4 The ability to suppress cytokines.

CHAPTER *12*

Multisystem

1. Before beginning any resuscitation efforts, the nurse must know the status of the patient's:
   1 Will.
   2 Advanced directives.
   3 Laboratory work.
   4 Disease state.

2. When managing a code using the American Heart Association's (AHA) secondary survey, the letter *D* stands for:
   1 Defibrillation.
   2 Drugs.
   3 Differential diagnosis.
   4 Death.

3. The most common arrest rhythm in adults is:
   1 Asystole.
   2 Pulseless electrical activity (PEA).
   3 Ventricular tachycardia (VT).
   4 Ventricular fibrillation (VF).

4. The most important treatment for VF is:
   1 Defibrillation.
   2 CPR.
   3 Drugs.
   4 Ventilation.

5. When you look at the ECG, how do you know that the patient is in PEA?
   1 You see VF on the monitor.
   2 There is no electrical activity on the monitor.
   3 The rhythm appears normal, but the patient is pulseless.
   4 The monitor shows tachycardia, and the patient has a weak pulse.

6. The first drug to be given in all three arrest rhythms is:
   1 Epinephrine.
   2 Lidocaine.
   3 Atropine.
   4 Aminodarone.

7. If you suspect a pulseless patient is in asystole, you must check to:
   1 Ensure that the code team is on the way.
   2 Determine whether the patient has an advanced directive.
   3 Ensure the patient has IV access.
   4 Ensure that the rhythm in another lead confirm the asystole.

8. Transcutaneous pacing is used for which arrest rhythm?
   1 VF
   2 Asystole
   3 PEA
   4 Pulseless VT

9. Nurses in ICUs are caring for more patients with multi-organ dysfunction syndrome (MODS), because:
   1 Patients with MODS require cardiac monitoring.
   2 Health care treatments and procedures are more effective; therefore more patients are surviving more traumatic insults.
   3 Only ICUs have adequate isolation facilities.
   4 The primary physicians order a transfer to the ICU on receiving laboratory results positive for MODS.

10. MODS is a progressive dysfunction of more than one organ in patients that are critically ill. A common cause is:
    1 Systemic infection.
    2 West Nile virus.
    3 Angioplasty.
    4 Hypertensive crises.

11. After a serious illness or injury, the critically ill patient may develop an uncontrolled inflammatory response. The by-products eventually cause:
    1 Rapid healing with abundant WBCs.
    2 Hyperoxygenation to the capillary beds.
    3 Mitral valve prolapse.
    4 Thromboxin, a vasoconstrictor, is released, and the synthesis of prostacycline, a vasodilator, is inhibited.

12. The prognosis for the patient with MODS:
    1 Is very good if the syndrome is promptly and adequately treated.
    2 Depends on the age of the patient.
    3 Is terminal in a high percentage of patients with MODS. Potential for recovery depends on the severity of the illness, the speed and adequacy of treatment, and the severity of subsequent complications.
    4 Mortality is the expected outcome for approximately 97% of the patients diagnosed with MODS.

13. Primary treatment goals for the patient with MODS include providing nutritional support. This will usually include:
    1 A 2500-calorie American Dietetic Association (ADA) diet.
    2 Encouraging the family to bring the patient's favorite foods from home.
    3 Replacing carbohydrates, proteins, and amino acids with IV or enteral feedings.
    4 A regular diet with high-protein shakes at bedtime.

14. Emergently placed lines can be a source of nosocomial infections. This may be avoided by:
    1 Replacing emergently placed lines as soon as possible.
    2 Changing central lines every day.
    3 Providing proper site care to emergently placed lines every 24 hours.
    4 Request that Emergency Response Personnel wait until the patient arrives at the hospital to place lines so that they may be placed in a clean environment.

15. What could place a patient receiving tube feedings at risk for developing MODS?
    1 The patient already has GI failure.
    2 Tube feedings do not provide adequate nutritional support.
    3 Increased potential for aspiration has occurred.
    4 Tube feedings cause diarrhea and dehydration.

16. The most effective tool in combating MODS in the at-risk population is:
    1 Early recognition of symptoms and appropriate treatment.
    2 A ventilator.
    3 Unknown. No population had been identified as being at risk for developing MODS.
    4 Antibiotics and dialysis are the best tools for combating MODS.

NCLEX® CHAPTER *1* ANSWERS

1.3   Contractility is the degree of ventricular stretch. Preload is the volume in the left ventricle at the end of diastole. Afterload is the resistance against which the left ventricle has to work. CO is the amount of blood ejected from the ventricles in 1 minute.

2.2   The electrical conduction system provides the stimulation for depolarization of cardiac cells, resulting in contraction. Right atrial filling results from venous return to the heart. Left atrial filling results from return from the pulmonary capillary bed via the pulmonary veins. SVR is reflective of afterload. Afterload is the resistance against which the left ventricle works.

3.1   The formula for CO is CO = stroke volume × HR. The CO formula does not include patient weight. Contractility is one of the parameters that influence stroke volume, and preload and afterload should also be considered. Stroke volume is included in the formula for CO, but contractility is one of the parameters for stroke volume.

4.3   HR is *not* a parameter of stroke volume; however, it is part of the formula for CO. Preload, afterload, and contractility *are* parameters of stroke volume.

5.3   Preload is a measurement of left ventricular–end diastolic pressure, which is reflective of left ventricular–end diastolic volume. Preload is a measurement of left ventricular end–diastolic pressure and is not the only parameter considered in CO.

6.4   Afterload is the resistance against which the left ventricle works and is measured by obtaining SVR. PCWP is reflective of preload. CO considers stroke volume and HR. Afterload is the resistance against which the left ventricle works and is measured by obtaining SVR.

7.2   Inotropic means affecting contractility. Chronotropic refers to affecting rate; vasoactive means affecting the blood vessels, and vasodilatory means causing dilation of the vessels.

8.2   A PCWP is reflective of left ventricular–end diastolic volume or pressure (or preload). SVR is reflective of afterload. LVSWI is reflective of contractility. Pulmonary artery systolic pressure reflects pressure in the pulmonary artery during systole when the mitral valve is closed, thus only reflecting left atrial pressure.

9.2   SVR is a reflection of the peripheral resistance during mean aortic pressure. PVR reflects the resistance against which the *right* ventricle works (the resistance from the lungs). MAP is a reflection of the perfusion pressure to vital organs. PCWP reflects left ventricular end–diastolic pressure.

10.3   Hypoxia, myocardial scar tissue, and parasympathetic stimulation *decrease* contractility. Miscellaneous influences that decrease myocardial contractility include hypoxia, hyperkalemia, hypercarbia, hyponatremia and myocardial scar tissue. Sympathetic stimulation increases contractility.

NCLEX® CHAPTER *2* ANSWERS

1.3   Although epinephrine is the hallmark of management for anaphylactic reactions, the first step in treating a suspected anaphylactic reaction is to discontinue the causative agent to prevent further degranulation of mast cells and the release of mediators. The priority should be placed on investigating the patient's complaint; you should never reprimand the patient. Your knowledge of the situation should make you think of an allergic reaction to the blood, and you should immediately discontinue the blood.

2.2   Your first steps in treating a patient with anaphylaxis are to discontinue the causative agent and then to assess the patient's respiratory system. Ensure that the patient can maintain his or her airway and provide supplemental oxygen if needed. After discontinuing the causative agent, the next step is to evaluate the patient's airway and provide oxygen. Severe mismatching of ventilation and perfusion may occur from bronchospasm, leaky capillaries, or pulmonary hypertension. These changes can take place for several hours, which produces hypoxia. Although establishing multiple large-bore IV lines is important to replace lost intravascular volume from leaky capillaries, establishing the patient's airway is more important. Remember the ABCs. Allergic reactions are not considered normal events; you should never falsely reassure the patient in any situation.

3.4 Anaphylactoid reactions represent IgE-independent activation of mast cells or basophils with resultant degranulation and mediator release. Anaphylactoid reactions may occur without prior exposure. Anaphylactic reactions are immune mediated and require prior exposure to a causative agent. The patient stated that he had not had that type of test before. Acidotic is not a type of reaction. Anaphylactic and anaphylactoid reactions produce lactic acidosis if allowed to progress untreated. Basophils and mast cells release mediators such as histamine, which causes an anaphylactic and anaphylactoid reaction.

4.2 Another nurse is already in the room evaluating the situation. You know that the patient is allergic to PCN and the antibiotic previously hung was a PCN. You should immediately suspect an anaphylactic reaction, and epinephrine should be brought to the room while other personnel are taking care of the patient. Morbidity and mortality decrease with faster treatment. You should never leave your patient in the time of a crisis; it is your responsibility to provide rapid direct treatment. The patient needs immediate intervention now.

5.1 Primary treatment for anaphylactic reactions includes discontinuing the causative agent, providing oxygen and administering epinephrine. If at any time the patient cannot maintain his or her own airway, you must support the respirations. Laryngeal edema obstructs the airway and makes it difficult for the patient to breathe. The patient needs immediate intubation. The patient probably needs cardiac resuscitative medications, but epinephrine, atropine, and lidocaine may be given via an ET tube. If there are extra people in the room, they may simultaneously attempt IV access, but the priority is to establish an airway. Although the patient is difficult to arouse, you must first check to see whether the patient has a pulse and BP. The patient is becoming hypoxic and progressing to anaphylactic shock. You do not want to slow the patient's HR because it is compensating for a lower intravascular volume and decreased tissue perfusion by increasing the rate.

6.3 The patient is experiencing severe hypoxia with anaphylactic shock. All attempts have been made to orally intubate; the patient is decompensating every second and needs an airway immediately. Laryngeal edema may be so severe that oral tracheal intubation can be unsuccessful. At this time, either cricothyroid ventilation or an emergency tracheotomy is required to maintain an adequate airway. Both can be performed by experienced personnel.

7.1 You must take immediate action with rapid intervention. Although the patient is probably hypovolemic and needs volume expanders, CPR must be established to generate circulation any time a patient loses his or her pulse. Although the patient is hypoxic and needs oxygen, the patient must also have circulation to deliver the oxygenated blood to the tissues.

8.3 The situation should remain as calm as possible at all times; this is not the time to voice opinions. Although establishing a new IV access is important, remember that cardiac "code" drugs such as epinephrine, lidocaine, and atropine can be administered via an ET tube while another person is establishing a new IV access. CPR must continue to circulate the medications and blood volume to keep the body perfused. At no time should CPR be discontinued for more than a few seconds unless the physician believes that every attempt has been made to save the patient and the physician is willing to stop the intervention.

9.3 Infection and embolus are not immediate problems. The patient does not have much forward flow if the pump fails. The patient can move.

10.4 Epinephrine is an extremely potent vasoconstrictor. Nitroprusside is a vasodilator, and dopamine is a vasodilator at lower doses, requiring higher doses for vasoconstriction. Dobutamine is a beta-1 stimulant.

11.4 It usually takes at least 40% ventricular damage to cause cardiogenic shock.

12.2 IABP has very little effect on preload and should cause a decrease in the heart oxygen demand by decreasing workload. When the balloon deflates, it creates a dead space of several inches into which the left ventricle pushes blood with almost no resistance to flow.

13.3 In cardiogenic shock the pump is damaged and cannot maintain adequate flow. This causes an increase in fluid (or blood) left in the heart. Hypovolemic shock is due to the loss of blood or fluid (or both) from the vascular space. The BP measurement is lowered, and the pulse rate is increased in both.

14.1 The prognosis increases with decreasing heart muscle damage. The patient may need an increased HR to maintain output. Decreasing the core temperature has negative effects, such as shivering, that increase oxygen demand and blood viscosity. which may decrease blood flow. The heart is already full of fluid and having a difficult time moving vascular volume forward; vascular volume needs to be decreased in this case.

15.4 Cardiogenic shock is a result of heart muscle damage. Blood loss is a sign of hypovolemic shock, and a high temperature is a sign of septic shock. Hives with breathing difficulty are hallmarks of anaphylactic shock.

16.3 Dobutamine is a positive inotropic agent that stimulates beta-1 receptors in the heart.

17.1 The hallmark of all forms of shock is inadequate tissue perfusion. Respiratory alkalosis is a compensatory mechanism to correct the acidosis that occurs from anaerobic metabolism. SVR increases in shock in response to the compensatory vasoconstriction of the arterial vascular bed. Although the basal metabolic rate (BMR) is increased, it is not the underlying pathologic result.

18.1 A suppression of antidiuretic hormone (ADH) occurs with DI, which causes the patient to have massive diuresis as does hyperosmolarity of the intravascular space from hyperglycemia. The patient is at risk for diuresing a very large amount of his or her intravascular volume. Hypotension is a clinical manifestation of shock, and sepsis and thermal injuries are categorized as relative or indirect losses. Protein albumin and magnesium are not direct losses.

19.1 A decrease in venous return to the right side of the heart, which leads to a decrease in filling pressure and volume, occurs with hypovolemic shock. Therefore the result is a decrease in CO and PCWP. This decrease in volume is sensed by the baroreceptors that stimulate the sympathetic nervous system (SNS) to release epinephrine and norepinephrine. The posterior pituitary responds to the shock state by releasing ADH to conserve water. Acidosis is a result of inadequate tissue perfusion that causes the cells to resort to anaerobic metabolism. Release of nosocomial infection mediators and APF are not related to hypovolemic shock.

20.2 Hypotension with a narrowed pulse pressure is a sign of the progressive stage of shock during which body systems become dysfunctional. The patient in this stage can lose up to or greater than 30% of his or her volume. The clinician must remember that hypotension is a late sign. In the compensatory stage the patient may have a normal BP and narrowed pulse pressure. In the refractory stage the patient has a volume loss greater than 40% and the compensatory mechanisms have been exhausted. Multiple-organ failure is not a named stage but an imminent outcome of the refractory stage.

21.1 Kidney perfusion is very sensitive to changes in blood volume and CO; therefore the patient's fluid status is reflected in urine output. BP can be normal in the compensatory stage of shock and the patient can be hypovolemic, which is exhibited as decreased urinary output. Further, by the time hypotension occurs, significant volume loss has taken place (30% to 40%), and the clinician must remember that hypotension is a late sign of shock. However, if volume loss is severe enough to produce hypotension, then the BP can be a valuable guide in the resuscitative efforts. CVP is not the best indicator because it shows a poor correlation with the extent of volume loss. CVP is normally a low pressure and does not produce a significant change until volume loss is severe—greater than 30%. The acidity or alkalinity of the skin is not an indicator.

22.2 The first-line treatment of hypovolemia is volume load. First, it is imperative to restore intravascular volume and tissue perfusion with crystalloids to sustain CO and MAP, thereby promoting tissue oxygen uptake and anaerobic metabolism. The effects of a low CO from low volume are worse than anemia. Vasopressor drugs such as dopamine can worsen capillary blood flow to tissues, leading to continued cellular hypoxia and anaerobic metabolism and organ death if adequate fluid volume replacement has not been initially performed. Blood transfusion is secondary; platelet transfusions are not necessary.

23.3 Volume load with crystalloids is the first-line and most important treatment of hypovolemia. Initial treatment is with a bolus of 1 to 2 L RL and evaluation of the patient's response. NS is used for blood and blood-product administration. Too much NS can contribute to hyperchloremic acidosis. Colloids are not a first-line treatment. Colloids are expensive compared with crystalloids and are effective once the patient has had fluid replacement with crystalloids. Mannitol 10% is an osmotic diuretic.

24.2   Hypothermia causes cardiac depression and can pre-dispose the patient to cardiac dysrhythmias. Cardiac depression can lead to a decrease in cardiac contractility and output. Hypothermia can also cause coagulopathies, which can cause further bleeding if hemorrhaging is a problem. The clinician must also remember that shivering increases the metabolic demand for oxygen by 400%, thereby worsening hypoxia. Colloid administration is part of the treatment of hypovolemic shock and can be beneficial in expanding plasma volume once crystalloids have been given. Elevating the HOB 30 degrees helps improve pulmonary ventilation and oxygenation; however, if the patient is unstable, a flat HOB is the best position. Urticaria is not a contributing factor.

25.3   Although the autonomic nervous system is part of the neurologic system, it is not directly involved with neurogenic shock. Disruption in the SNS impulses causes neurogenic shock. The reticuloendothelial system is primarily involved with fighting infection; central third ventricular has nothing to do with neurogenic shock.

26.4   A spinal cord injury, especially above T-6, is a common cause of neurogenic shock. The head is not part of the spinal cord; diabetes mellitus and HTN have nothing to do with neurogenic shock and the spinal cord.

27.3   Bradycardia occurs as a result of influences of a parasympathetic response. BP and temperature show hypotension and hypothermia if the patient is in neurogenic shock. The respiratory system is not directly involved; neurogenic shock primarily involves the cardiovascular system.

28.2   Decreased CO causes decreased tissue perfusion along with decreased pulmonary artery pressure (PAP) and PCWP.

29.4   Vasodilation is the causative factor of hypothermia. hypertension (HTN), tachycardia, and vasoconstriction do not cause or contribute to hypothermia and are not related to neurogenic shock.

30.3   The primary goal is to improve tissue perfusion, which may include treating cardiac instability.

31.2   A pulse oximeter measures percent of oxygen and assists in monitoring the patient for the development of hypoxia. Serum glucose levels are not used to monitor for hypoxia. ECG monitors cardiac rhythms, not hypoxia. Tidal volume calipers measure tidal volume and are not a frequently used measurement and do not directly indicate hypoxia.

32.1   Tissue perfusion is managed by IV fluids because it assists in managing and maintaining the cardiovascular status of the patient. HTN is not a problem in neurogenic shock, but hypotension is, which is the reason for administering IV fluids. DI has nothing to do with neurogenic shock; increased ICP has to do with the head, not the spinal cord.

33.3   Although fluid replacement is important, and isolating and identifying the causative agent are critical steps in the treatment of sepsis, respiratory status is always addressed first. Oxygen supplementation is important in that the patient's respiratory status is obviously compromised with the tachypnea and pulse oximetry. Patient comfort is always a consideration and should be incorporated, but it is not as important as respiratory status.

34.1   Fluid replacement should be in the form of crystalloids because hypoperfusion is caused by vasodilation and increased capillary permeability. Beta blockers cause a decrease in myocardial contractility. Colloids are more prone to leak through the capillary wall and take more fluid with them; they are not the best choice.

35.4   Septic encephalopathy occurs in response to decreased oxygenation to cerebral tissues. Complete reversal of septic encephalopathy depends on eradicating the offending organism. Although CNS infection should be suggested in all patients with an altered level of consciousness, few patients with septic encephalopathy actually have a CNS infection. The alteration in the level of consciousness stems from the decreased perfusion of oxygen to the cerebral tissues. A possible lumbar puncture can be anticipated for cultures as part of the septic work up; however, this intervention alone does not help alleviate any of the signs of septic encephalopathy. Although fever can produce some change in the level of consciousness (e.g., lethargy), the dramatic changes seen in septic encephalopathy occur as a result of decreased oxygenation of the brain. Oxygenation always takes precedence over fluid replacement.

36.3 A patient with an already severely compromised respiratory status who is complaining of tiredness may have ensuing respiratory collapse. Although oxygen by 100% nonrebreather may increase the arterial oxygen content, it does not help increase ventilation. A breathing treatment may be a first-line choice in a patient with respiratory compromise; however, the patient in septic shock with the same ABGs has depleted the patient's reserve. A breathing treatment does not maintain the airway and intubation. Placing the patient in an upright position and administering supplemental oxygen and anxiolytics can support both oxygenation and ventilation, but the patient's compensatory mechanisms have already failed.

37.2 The patient in choice 2 is older, chronically ill, and has multiple sites for entry of microorganisms. Although patients in choices 1, 3, and 4 are at risk for sepsis, they are not as much at risk as the patient in choice 2.

38.4 Cellular mediators such as cytokines, nitric oxide, and down regulators of peripheral catecholamines cause vasodilation and decreased SVR. Fever may cause a slight vasodilation, but it is not the primary vasomediator in septic shock. The CO actually increases with a decrease in SVR as long as myocardial contractility remains constant. Respiratory acidosis may cause a vasodilation but not profoundly.

39.1 The end result of septic shock if left unmanaged (and sometimes even when properly managed) is tissue hypoperfusion and end-organ failure. Although hypotension is a major complication and a cause of hypoperfusion, it alone is not the terminal result. Respiratory acidosis is a symptom of inadequate ventilation; coma is a symptom of altered metabolic imbalances and cerebral hypoperfusion.

40.2 Administration of positive inotropes increase the contractility of the heart, which counteracts the myocardial depression that occurs during septic shock. Positive ionotropes increase contractility of the heart and thus increase the force of contraction, which leads to an elevation of BP; they do not have anxiolytic properties. An increase in the calcium pump of the heart does not occur.

NCLEX® CHAPTER 3 ANSWERS

1.3 Emergencies and labor and delivery cases both assume a "full stomach" and call for aspiration precautions. Routine intubations do not require a rapid sequence and allow for a "test breath" before neuromuscular blockade. Some cases of airway trauma require a tracheostomy, and patients with limited range of motion (ROM) of the neck are candidates for awake fiberoptic intubations.

2.4 Three-to-five vital capacity breaths of 100% oxygen are adequate in most cases. Some unconscious patients are not preoxygenated, whereas almost all awake patients are. Preoxygenation requires 3 to 5 minutes, not 2, and requires 100% FIO_2.

3.1 Excessive pressure may hinder intubation. Cricoid pressure may result in an esophageal tear. Cricoid cartilage fracture is limited to 0.5 to 8.0 pounds of pressure and is applied at the cricoid cartilage, below the cricothyroid membrane.

4.2 The short duration of action allows for the return of spontaneous ventilations. Although the "gold standard" for RSI, many contraindications exist for succinylcholine; it does not cause precipitation in the IV line.

5.4 Lack of positive pressure to the stomach helps prevent regurgitation and aspiration. No difference in time occurs, whether a test breath is made or not; most patients are apneic during RSI, and there is no such thing as laryngeal distention.

6.4 After the BURP acronym. Cricoid pressure should be backward, slightly upward with a slight right displacement. Pressure is not removed until the ET tube has been inserted and placement is verified by chest auscultation or end-tidal carbon dioxide ($ETCO_2$).

7.3 Neuromuscular disorders such as spinal cord injuries predispose patients to dangerous hyperkalemia when succinylcholine (Anectine) is used. CRF has minimal effects on the onset times of the induction and paralytic medications. Many factors affect the need for fiberoptic intubation. Quadriplegia alone is not sufficient reason. Patients with spinal cord injuries do not routinely require more induction medications.

8.1 This is the anatomic description of the cricoid cartilage; the cricoid cartilage lies below the larynx. Cricoid pressure is used to occlude the esophagus and may be released after verification of ET tube placement by $ETCO_2$ or bilateral breath sounds (BBS).

9.2 Placement of an oxygen mask allows for diffusion of oxygen during apnea. RSI requires no ventilation between administration of medications and laryngoscopy and does not allow for a test breath. The patient's eyelids are taped shut during routine inductions for anesthesia.

10.3 Volume divided by pressure are the concepts for intracranial compliance. RR and BP might contribute to compensation; however, they are not directly involved with intracranial compliance. Temperature and CO are not directly involved with intracranial compliance.

11.4 High elastance means intracranial volume is high, and the ability to distend is limited. Normal compliance means that everything is normal and that no problem exists. High compliance and low elastance cause a normal or decreased ICP.

12.2 A decrease in both brain volume and blood volume compensates for increased CSF. Blood viscosity is not directly related, and BP is not one of the components in the Monroe-Kellie hypothesis. An increase in brain volume further accentuates the problem.

13.4 Cerebral perfusion pressure (CPP) is a pressure gradient across the brain. CBF maintains cerebral perfusion; CO is stroke volume × HR, and brain volume is an intracranial component.

14.1 Autoregulation controls ICP fluctuations in healthy individuals. Perfusion directly affects ICP and can make it worse or better but does not automatically correct. Hypoxia can contribute to further ICP problems, and thermal dilation could be a response from the hypothalamus; however, it does not have an autoregulation component.

15.2 Cerebral edema can occur secondary to surgery and with space-occupying lesions such as a tumor. An extremity fracture is not directly related to the head; consequently, this patient is not at risk for increased ICP, and the sinus cavity is a hollow cavity that has no direct relationship to the components (brain tissue, blood, CSF) within the intracranial cavity. A diabetic patient with blood sugar of 138 mg/dl does not present a risk of developing increased ICP.

16.3 Herniation of the brainstem causes immediate death. Although some of the late signs of increased ICP mimic stroke, stroke is not the outcome of brainstem herniation. Possible seizure activity is a possible late sign of increased ICP; however, stroke is not the outcome of brainstem herniation. Headache is a possible early sign of increased ICP and is not the outcome of brainstem herniation.

17.4 The best position to use on a patient with an increased ICP is to slightly elevate the HOB to less than 30 degrees. Prone positioning alone does not decrease ICP. If using the prone position, then the hips should be flexed. Trendelenberg positioning can further increase ICP. The body should be in a neutral position with little flexion.

18.2 Disability focuses on the CNS; assessing mental status and physical findings involving brain or spinal cord injuries. Each stage of resuscitation requires a decision as the assessment is conducted; decision time is not unique to *D*. Dextrose is not a standardized step in the stabilization process, although it may be needed if the patient is hypoglycemic. Deep tendon reflexes may be a part of the *disability* examination; however, it is not the key factor of this resuscitative step.

19.3 Eye opening (2) + motor (4) + verbal (1) = 7.

20.4 A late sign of ICP has an associated syndrome of hypertension and bradycardia. Different syndromes are assigned to cardiac tamponade and tension pneumothorax. An increased risk of fracture is associated with TBI; however, it is not the Cushing response.

21.2 The patient *most* likely sustained a minor head injury. The normal neurologic examination with the noted limited amnesia is a likely symptom associated with minor head injuries. No indications of a basilar skull fracture exists in the scenario. Diffuse axonal injury is a brain injury involving deep axonal neurologic pathway damage. The potential for a slow bleed is a possibility but is not the *most* likely injury.

22.3 The symptoms described are accurate for a classic presentation for this cranial fracture. Although linear is the most common type of skull fracture, this is not a typical presentation. For drainage to be present, a break in the integrity of the cranium needs to occur. No indications to either confirm or rule out ICP is found in this question.

23.1 The mechanism of action helps reduce ICP by drawing fluid off the brain. Morphine and Versed are regularly used in TBI management to sedate the patient. Epinephrine is harmful; its mechanism of action exacerbates ICP.

24.3 Because the cranial nerve III does not decussate, the pupil on the opposite side of the brain injury is not involved; pupil response correlates with the same side of the brain injury. The compression causes the muscle tone to be lost, resulting in dilation.

25.3 Denial is the first stage; it is an inability to comprehend the reality of the situation. Grieving takes approximately 1 year; anger reflects stage II crying. Resolution is too early in the sequence of stages in the grieving process.

26.2 Symptoms of a TIA resolve quickly. CVA symptoms last long and do not resolve quickly. Brain herniation result in death; peripheral neuropathy is usually a long-lasting condition.

27.3 Heart disease, high lipids, prior stroke, and smoking make this patient at very high risk. Although diabetes is a modifiable risk factor, Patient 1 is young and not at the greatest risk compared with the other patients listed. Obesity is a risk factor, but Patient 2 is also not at the greatest risk. Patient 4 has the age risk factor, but his low BP does not place him at the greatest risk.

28.3 Facial droop indicates stroke and is assessed by having the patient smile or show his or her teeth. Assessing the patient's smiling ability has nothing to do with hearing loss. Although speech is an important assessment for acute ischemic stroke, speech cannot be assessed because the patient is asked to smile, not speak. Assessing drift of the upper extremities is also an important assessment for acute ischemic stroke; however, it has nothing to do with the smile assessment.

29.2 An abnormal motor arm drift is when one arm drifts down lower than the other. Both arms equal in height indicate normalcy. The leg and pupil reaction are not being assessed with the arm drift assessment.

30.3 The window of time is 3 hours from onset of symptoms to the institution of thrombolytic therapy for brain attack. The timeframes of 30 minutes and 1 hour are too short; it is unlikely that the patient can be seen in 30 minutes, let alone initiate treatment. A 24-hour timeframe is too long.

31.3 Weight determines the dose for rt-PA. Although age is an inclusion-and-exclusion criterion and height is important in calculating the body surface area (BSA) of a patient, the dose for rt-PA is not calculated on the basis of either. Temperature has nothing to do with the dosing of rt-PA.

32.4 A GI bleed within the last 3 weeks makes this patient ineligible to receive rt-PA. Patients with lupus erythematosus and who are older than 18 years of age are eligible. An MI 3 years ago indicates a timeframe that makes this patient eligible for rt-PA.

33.2 Airway must be patent for respiratory status and to avoid aspiration because the patient is dysphagic. Although circulation is important and a part of the ABCs, it is not the most important consideration in this case. Incontinence is not a priority and does not relate to dysphagia. Communication is important with a patient; however, the ABCs are the priority, with airway being the first priority.

34.3 Between 1500 and 2000 ml blood loss is characteristic of a Class III hemorrhage. Up to 750 ml characterizes a Class I hemorrhage, and 1200 ml characterizes a Class II hemorrhage (750 to 1500 ml). Approximately 3500 ml of blood loss qualify as a Class IV hemorrhage (greater than 2000 ml).

35.3 The American College of Surgeons recommends that each milliliter of blood loss be replaced with 3 ml of crystalloid, either NS or RL. This is known as the 3-to-1 rule. The other ratios are incorrect.

36.3 Between 20% and 30% describes a Class III hemorrhage. Ten percent loss of blood volume is a Class I hemorrhage (up to 15%); 45% is a Class IV hemorrhage (greater than 40%), and 35% represents a Class III hemorrhage (30% to 40%).

37.4 According to the American College of Surgeons, 0.5 ml/kg/hr in an adult indicates the minimum output for adequate renal perfusion. The other levels are less than adequate.

38.4 Left ventricular dysfunction is a contraindication for MAST or PASG. Compression to the lower extremities and abdomen increase intrathoracic pressure and compression of lower body vasculature, causing increased work for the poorly functioning left ventricle.

39.2 The ABCs have been followed and you have recognized that the patient's injuries are too extensive to be controlled in the ED. The only chance for survival for this patient in a Class IV hemorrhage is to control the bleeding and provide aggressive volume replacement, both of which may be accomplished in the surgical unit. Hypovolemic shock and septic shock are both indications for MAST or PASG. They increase venous return and support BP. Pelvic or lower extremity fractures may also be indications for MAST or PASG.

40.3 O negative blood can be administered; men may also receive O+ blood if necessary. O blood is universal and can be received by all blood types. All other types need to be typed and crossmatched before using.

41.1 Improving oxygenation and ultimately tissue perfusion increases the patient's chances for survival. Hemoglobin probably varies from patient to patient. Although an oxygen saturation of 100% is preferable, the aim is to maintain oxygen saturation of approximately 93%. Equalizing blood into blood lost is a never-ending battle. Blood loss must be stopped to stabilize the patient, which can be accomplished with either a transfusion or surgical intervention.

42.3 The increased fluid in the pericardial sac results in muffled heart tones. Crackles in lung fields do not indicate cardiac tamponade. Bradycardia is a sign of tamponade in infants, not in a 65-year-old patient. Hypotension is more commonly associated with tamponade.

43.3 Bradycardia accompanies hypotension in cardiac tamponade in premature infants. Urine output does not increase in cardiac tamponade; it may be decreased as a result of hypoperfusion of the kidneys because of decreased CO. Fever is not a common sign of tamponade, although it may be related to an underlying condition. Central venous pressure is more likely elevated in cardiac tamponade.

44.2 The greatest risk for developing tamponade is during the first 24 hours after the procedure. Additionally, women and the older adults are more likely to develop tamponade after a revascularization procedure. Although a slow tamponade is possible, it is not likely. Tamponade is more commonly associated with insertion—not removal—of central lines. Although acute pericarditis is associated with tamponade, the patient does not currently have the illness.

45.1 Anticoagulants predispose patients to bleeding. The other classes of medications are not commonly associated with cardiac tamponade.

46.3 Tamponade is caused by the accumulation of fluid, clots, gas, or pus in the pericardial sac. The ability of the ventricles of the heart to fill and contract is diminished in cardiac tamponade. Decreased venous return can be a sign of cardiac tamponade, but it is not a cause. CO decreases as a result of cardiac tamponade.

47.3 Administering oxygen helps maintain oxygenation while waiting for other procedures to take place. Heart catheterization can confirm the presence of tamponade; however, catheterization is not always performed and surgery is not always the treatment of choice. Nitroglycerin administration is contraindicated because it is a vasodilator.

48.4 Entering the pericardial space with a needle may induce arrhythmias; hypokalemia increases the possibility of an arrhythmia occurring. Although fluid may contain potassium, the amount does not result in hypokalemia; hyperkalemia is not a direct cause of cardiac tamponade. The fluid is removed from the pericardial space, not inserted.

49.1 ECG abnormalities occur in only 20% of cardiac tamponade cases. Alterations in BP, jugular vein distention (JVD), and muffled heart tones are more commonly present.

50.2 Osteoporosis is considered a spinal, degenerative disease and can result in pathologic fractures or vertebral collapse that compresses the spinal cord. Onycholysis is a nail disorder, and melanoma is a type of skin cancer. Meningitis is an inflammation of the brain and spinal cord and does not result in fracture.

51.4 A compression in the lumbar spine region disrupts the nerve innervation to the bladder and bowels. Constipation, diminished urge to defecate, incomplete voiding, and urinary retention are all initial signs and symptoms that the patient is having a bowel or bladder problem. Loss of buttock sensation can result from a disk or thoracic spinal cord dysfunction; quadriplegia and diaphragm paralysis results from cervical spine trauma.

52.3 Back pain is the initial and most common symptom and complaint of a patient with spinal cord compression. Weakness has multiple causes such as diabetes, dehydration, and sleep deprivation. Paresthesia is related to hypocalcemia, diabetes, or other causes. Ataxia is usually related to brain (not spinal cord) dysfunction and is a late symptom.

53.1 Rheumatoid arthritis is a connective tissue disease that destroys the joints and may cause pathologic fractures or collapse (or both) to the vertebral bodies and shift, compress, or occlude the spinal canal and the integrity of the spinal cord. Metastasis usually occurs first in the lower spine in the lumbar and sacral regions. Spinal cord compression is not a risk factor in breast cancer; SLE is an inflammatory connective disease that leads to kidney dysfunction.

54.4 The autonomic symptoms that are exhibited in a patient with spinal cord compression are bradycardia and hypotension. AD lowers HR and BP. Confusion is not a symptom of AD.

55.4 AD symptoms are most commonly bowel and bladder dysfunction. Therefore the patient and family are taught how to perform self-catheterization to empty the bladder adequately and to prevent urinary retention and a possible urinary tract infection. Transferring is not associated with AD. Application of a brace or splint does not affect AD, and correct administration of antidepressants does not affect the management of AD.

56.3 A patient with spinal cord compression in the cervical spine is at risk for developing breathing problems because the diaphragm might be involved. Maintaining the patient's airway is the priority. Immediate assessment is required for any neurologic symptom. The arm exercises can increase problems, and pain medications can mask signs and symptoms.

57.2 An MRI precisely identifies the location of the spinal cord compression lesion and is also able to distinguish whether the lesion is extradural, intradural, or extramedullary. An MRI is a diagnostic test of soft tissue, not CSF. Injecting dye into the epidural space is used for a myelogram; nerves are only visualized with microscopic surgery.

58.3 Hypothermia is defined as a core temperature below 35° C. The 12-lead ECG may show a J or Osborne wave, but that alone is not diagnostic. Axillary temperature is not a measurement of core temperature. Shivering stops below a core temperature of 32° C, and bradycardia is present but also a nonspecific sign of many clinical problems. It may even be a normal variant.

59.1 Paraplegia and quadriplegia produce vasodilation of the peripheral thermal compartment below the lesion, which increases heat loss. Thin, malnourished patients, rather than obese patients, are at increased risk of hypothermia. Hypothyroidism produces hypothermia as a result of the reduced metabolic rate; respiratory failure does not have a significant influence on body temperature regulation.

60.3 The four methods through which the human body loses heat are convection, conduction, evaporation, and radiation. The other mechanisms are not related to heat loss.

61.4 Hemodialysis, with a potassium-free dialysate heated to 43° C is the appropriate method to provide active core rewarming. This patient is severely hypothermic. Warmed blankets does not add heat to the core. A room temperature Hubbard tank immersion cools the patient further. Warm oral fluids are not acceptable because the patient is mentally obtunded to the point of coma with a core temperature of 27° C.

62.3 Coagulation enzymes are temperature sensitive, and coagulopathies occur during hypothermia. The hemoglobin rises as a result of hypovolemia. Both hypokalemia and hyperkalemia occur during an episode of hypothermia, and both hypoglycemia (caused by shivering) and hyperglycemia (caused by impaired insulin function) can occur.

63.1 A hypothermic patient may exhibit pronounced bradycardia, and more time is needed to detect the presence of a slow pulse. Defibrillation is rarely successful in the patient with a core temperature under 30° C. The hypothermic patient in cardiopulmonary arrest should receive the initial three shocks as per the BLS protocol, but no further shocks should be delivered until the patient's core is warmed above 30° C. Patients may sustain cardiopulmonary arrest as a result of an MI or a CVA in a cold environment and become rapidly hypothermic. However, because no hypothermia existed before the arrest, some CNS protection from hypoxic damage may have occurred.

64.4 The patient intoxicated with alcohol exhibits peripheral vasodilation, which causes more rapid heat loss. Alcohol impairs shivering and the hypothalamic temperature that regulates the center. Intoxicated patients are not able to recognize and avoid situations appropriately, placing them at risk for hypothermia.

65.4 Vasoconstriction of the peripheral vasculature is an important mechanism for preserving and maintaining core temperature. Metabolic heat is generated in the core. The core temperature is tightly controlled within a narrow range, and almost all heat is eliminated from the body through the skin.

66.2 Dry drowning occurs after immersion in cold water, which causes laryngospasm and vagal stimulation. The laryngospasm causes the larynx to become occluded, which leads to asphyxiation, hypoxia, and cardiac arrest. A little water may have entered the lower airway and lungs; a diminished loss of conscienceness (LOC) usually causes relaxation.

67.3 Wet drowning is caused from drowning and near drowning. When victims are immersed in water, they first hold their breath and then are forced to inhale as the body attempts to attain oxygen. However, because the victims are under water, they inhale and aspirate fluid into the lungs. Laryngospasm leads to asphyxiation, hypoxia, and cardiac arrest. Glottic closure can result in aspiration and suffocation.

68.1 Drowning deprives the body of oxygen, which results in hypoxia and carbon dioxide build-up, causing an acidotic response. Respiratory acidosis and hypercarbia are present.

69.1 Tachypnea is the most frequent finding in a near-drowning patient because it is the normal compensatory mechanism of the body in an attempt to increase the amount of available oxygen to be delivered to the tissues. Apnea, Cheyne Stokes, and Kushmal breathing are not typical findings.

70.4 Immediate and quality CPR is necessary to increase the chance of survival. Cold water slows the metabolism and bodily functions, which then increases the chance of survival. A spinal cord injury complicates matters. Muddy water increases the chance of infection and complication.

71.2 Because of the decrease in tissue oxygen, hypoxemia results, which makes the heart irritable and causes arrhythmias to occur. Hypothermia and acidosis are usually present. Renal failure is a complication if developed.

72.3 Cardiac arrhythmias are due to hypothermia, acidosis, or hypoxemia of the patient. Rewarming is instituted on hypothermic patients to prevent such arrhythmias as VF, which could ultimately result in death. Anoxic encephalopathy is usually a result of apnea and the patient being hypoxic for a long period. Both ARDS and DIC are complications that can develop no matter whether the patient is rewarmed.

73.2 When the patient is unable to provide information and no significant others can be contacted, the emergency medical technician becomes the primary source of information. The emergency medical technician has valuable information regarding the condition of the patient when he or she was found that will help make medical decisions. The ED nurse and physician are just beginning to care for the patient.

74.3 The utmost concern for a patient brought to the ED with a suspected drug overdose is to ensure the physical stabilization. Research and ongoing medical management (although important) are not the focus of the treatment for this patient. Rehabilitation is more of a discharge planning item.

75.1 Once the patient has been physically stabilized, the focus then turns to reducing further drug absorption and eliminating drugs from the body. Locating the patient's family, although important, is not the main focus. Calling the police and sending the patient for a CT scan have nothing to do with the current treatment for this patient.

76.1 Although a side effect from drug overdose might be unsteadiness, suicide precautions provide procedures that are enacted to protect the patient from further self harm. Universal precautions should be instituted for all patients; delirium tremens precautions are not the primary safety measure in this case.

77.2 Gastric lavage is the method of choice to remove the contents in the GI tract. It is most effective if performed within 1 hour of ingestion.

78.1 Sorbitol is a fast-acting and potent cathartic. Magnesium citrate is not the fastest cathartic. Ipecac induces vomiting, and nalmefene is a reversal agent, not a cathartic.

79.3 The patient needs further evaluation and possible treatment. A psychiatric consultation is necessary. In response to the history of mental health issues and the present identification of suicidal ideations, a consult is necessary to determine the need for continued inpatient care.

80.2 Intubate with a cuffed ET tube to provide protection to the patient's airway and to allow for rapid intervention. Hemodialysis takes a long time and is quite involved. Forced diureses are not the safest nor the most effective treatment for this patient; Trendelenburg positioning is not a safe intervention to perform on this patient.

NCLEX® CHAPTER 4 ANSWERS

1.2 Arterial blockage causes angina. Coronary artery vasospasm and congenital heart defects are not common. Mitral valve stenosis is rare.

2.3 The patient cannot change his or her age. Smoking is modifiable by quitting; diabetes is modifiable through diet and exercise; and malnutrition is modifiable by increasing specific intake.

3.4 Demand exceeds supply concerning oxygen during work and increased activity. Narrowing or constriction is the problem in angina; not enough oxygen is supplied during an angina episode. The contractility is usually normal.

4.2 Predictability is the key to stable angina. Chest pain that occurs predominantly at rest is a result of a blockage. Chest pain that is relieved with nitroglycerin is a sign of unstable angina. Lack of prediction is caused by factors other than the narrowing of the arteries.

5.1 Elevated ST segment indicates Prinzmetal's angina. Inverted T waves, Q waves, and ST-segment depression are not signs of Prinzmetal's angina.

6.4 Dilatation of both artery and venous paths increase oxygenation to the myocardium, thereby decreasing anginal pain. Venous constriction decreases oxygen concentration, whereas artery constriction increases anginal pain.

7.2 Increased HR increases oxygen demand. The hemoglobin count is within normal range. Low HR and low RR decrease oxygen demand.

8.4 Morphine relieves anxiety and reduces left ventricular work by reducing preload pressure. Demerol is prescribed for acute pain and does not dilate coronary arteries. Lasix reduces edema, and Ancef is an antibiotic.

9.3 Emboli are common causes of AMIs. Vasospasm results in angina. Electrocution is a rare occurrence of cardiac standstill. Blunt trauma is not a causative factor but can be, depending on where the trauma is anatomically.

10.1 Inflammation of the myocardial muscle leads to increased WBC count. An infection causes a change in the differential as well. Circulating catecholamines are not associated with leukocyte count; glycogenesis is not directly related to leukocytes.

11.2 Dysrhythmia is the most common complication after an AMI. Cardiogenic shock is not common, and rupture of the myocardial wall is a rare occurrence. Congestive heart failure is not a complication but a co-morbid disease.

12.4 Women have atypical symptoms, usually not chest pain but rather GI distress. Patients with renal dysfunction have symptoms that are typical of any other patient. Race is not a factor with symptoms, and alcohol does not cause atypical clinical presentation.

13.3 Alteration in the membrane potential leads to electrical conduction abnormalities. Aerobic metabolism is the result of a lack of oxygen. AMI is not overexcitation, and the heart cells do not contain excess potassium that results in dysrhythmias.

14.2 ST elevation is classic for AMI as confirmed with an ECG. The other three are not observed in an AMI.

15.1 Leads II, III, and aVF are associated with the inferior aspect of the heart.

16.4 Troponin is a specific cardiac marker for diagnosing AMI. Myoglobin is often the cause of a urinary dysfunction. CK is a nonspecific test with multiple causes for increased values. LDH is an enzyme that is found in all body tissues.

17.1 Systolic dysfunction occurs during systole when the heart is pumping or emptying, which is the definition of systolic heart failure. The inability of the ventricle to relax during filling causes increased BP. Additionally, bradycardia is not systole, and two ventricles are found in the heart. Atrial fibrillation is not a dysrhythmia, and an increase in ventricular filling pressure with normal EF is not systole.

18.3 Left-sided heart failure causes fluid to back up into the lungs, which causes pulmonary resistance to blood that is trying to exit the right ventricle. Blood backs up into the right atrium and further backward into the systemic circulation, causing symptoms of right-sided heart failure. ARDS is a form of respiratory dysfunction that often leads to respiratory failure. JVD is a symptom of right-sided ventricular failure. Systemic hypertension is a sign of many diseases and conditions and is not a common cause of right-sided heart failure.

19.1 Systolic heart failure is defined as an EF of less than 40%; echocardiography can quantify the EF. Chest x-ray studies evaluate the lungs and size of the heart. An ECG evaluates electrical activity of the heart. A BNP test evaluates acute heart failure.

20.2 ACE inhibitors and beta blockers can help prevent compensatory mechanisms from causing the permanent cellular changes of ventricular remodeling. Digitalis and diuretics do not decrease ventricular remodeling but affect CO and edema. Natriuretic peptides and phosphodiesterase inhibitors are not intended to be used in chronic heart failure but in acute heart failure. NSAIDs are administered for pain and are used as antiinflammatory agents.

21.4 Natrecor does not increase the preload of the heart.

22.3 Primacor is a phosphodiesterase inhibitor that is used intravenously in acute exacerbations of heart failure to strengthen the contractions of the heart. Primacor does not decrease venous return or dilate arteriolar beds. Remodeling is accomplished by using ACE inhibitors and beta blockers.

23.1 Potassium is lost in the urine with diuresis. Low potassium can cause life-threatening dysrhythmias. Hyponatremia is most likely due to sweating or diaphoresis. The probable causes of hypocalcemia include renal dysfunction and malabsorption. Phosphorus balance and calcium balance are intertwined.

24.3 It appears that the current dose of diuretics is insufficient. If the fluid is allowed to accumulate, then shortness of breath occurs. The patient is also exhibiting signs of digitalis toxicity—nausea and dysrhythmias. No signs of coagulation dysfunction are exhibited.

NCLEX® CHAPTER 5 ANSWERS

1.2 Pressure-cycled ventilation delivers a breath until a preset pressure is reached. Tidal volumes vary. Volume-cycled ventilation delivers a breath until a preset tidal volume is reached. Airway pressures vary. Flow-cycled ventilation delivers a breath until a preset flow rate is reached. Time-cycled ventilation delivers a breath over a preset period.

2.3 Synchronized intermittent mandatory ventilation delivers a preset volume at a preset rate and allows the patient to take spontaneous breaths between ventilator breaths. Controlled ventilation delivers a preset volume or pressure at a preset rate but does not allow the patient to breathe spontaneously. ACV delivers a preset volume or pressure whenever the patient initiates a breath. The ventilator only gives a breath if the patient does not breathe within a certain time. Pressure-controlled ventilation delivers a preset amount of positive pressure during each breath. The amount of tidal volume is not constant.

3.4 The decrease in CO causes the BP to decrease. The addition of PEEP increases intrathoracic pressures, which causes a decrease in venous return, leading to a decrease in CO.

4.2 The normal inhalation/exhalation (I/E) ratio is 1:2.

5.1 High airway pressures cause over distention of the alveoli, causing them to rupture and leak air. Barotrauma occurs because of leakage of air from the alveoli and causes air to leak under the mediastinum. Pneumothorax is a complication of barotrauma.

6.2 The ventilation rate is gradually decreased during weaning to allow the patient to breathe more on his or her own. Tidal volume remains unchanged.

7.3 Moisture accumulation impedes the flow of oxygen, causing less to reach the patient; it also provides a medium for bacterial growth. Carbon dioxide is removed and flows out of the circuit before reaching any moisture accumulation.

8.1 Flow rate determines how fast the tidal volume is delivered. RR is the number of breaths per minute delivered to the patient. I/E ratio is the duration of inspiratory time to expiratory time for each breath. Tidal volume is the amount (volume) of oxygen delivered to the patient with each breath.

9.4 Atrial fibrillation is a risk factor for PE development because of the turbulent blood flow and the inability of the atrium to expel all of its blood. Blood that is not coagulated is a risk factor for PE. Anticoagulation is a treatment for the prevention of PE development. Bedrest and immobility are risk factors for PE. Early ambulation helps prevent PE. The use of pneumatic stockings decreases venous stasis and decreases the change of PE development.

10.1 When a PE occurs, alveoli distal to the occlusion are ventilated but not perfused. Carbon dioxide decreases and causes bronchoconstriction, which shunts blood to ventilated areas of the lungs. Bronchoconstriction increases pulmonary resistance when blood is shunted to more ventilated areas. Oxygenation actually decreases because there is less area for gas exchange to occur. Blood is shunted to unaffected areas that have perfusion and ventilation.

11.4 Shortness of breath is the most common clinical manifestation and usually has a sudden onset or occurs on exertion. Chest pain with PE occurs on inspiration with a deep breath. PE can cause hypotension related to increased pulmonary pressures, leading to a decrease in CO. Wheezing does not occur with PE development.

12.3 The therapeutic range is 1.5 to 2.0 times normal.

13.2 ABG results show respiratory alkalosis from a low pCO_2 level.

14.3 Pulmonary angiography is the most definitive test for the diagnosis of PE. V/Q scans are rarely diagnostic for PE; echocardiography cannot diagnose PE, but it can rule out other diagnoses. Spiral CT scanning is the most common approach for diagnosis but not the most definite.

15.2 Urokinase is a thrombolytic therapy agent that can be used for major PE. Thrombolytic therapy may be used for patients with a major PE. Heparin therapy is initiated within 24 hours after thrombolytic therapy is initiated. Coumadin is used after heparin therapy at therapeutic levels to prevent further PE development. Protamine is the reversal agent for heparin therapy.

16.1 Inferior vena cava is the most accessible placement location to prevent any potential thrombi from reaching the lungs. Placement in the iliac artery leaves too much distance from the lungs for thrombi to form and travel to the lungs. The superior vena cava does not prevent thrombi from traveling from the lower parts of the body, where most thrombolytic thrombi develop. The pulmonary artery is not accessible to the placement of an umbrella filter.

17.2 Hyperventilation develops in response to acidosis and increasing hypoxia. Hypoxia related to ARDS causes acidosis and pulmonary vasoconstriction.

18.1 Despite increased supplemental oxygen, ABG results that reveal a low PaO_2 are defined as refractory hypoxia and are important in the diagnosis of ARDS. $PaCO_2$ levels initially decrease during hyperventilation. Oxygen concentration is not a factor in $PaCO_2$ levels.

19.3 IRV is the mode of ventilation that can be used in the treatment of ARDS, allowing alveoli to open and airway pressures to lower. Constant positive airway pressure (CPAP) allows alveoli to open, but it is not used as treatment for ARDS. PSV allows the patient to breathe easier by decreasing airway resistance, but it is not used as a treatment for ARDS. The goal of ventilator management in ARDS is to decrease the work of breathing for the patient until the underlying cause can be treated. ACV is used for patients with normal breathing who cannot achieve a desired tidal volume.

20.1 Dobutamine is a positive inotropic drug that increases contractility, thus increasing CO and BP for tissue perfusion. Neosynephrine is a vasoconstrictor that increases BP by increasing SVR. Nitroglycerine and Nipride are vasodilators that are used to decrease BP.

21.4 Corticosteroids decrease the permeability of the alveolocapillary (respiratory) membrane and prevent leakage of fluid into alveoli. The best benefits are seen when given several days after onset. Corticosteroids increase the risk of nosocomial infections by decreasing the immune response.

22.3 Confusion is an indicator of increasing hypoxia. Tachypnea is what occurs with the progression of respiratory distress. Tachycardia may develop in response to the increase in anxiety related to respiratory distress. Pale mucous membranes signify increased respiratory distress.

23.2 Increasing PCWP signifies an increase in the pulmonary pressures and may lead to right ventricular dysfunction. A decrease in CVP or PCWP readings may be significant if coupled with decreasing BP and the need for volume administration; however, a decreasing CVP or PCWP alone should not alert you to call the physician. Increased CO does not signify problems unless a decrease in vascular resistance results in a low BP.

24.4 Symptoms of respiratory distress usually begin to appear 24 to 48 hours after insult or injury to the lungs.

NCLEX® CHAPTER 6 ANSWERS

1.4 Initially, the patient's airway, breathing, and circulation are the priorities, followed by seizure assessment and treatment.

2.1 Flumazenil is a benzodiazepine antagonist that reverses the effects of diazepam. It should be administered if respiratory distress is noted, secondary to an overdose of diazepam (valium). Although Phenobarbital can effectively control seizure activity, the nurse must be aware of the amount of medication that has already been given because this medication may further suppress respiration. Naloxone is used to reverse the effects of opioids. Phenytoin does not reverse the effects of benzodiazepines.

3.4 Airway, breathing, and then circulation are the priorities in patient care. Padding the bed's siderails is a controversial nursing intervention because of the social stigma associated with seizures. Ensuring that the patient is never alone is not necessary. Although a padded tongue blade is used before a seizure starts, it is not a priority for patient care.

4.2 An EEG requires a clean, oil-free surface for recording the electrical activity of the brain. The nurse must wash the patient's hair so that it is clean and oil free. The patient should not be sedated, and dilantin is often withheld to ensure that maximal seizure activity is recorded. Sometimes the patient is kept awake for 24 but not for 48 hours.

5.1 Protecting the head from trauma and decreasing the risk of aspiration are the priorities for patient safety. Forcing something into his or her mouth after the seizure has begun is also likely to cause injury; a piece of tooth may break off and be aspirated. Restraints and holding the patient down may cause any injury that may occur to become more serious.

6.4 Anticonvulsant medications administered as scheduled help prevent further seizures. Bedrest and closing the door are not interventions that help minimize the risk of seizures. Sedation is also not an intervention that helps minimize the risk of seizures.

7.1 A patient is often drowsy after a seizure. Despite this drowsiness, the patient is usually able to move and speak. Hypotension is not a frequent problem after a seizure. The patient may not remember what, if anything, triggered the seizure.

8.3 A common side effect of long-term phenytoin (Dilantin) therapy is an over growth of gingival tissues; problems may be minimized with good oral hygiene. Dilantin should always be taken with meals to decrease GI upset; however, diarrhea is not a frequent side effect. Hyperactivity is not a common early side effect; rather, drowsiness may occur but may decrease with time.

9.1 With the photosensitivity and irritability exhibited in meningitis, the environment should be as controlled and calm as possible.

10.3 Cool compresses or ice bags to the forehead help relieve febrile delirium. Warmth may increase the fever, and restraints often cause injury to the patient. Fluid intake does not relieve the fever, although it may help prevent dehydration.

11.2 In acute bacterial meningitis, the CSF analysis reveals increased protein (100 to 500 mg/dl); normally CSF protein is between 15 and 45 mg/dl. Glucose is usually decreased (40 mg/dl); normally CSF contains glucose levels between 60 and 80 mg/dl. The CSF will reveal an increase in WBCs (1000 to 2000 mm^3 or more); normally, CSF WBCs is between 0 and 5 mm^3. The CSF is also cloudy; normally, specific gravity of CSF is 1.007.

12.4 Pulmonary embolus is not a complication of fulminating meningococcal meningitis. Waterhouse-Friderichsen syndrome, DIC, and encephalitis are all complications associated with fulminating meningococcal meningitis.

13.3 Trousseau's sign is carpopedal spasms when an arm tourniquet is inflated; it is present in hypocalcemia. Nuchal rigidity and headache are both classic signs of meningeal irritation. Kernig's sign is an indication of meningitis; it is elicited with the patient supine. The examiner flexes the patient's hip and knee and then straightens the knee. Pain or resistance on knee straightening (Kernig's sign) suggests meningeal irritation.

14.2 Persistent neurologic deficits may occur with meningitis. If the VIII cranial nerve is involved, deafness may result. Cerebral edema occurs rather than dehydration. Hyperthermia, not hypothermia, may result. Hypervigilance is a sign found in selected psychiatric disorders.

15.3 The child needs to be comforted after an invasive procedure by individuals he or she trusts. Little discomfort is experienced at the insertion site after a lumbar puncture. Narcotics are not the drugs of choice because they hinder the assessment of neurologic status. A young child does not need to lay flat for any length of time after a lumbar puncture; it is difficult to persuade a 4 year old to lay fat for any period. Applying a small bandage after applying pressure for a short time is usually sufficient to stop any leaking and to prevent infection of the site.

16.1 Viral meningitis is not expressed with a positive Kernig's sign. Patients with a mild case of meningitis, and particularly with viral meningitis, may exhibit few symptoms, including muscle aches and pains, severe headache, and abdominal and chest pain.

17.4 Because of the presence of ipsilateral loss of motor function with contralateral loss of pain and temperature sensations, the nurse can assume that laceration or hemisection of the spinal cord has occurred in this patient. The corticospinal (motor) tracts cross at the level of the medulla. Thus the decussation results in left-sided motor deficits. However, the spinothalamic (sensory) tracts cross at the level of entry into the spinal cord. Trauma to the left side of the spinal cord results in right-sided sensory deficits. Posterior spinal cord injury associated with hyperextension are rare and generally occur with hyperextension. Damage affects the posterior horns of the spinal cord; proprioception and light touch are impaired bilaterally, but motor function remains intact bilaterally. Upper extremity motor function is lost with an accompanying but less significant loss of lower extremity motor function. Some patients do not experience a loss of lower extremity motor function. Varying degrees of sensory function remain intact. Motor function, pain, and temperature sensations are lost with anterior spinal cord syndrome associated with dislocation.

18.2 When a patient suffers a spinal cord injury, it is important to determine the level of injury to anticipate probable complications. Loss of speech is more likely to occur with head injury than with spinal injury. Loss of perspiration and loss of sensation below the level of the injury and the presence of spontaneous respirations are vital considerations for the nurse when assessing spinal cord injury.

19.2 Bradycardia, not tachycardia, is a symptom of autonomic dysreflexia. Severe headache is a typical symptom of autonomic dysreflexia from the increased BP. Rapidly increasing BP is a cardinal symptom of autonomic dysreflexia. Profuse sweating is another typical symptom of autonomic dysreflexia.

20.1 If the patient is prone, pressure on the penis or catheter is likely, which leads to dysreflexia. All other responses are appropriate ways to prevent autonomic dysreflexia.

21.4 Supporting the back and body as an immovable whole is the principle of logrolling. If the spine has been injured, it is important to move the patient as a single unit.

22.4 Immobilization of the cervical spine is the priority of care to avoid causing more damage to the spine. All other responses are important but not the priority of nursing care.

23.4 Ineffective airway clearance as a result of a high cervical spinal cord injury is the priority of care for Jack. Remember the ABCs.

24.3 An assessment of leg strength, motion, position sense, and sensation, as well as checking the dressing, are essential in the assessment of a lumbar injury and postsurgical intervention. Assessing arm strength and arm sensation are appropriate steps for the patient who has undergone cervical neck surgery. Checking for bladder distention is appropriate for the patient with a lumbar injury, but assessment of the pupils and cranial nerves II, III, IV, and VI are appropriate for the patient who has undergone a craniotomy.

NCLEX® CHAPTER 7 ANSWERS

1.1 Complications of peptic ulcer disease include hemorrhagic shock, perforation, and obstruction. Perforation occurs when an erosion of all the layers of the GI wall occur and the contents of the GI tract spill into the peritoneum. The result is an inflammatory process known as peritonitis. Sudden onset of abdominal pain; a rigid, boardlike abdomen; nausea and vomiting; fever; tachycardia; hypotension; and paralytic ileus can result. No signs of hemorrhage or bleeding are observed to indicate hemorrhagic shock. An obstruction has no bowel sounds.

2.4 Patients with *Heliobacter pylori* infection are treated with antibiotics. Antibiotics are used in combination to minimize the potential for bacterial resistance. Antacids, mucosal protectant agents, and histamine 2–receptor antagonists are used in the pharmacologic management of peptic ulcer disease. However, when *H. pylori* is identified as the cause of the ulcer, antibiotics are the most appropriate therapy.

3.1 Endoscopy is the diagnostic tool that provides direct visualization of the GI tract and bleeding site. Radiographic studies such as barium enemas do not allow for direct visualization of the GI tract. Angiography and radionuclide scanning are used to identify the site of a bleeding vessel.

4.4 Metabolic alkalosis results from the loss of hydrogen ions when vomiting. Metabolic acidosis, respiratory acidosis, and respiratory alkalosis are not associated with vomiting and the loss of hydrogen ions.

5.3 Hematemesis is bright red, bloody vomitus or vomitus with a coffee-ground appearance. Hematochezia is a bright red or maroon blood passed via the rectum. Occult blood can be found in gastric contents or stool and is not identifiable on visual examination. Melena is black, tarry stool passed via the rectum.

6.2 When a patient is recovering from a GI bleeding episode, the diet is prescribed as tolerated. No specific diet prescriptions are recommended for patients who are recovering from GI bleeding. The diet is geared to the treatment of the underlying cause of the bleeding.

7.4 The symptoms of tachycardia—decrease in urine output to less than 30 ml/hr, skin cool to the touch, confusion, and pallor—are indicative of hemorrhagic shock. Hemorrhagic shock is characterized by a decrease in preload to the heart (as a result of massive blood loss) and an associated reduction in CO. Hemorrhagic shock results in the inability of the body to meet cellular needs. The body responds by increasing the HR (tachycardia), shunting blood to the cerebral and cardiovascular systems (and away from the integumentary system), cooling the skin, producing a pallor to the skin, and decreasing urine output. Cardiogenic shock is caused by direct pump failure, neurogenic shock is paralysis and bradycardia, and distributive shock occurs with sympathetic stimulation causing vasodilation.

8.3 Parietal cells are found in the stomach and are responsible for the production of gastric acid. Receptors on the parietal cells respond to three stimuli that promote hydrochloric acid secretion: (1) acetylcholine, (2) histamine, and (3) gastrin. Chief cells release pepsinogen, which is then converted to pepsin in the presence of hydrochloric acid. G cells secrete gastrin, which is a stimulus for hydrochloric acid release. Mucosal cells secrete mucus, which is a defensive factor of the stomach.

9.2 No bowel sounds are heard directly over the intestinal obstruction. The site proximal to the obstruction may have bowel sounds. A 45-degree angle 2 inches from the midclavicular line is not anatomically over the intestines; neither are the inguinal lymph nodes.

10.4 An increased hematocrit indicates dehydration because hematocrit is based on total blood volume. Serum magnesium measures metabolic activity and renal function. BUN measures renal function. Platelets measure clotting ability.

11.3 A CT scan of the abdomen differentiates cause and location of bowel obstructions. X-ray, Doppler, and gastroscopic studies reveal general location and gastric area only.

12.2 The large bowel is anatomically able to accept a rectal tube. The small bowel, appendix, and stomach are too far from the rectum.

13.2 Intake and output (I&O) is essential to monitoring hypovolemia. Calcium does not measure volume. Serum WBC count measures infection-fighting ability. Bowel sound auscultation does not assess hypovolemia but rather bowel activity.

14.4 A large nonmovable tumor needs to be surgically treated to avoid complete obstruction or bowel necrosis. Hemoptysis (blood in the sputum) and bradycardia (cardiac-related) are not indications for surgical treatment of bowel obstruction. Intermittent abdominal pain may be referred from another area and is not a sign of a complete obstruction because of the intermittent nature of the pain.

15.3 Auscultate the abdomen before palpation or percussion to avoid altering the bowel sounds. Percussion can cause sounds and palpation can cause abdominal distress, making auscultation inaccurate. Digital rectal examination is not appropriate for abdominal problems.

16.4 Oral care is best because giving fluids or increasing saliva production are contraindicated. Ice and the liquid produced by candy and a liquid diet increases obstructive symptoms.

17.2 Endocrine cells, found in the islets of Langherhan, produce several hormones that pass directly into the bloodstream. Exocrine secretions are produced by the acini cells, which are then received by the duodenum. The liver drains bile into the bowel.

18.2 Demerol does not cause spasm of the sphincter of Oddi. Dilaudid increases bile obstruction, and Sublimaze is not a drug of choice for pancreatic pain. Morphine causes spasm of the sphincter of Oddi, which increases bile obstruction.

19.2 The main symptom is found in one of four patients with acute pancreatitis. Nausea and vomiting are specific to many GI disorders. Normal levels of lipase and amylase serum appear in chronic cases of pancreatitis; consequently, elevated lipase and amylase serum levels are not specific for diagnosis. Hypocalcemia and hypercalcemia are found in chronic pancreatitis when islets of Langerhans cells malfunction and sugar levels are unable to be maintained.

20.1 Calcium gluconate combats deficiency of calcium found in cases of shock. Atropine is an anticholinergic. Cotazym is used to replace enzymes in cases of pancreatic insufficiency, and Tagamet is used to decrease acid production.

21.2 Chronic pancreatitis does not resolve itself and causes permanent damage to the gland. The sudden onset of symptoms resulting in acute pancreatitis may last for a short time; if promptly treated, the patient will have a full recovery. Pseudocysts may spontaneously resolve. Pancreatic sufficiency is one of several complications of chronic pancreatitis.

22.3 Contrast-enhanced CT provides the best image of the pancreas and surrounding structures and may reveal fluid accumulation and inflammation of the gland. Plain radiographic films are only helpful in revealing gallstones and areas of calcification. ERCP is indicated when biliary pancreatitis is suspected. Ultrasound studies are used in suspected cases of biliary causes.

23.4 As the pancreas digests itself, bleeding results and the patient has the potential to exhibit signs and symptoms of hypovolemic shock. Nutrition at a level that is less than the body requires occurs as a result of enzymatic dysfunction. No hypovolemia occurs as a result of hemorrhage. No peripheral tissue perfusion is found in the patient with pancreatitis.

24.2 Diabetes develops when the islets of Langerhans are no longer able to produce hormones necessary to maintain proper sugar levels. Shock occurs when circulating blood volume is low. Because of a susceptibility of infection as a result of pancreatic necrosis, secondary infection may appear after the acute attack subsides. The formation of fibrous tissues that replaces healthy acini tissue refers to the formation of pseudocyst structures.

25.2 The nurse monitors the patient for a decrease in the level of consciousness. Hepatic encephalopathy is thought to be caused by the inability of the liver to convert ammonia to urea. When the liver is unable to perform the conversion, the levels of ammonia build. The elevated ammonia levels have a neurotoxic effect on the CNS and can result in symptoms ranging from confusion to coma. A decrease in urine output can be associated with the liver's ability to inactivate aldosterone and ADH and hepatorenal syndrome. Upper GI bleeding is associated with esophageal varices. Shortness of breath can be a symptom of increased pressure on the diaphragm associated with ascites.

26.1 Hepatorenal syndrome is caused by a decrease in renal blood flow, which results in a decreased glomerular filtration rate and an increased level of aldosterone. The accumulation of unmetabolized wastes results from a decrease in glomerular filtration rates but is not the cause of hepatorenal syndrome. The kidneys and ureters are retroperitoneal organs.

27.4 Diseases that can lead to liver failure are hepatitis and biliary atresia. Hepatitis is an inflammation of the liver cells caused by a viral or bacterial infection or toxic substance. Biliary atresia is the congenital absence or underdevelopment of one or more of the biliary structures. Glomerulonephritis, renal carcinoma, abdominal aortic aneurysm, arteriosclerosis, GI bleeding, and bowel obstruction are not commonly causative diagnoses associated with liver failure.

28.2 Nitrates can be used to reduce portal pressures in patients with portal hypertension. Nitrates act primarily in veins and promote smooth muscle vasodilation. Nitrates have no effect on the development of hepatic encephalopathy, which is caused by the inability of the liver to convert ammonia to urea. Nitrates also do not promote the excretion of ascitic fluids that are found outside the vascular space.

29.3 Lactulose creates an acidic environment in the bowel that prevents ammonia from leaving the colon and entering the bloodstream. It also has a laxative effect and eliminates ammonia from the GI tract. An expected outcome associated with the administration of lactulose in a patient with hepatic encephalopathy is a decrease in serum ammonia levels and a resulting improvement in the patient's hepatic encephalopathy. Creatinine is a nonprotein endproduct of skeletal muscle metabolism and is used in monitoring renal function. Albumin is a plasma protein and responsible for maintaining plasma oncotic pressures and is a contributing factor in the development of ascites. Bilirubin is a product of hemoglobin breakdown, and elevated levels are associated with jaundice.

30.1 Hypoalbuminemia, jaundice, loss of appetite, and coagulopathies are symptoms associated with liver failure. The liver's functions include the metabolism of carbohydrates, fat and proteins, the elimination of bilirubin, and the production of clotting factors. When the liver is unable to metabolize the plasma protein albumin, hypoalbuminemia results. No means exist for creating energy stores, which results in malnutrition. Bilirubin stains the tissues and causes the yellowish discoloration of the skin, mucous membranes, and sclera, which is known as jaundice. An increased bilirubin level (hyperbilirubinemia) is the cause of jaundice. Coagulopathies develop when the liver is unable to produce the clotting factors II, V, VII, VIII , IX, and X.

31.1 Ascites is the accumulation of fluid in the peritoneal cavity. Significant accumulations of ascitic fluids in the peritoneal cavity can cause abdominal organ compression and discomfort, respiratory compromise as a result of pressure on the diaphragm, and impaired skin integrity. In severe ascites, the patient is placed in a Fowler's position to promote ventilation and to relieve pressure on the diaphragm. The other positions do not relieve the pressure caused by the ascitic fluid.

32.2 Clotting factors are not synthesized by a failing liver. Patients with liver failure can exhibit a range of symptoms from petechiae, ecchymosis, bleeding from the oral mucosa, and nosebleeds to massive hemorrhaging. The stool and gastric contents should be monitored for evidence of bleeding. Urine output, assessment for changes in level of consciousness and the elimination of hepatotoxins are all interventions associated with the care of a patient with liver failure but are not specifically related to the problem of coagulopathies.

NCLEX® CHAPTER 8 ANSWERS

1.1 Urinary output is dependent on glomerular filtration rate (GFR). The GFR decreases, which causes a decrease in urinary output. Uremic levels are not high enough to produce ATN. Chills and fever should not be present unless the patient has an infection or is septic. Cardiac friction rub has nothing to do with ATN.

2.2 Heart failure is ischemic in nature and is considered prerenal; it contributes to decreased blood flow to the kidney. Aminoglycosides and iodinated contrast dyes are endogenous nephrotoxins and affect the inside (intrarenal) of the kidney. BPG is considered postrenal in nature.

3.3 Azotemia is the presence of nitrogenous waste products (creatinine and nitrogen) in the blood.

4.2 Urine production increases during polyuria; however, BUN and creatinine continue to remain elevated as a result of increased GFR.

5.4 A 75-year-old patient with BPH is at greatest risk for developing postrenal failure because of the problem with the urine flow after it leaves the kidney. A 29-year-old woman who smokes is not at risk for developing postrenal failure. Although the 15-year-old adolescent with diabetes may have cellular membrane changes that could contribute to postrenal failure later in life, he is not the patient most at risk in this group. Age may certainly be a factor with the 10 year old; however, this patient is young and a problem with their postrenal function should not develop.

6.2 The amount of insensible losses that the nurse should include is 500 to 800 ml.

7.2 An increased potassium can be attributed to irritability of the heart and should be monitored closely. Although sodium, chloride, and phosphorus are important electrolytes, they are not the most important for heart conduction (dysrhythmias) problems.

8.4 Negative JVD is found in a status of fluid volume deficit. The others are found in fluid volume excess.

9.3 A bruit and thrill indicate adequate blood flow through a fistula. Redness is not an expected finding, and no skin discoloration at the site should be found. A loss of pulse is indicative of circulatory compromise and needs to be reported to the physician immediately.

10.1 The patient should have a thorough understanding of dialysis and its implications and should be taught to weigh him or herself daily. The patient is not expected to access a catheter, fistula, or graft. The question is about dialysis, not about specific medications.

11.4 The patient should be taught to avoid the use of tight or restrictive clothing around the affected arm. A bruit is heard, not felt, and a thrill is felt, not heard. Care must be taken to never apply pressure to the site. The patient should never sleep on the affected arm.

12.1 Azotemia refers to elevated serum BUN and creatinine levels. Itching caused by uremic frost is pruritus, and an increase in creatinine clearance levels indicates improved renal function. A decrease in erythropoietin secretion leads to anemia.

13.2 The progression of renal disease is variable but can slow with an adherence to prescribed diet and fluid restrictions. Dialysis and a kidney transplant are not indicated for renal insufficiency. Telling the patient, "Don't worry about dialysis; you'll probably never need it!" is an inaccurate and a patronizing statement.

14.3 An increase in urinary frequency is not a sign of renal failure and indicates a need for further patient teaching. Anorexia, fatigue, and fluid retention are all signs of renal failure.

15.2 African-American men with hypertension are among the highest group for developing renal disease. Osteoporosis is not a risk factor for renal disease. Age may contribute to the development of renal disease but not to the extent of hypertension. Obesity is a risk factor for hypertension but not necessarily renal disease. Cerebral palsy is not a risk for renal disease.

16.1 The use of acetaminophen is contraindicated in the patient with renal disease. Epogen is commonly used to treat anemia; calcium carbonate is commonly used to treat hypocalcemia; and Phos-Lo is commonly used to treat hyperphosphatemia in the patient with end-stage renal disease (ESRD).

17.2 Mean arterial pressure must be at least 60 mm Hg for CRRT to be effective.

18.3 Trisodium citrate may be used to prevent clot formation in the extracorporeal circuit. Vitamin K is an antagonist of Coumadin. Coumadin, although an anticoagulant, is not indicated to prevent clot formation during CRRT. Protamine sulfate is an antagonist of heparin.

19.4 Calculating amount of fluid replacement based on hourly and cumulative intake and output and fluid balance goals are nursing functions. Selection of the composition of dialysate is made by the physician, as are the fluid balance goals. Electrolyte levels should be monitored every 4 to 6 hours.

20.4 CRRT provides better azotemic and uremic control than ischemic heart disease (IHD) and can be used in unstable patients; it decreases fluid volume and improves electrolyte balance.

21.1 Once pressure stabilizes, flow rate is gradually increased. Aggressive fluid replacement and the use of vasopressors are typically not indicated. CRRT typically does not need to be discontinued.

22.1 An in-line fluid warmer helps control hypothermia. The complete circuit, including the access site, must remain visible. Do not cover the access site with a blanket or pajamas. The use of warm compresses at the vascular access site is not appropriate.

23.4 The blue line is the venous or return line. The red line is the arterial or outflow line. No yellow or green lines exist.

24.3 CRRT should only be performed in a critical care setting.

NCLEX® CHAPTER *9* ANSWERS

1.4 DKA occurs in patients with type I diabetes who lack any production of endogenous insulin. Lack of endogenous insulin leads to hyperglycemia; if left untreated, it can lead to DKA, which results in metabolic acidosis. Hypotension is not a direct result of a lack of endogenous insulin. HHNK coma is commonly associated with type II diabetes, in which there is a relative but not total lack of insulin.

2.2 HHNK coma is usually accompanied by blood glucose levels greater than 1000 mg/dl and severe dehydration that is the result of hyperosmolarity and osmotic diuresis. Causes of metabolic alkalosis include loop diuretics, antacids, hypokalemia, blood products, lactate administration, nasogastric suction, and H2-blockers. DKA is commonly associated with blood glucose levels greater than 250 mg/dl but usually less than 1000 mg/dl, as well as dehydration, hyperosmolarity, and acidosis. Adrenal insufficiency from glucocorticoid insufficiency results in fever, nausea and vomiting, abdominal pain, hypotension, and altered mental status. Adrenal insufficiency caused by mineralocorticoid insufficiency results in hyponatremia and hypokalemia.

3.2 Type I diabetic patients who are hyperglycemic become dehydrated because of an osmotic diuresis from hyperosmolarity. Administration of IV fluids helps rehydrate the patient and decreases blood glucose levels. Administration of insulin allows the cells to use the available glucose, avoiding the breakdown of fats and ketosis. Monitoring blood glucose levels and replacing electrolytes and fluids are important, but if serum glucose levels are elevated, then they should be treated with a form of rapid-acting insulin, and the patient should be rehydrated. Administration of glucose is avoided in patients with elevated serum glucose levels. In the patient with DKA on an insulin drip, glucose can be added when the serum glucose level approximates 150 to 300 mg/dl.

4.4 The primary cause of dehydration in patients with DKA and HHNK is osmotic diuresis. Because the serum is hyperosmolar, water is pulled from the cells into the serum and then eliminated through the kidneys as urine. Normal serum levels are 136 to 145 mEq/L. Although this value represents hyponatremia, it is not the primary cause of this patient's dehydration. This patient is hyperthermic. Often patients with DKA have an underlying infection that may be responsible for the temperature elevation. Ketosis results from the formation of ketone bodies with the breakdown of fats for fuel. This promotes acidosis.

5.2   The administration of IV fluids based on estimated fluid volume deficit rehydrates the patient and alone decreases serum glucose levels. Rapid decrease of serum glucose levels can cause insulin shock. Restoring serum potassium to normal is essential in the treatment of the patient in a diabetic crisis, but it is not the initial primary goal. Identifying the precipitating problem is also essential in a patient with HHNK. Often patients have underlying infections as a precipitating cause; however, this, again, is not the initial treatment for this patient.

6.4   The brain has a high requirement for glucose for metabolism. Prolonged hypoglycemia can cause the death of brain cells and result in irreversible brain damage. Insulin results in a decrease of serum glucose levels by allowing glucose to enter the cells. The primary danger of too much insulin is low serum glucose levels and irreversible brain damage. Hyperglycemia results in osmotic diuresis, dehydration, and hypovolemia. Hypoglycemia causes poor concentration, irritability, tremors, and coma.

7.4   Insulin is a hormone released from the pancreas by beta cells. It allows glucose to enter the cells for metabolic fuel. Somatostatin is secreted by the delta cells in the pancreas; it inhibits growth hormone, thyroid-stimulating hormone (TSH), insulin, glucagons, and other GI hormones. Glucagon helps maintain normal blood sugar levels through the breakdown of glycogen and the formation of glycogen from fats and proteins. It is released by alpha cells. Gastrin is synthesized and released by the pyloric gland mucosa in the antrum of the stomach. Gastrin decreases the pH of gastric juice and assists in the digestion of food.

8.1   Hypoglycemia causes activation of the sympathetic nervous system. Signs and symptoms of hypoglycemia include irritability, nervousness, tachycardia, palpitations, pallor, diaphoresis, fatigue, headache, hunger and general weakness. Causes of seizures include prior seizure disorder exacerbated by drugs, sleep deprivation or fever, metabolic abnormalities, drug toxicity, focal brain disease (encephalitis, meningitis), and head injury or trauma. Patients with DKA often complain of abdominal pain. Patients with hypoglycemia often have normal serum sodium levels.

9.2   Insulin is released form the pancreas by the beta cells. The alpha cells produce glucagon; the delta cells secrete somatostatin; and the other pancreatic cells are responsible for the release of enzymes used in digestion.

10.4   In critically ill patients, stress causes the glucoregulatory hormones, such as cortisol and epinephrine, to be released, thereby promoting hyperglycemia. In addition, administration of hyperalimentation, enteral feedings, and corticosteroids can cause an increase in serum glucose levels. If not closely monitored, these levels, in addition to the stress response, will cause hyperglycemia.

11.3   Initially, isotonic (not hypotonic) fluids (0.9% NS) are used as replacement fluids in patients with DKA and HHNK. Once the patient's BP stabilizes, IV fluids may be changed to hypotonic solutions. Adding hypertonic dextrose solutions further promotes the hyperosmolar state. Hypertonic fluids increase hyperosmolarity.

12.2   Inappropriate secretion of ADH causes increased permeability of the distal tubule of the kidney to water. Extracellular water levels rise, diluting serum sodium. Small increases in BP cause sodium to be lost in the urine through pressure natriuresis, and urine-specific gravity is elevated.

13.2   ADH hormone causes water reabsorption and decreases urine volume. ADH secretion is in response to increased osmolarity and increases the permeability of distal tubules of the kidney to water.

14.1   Inappropriate secretion of ADH causes increased permeability of the distal tubule of the kidney to water. Extracellular water levels rise, diluting serum sodium. Urine output is diminished. Serum hypoosmolality results from water retention. Small increases in BP as a result of extracellular water expansion cause sodium to be lost in the urine through pressure natriuresis. Urine hyperosmolality is the result.

15.3   Confusion is associated with sodium levels below 115 mEq/L. Hyponatremia is a clinical manifestation of SIADH. The potassium level is normal in patients with SIADH. Although fluid intake and output is monitored in patients with SIADH, this is not the most appropriate answer.

16.4   The most common malignancy associated with SIADH is small-cell lung cancer. Diagnostic evaluation includes urine hyperosmolarity and serum hyponatremia. Muscle cramps are associated with hyponatremia. Although CNS injury and certain medications including diuretics can cause SIADH, this is not the best answer. Transient SIADH can result from surgery, but hyponatremia is a clinical manifestation. During pregnancy, women may develop hyponatremia (as low as 130 mEq/L) because of the release of the hormone, relaxin. This is a normal change.

17.1 Hyponatremia is a clinical manifestation of SIADH and can be exhibited as confusion in patients with severely low serum levels. Potassium levels and pH are normal in patients with SIADH. Water intoxication is also associated with SIADH.

18.4 Fluid restriction is a treatment of choice in SIADH because water intoxication and dilutional hyponatremia are manifestations of SIADH. "The physician has prescribed it" is not an appropriate answer. Fluid, not sodium restriction, is the treatment of choice. Potassium levels are normal in patients with SIADH.

19.1 The normal adult values of serum sodium are 136 to 145 mEq/L. Low serum sodium levels characterize hyponatremia. Although hyponatremia can cause CNS changes, many other diseases can also cause these symptoms.

20.4 ADH is deficient in patients with DI. Testosterone, estrogen, and insulin (secreted from the pancreas) have nothing to do with DI.

21.2 Polyuria is excess urination as a result of insufficient ADH. Tachycardia develops as a result of the loss in volume from polyuria. Mucous membranes are dry, and the patient becomes dehydrated. The patient has polydipsia, not polyphagia.

22.1 Renal disease is a common cause of DI. Syphilis, hypotension, and carotid stenosis have nothing to do with DI.

23.4 Hypotension and tachycardia indicate DI. Usually the patient becomes hypotensive as a result of the loss of fluid. The patient is usually tachycardic, and temperature may be affected. RR may vary, depending on the acid-base balance.

24.2 Loss of water in polyuria results in constipation. The patient becomes dehydrated; no extra fluid is available. Hemorrhage and ulcerative colitis do not relate to polyuria and the GI tract in the patient with DI.

25.3 Urinary osmolity is lower in DI because of polyuria. Sodium and potassium are important serum findings. Casts is a finding on urinalysis and is not related to DI.

26.4 Vasopressin is the exogenous hormone supplement of choice to replace ADH in patients with DI. Lasix further increases urine output, thus making the situation worse. Nipride vasodilates and makes the hypotension worse because the patient is already dealing with a fluid deficit. Mannitol is an osmotic diuretic and further increases urine output, also causing the situation to worsen.

27.3 Fluid volume status is directly associated with ADH, and neurologic status changes are clinically indicative of DI. The cardiac rate is important to assess in DI, but the patient's psychologic status is not considered crucial at this time. Airway is always an important assessment point, but in DI the GI loss is not crucial. Pain and pulmonary status are important assessment areas; however, when suspecting DI, these assessment points are also not crucial.

28.3 Hyponatremia is characteristic of CSW. Potassium is not a component of CSW. Sodium is an important component to assess CSW; however, CSW is characterized by low sodium (hyponatremia).

29.2 Hypovolemia is characteristic of CSW; the patient has polyuria.

30.3 SIADH shows weight gain as a result of large amounts of water being reabsorbed. CSW and DI cause a decrease in weight as a result of fluid loss. Increased ICP does not have any relevance to weight gain or loss.

31.4 CSW is a failure of the CNS to regulate sodium. Hypotension is a symptom of CSW. SIADH and DI are directly related to ADH and respond through the renal system.

32.2 IV fluid replacement is most accurate. Nasogastric tube replacement of sodium is not usually performed and tends to be inaccurate. Replacement of fluid through a PEG tube in the stomach is also a method that is not usually used; it tends to be inaccurate and takes longer. An enema is not relevant in this situation.

33.1 NS or hypotonic saline is used for fluid replacement. $D_{10}W$ is too hypertonic and does not replace the much-needed sodium. LR is isotonic; although it contains some sodium, the amount is small. $D5_{1/2}NS$ with 40 mg KCl does not contain the appropriate amount of sodium required in this case.

34.1 Volume replacement should equal volume output.

35.2 Rapid correction leads to problems in the pons of the brain. Pontine myelinolysis or loss of myelin on the nerve fibers can occur if hyponatremia is corrected too rapidly.

NCLEX® CHAPTER *10* ANSWERS

1.2 This patient is older and has diabetes that places her at risk because of the chronic nature of the disease. Although the 46-year-old man had abdominal surgery for an infectious process, he has no predisposing factors that place him at higher risk for sepsis. The 66-year-old woman also has no predisposing factors that place her at risk for sepsis. Although the 5-year-old girl is a young patient with an infection, she is not as much at risk as the older patient with a chronic illness.

2.1 Abdominal rigidity is a sign of peritoneal inflammation. The increased temperature is an indicator of infection and the decreased BP is a sign of decreasing SVR. The increased pulse and RR are early signs of sepsis. Although the 35-year-old woman has an elevated temperature, the rest of her vital signs are stable. The infant has only one instance of vomiting and has normal vital signs with no indication of infection. The teenager's vital signs are within normal limits; although her back pain and hematuria may be indicative of a urinary tract infection, no evidence of sepsis exists.

3.3 Mental clouding is an early symptom of sepsis because of the hyperdynamic state and increased oxygen demand. Decreased BP with narrowed pulse pressure occurs in late sepsis. Although rales associated with pneumonia may be heard, they are not a typical symptom of sepsis. Respiratory acidosis may occur if sepsis develops into septic shock, but it is not the earliest sign and symptom of the listed choices.

4.2 The priority is obtaining cultures to identify properly the offending organism. Anticipate treatment with broad-spectrum antibiotics but not until the cultures are obtained. Starting antibiotics before obtaining cultures negates the cultures. Fluid resuscitation is a priority if the patient exhibits signs of septic shock, not sepsis. Unless respiratory distress occurs, mechanical ventilation is not needed.

5.4 Although a transient increase in urine output may occur in the early stages of sepsis related to the hyperdynamic state, further progression of the disease results in suppression of cardiac function and thus decreased renal perfusion. The septic process is initiated by the launch of immune mediators that are part of the inflammatory reaction. This process starts a chain of events that are controlled by numerous feedback mechanisms. Eventually the immune system is overwhelmed, and the process actually harms the body. Stimulation of the inflammatory response leads to the formation of biochemical mediators that stimulate coagulation. This stimulation leads to microscopic emboli and end-organ damage.

6.1 The use of invasive hemodynamic monitoring allows for a port of entry for organisms. This is especially concerning because of the antibiotic-resistant strains that exist in the hospital (i.e., nosocomial infections). By sending a patient home for minor procedures, they are less likely to be exposed to microorganisms that normally exist in the hospital setting. In addition, a patient at home is less likely to have an indwelling device that provides a port of entry for microorganisms. Handwashing decreases the likelihood of microorganism transmission. The use of appropriate antibiotics eliminate possible sepsis-causing microorganisms.

7.3 Antibiotics are used to eradicate the offending microorganism. Although the hypovolemia associated with advancing sepsis has occurred, the hypovolemia is disruptive and not related to blood loss; therefore you do not anticipate a blood transfusion. Vasopressors may be used if the SVR causes profound hypotension, but it is used in later stages of shock. Respiratory failure may occur in advanced septic shock and may be needed if respiratory alkalosis occurs; however, treatment for acute sepsis depends on identifying and treating the offending organism with the appropriate antibiotics. Intubation is only necessary if the patient's status declines.

8.1 Presence of fever, tachycardia, tachypnea, and overwhelming infection are characteristics of sepsis. Hypotension and respiratory acidosis are characteristics of advancing septic shock. Identification of an infective microorganism through blood cultures merely indicates bacteremia. Chest x-ray and CBC can indicate infection of pleural infiltrates but not adequately diagnose the presence of sepsis.

9.1 This deficiency causes low production of platelets by the body. Hyperspleenism produces abnormal distribution of platelets, not low production of platelets. Hypothyroidism and hydrocephalus have nothing to do with platelets.

10.3 The average lifespan of a platelet is 10 days. The average lifespan of an RBC is 120 days.

11.4 A total platelet count of 20,000 cells/mm^3 is low enough for hemorrhage.

12.3 Low BP and increased HR are associated with low amounts of circulating platelets. Extremely low respirations and slow pulse rate are not associated with a low platelet count. A high level of pain is not a factor in thrombocytopenia.

13.2 Hemorrhage occurs as a result of low platelet count. A yellow sclera is associated with liver problems. Encrusted eyelashes occur with infection. Pupils that react to light are normal.

14.4 Increased ICP can lead to bleeding in the brain of patients with thrombocytopenia. Vomiting leads to increased ICP. The spleen can release large amounts of platelets in the bloodstream. Aspiration is not associated with thrombocytopenia or hypoglycemia.

15.2 Alloimmunization is the development of antibodies against HLA antigens from the transfusion of blood products. Leukocytosis is an increase in the number of WBCs. Autoregulation is the control of blood flow through the tissue. Red cell lysis syndrome is the destruction of RBCs.

16.1 Hemolytic transfusion reactions can occur from blood-product transfusions, including platelet transfusions. Amnesia is a loss of memory. Pneumonectomy is a surgical procedure to remove a lung. Sickle cell disease is a disease of RBCs.

17.2 Enlargement of spleen can cause thrombocytopenia through abnormal distribution of platelets. Sleep apnea is an alteration in respiratory patterns. Anxiety does not significantly relate to platelet production or destruction. Chronic scoliosis is a curvature of the spine.

18.3 Microthrombi production is noted in the first stage of DIC, which is precipitated by other causes such as cancer. Profuse bleeding is not immediate. Heparin and antifibrinolytic therapy is not an immediate treatment.

19.3 Kidney, skin, and lungs are especially at risk from ischemic damage from microthrombi. Neither the GI tract nor the liver are especially at risk for microemboli. CNS is a system not an organ.

20.1 Altered tissue perfusion is the best diagnosis to describe the spread of microthrombi throughout systemic circulation, resulting in tissue and organ ischemia or infarction.

21.3 Hemorrhaging occurs as the second phase of DIC as a result of consumption of coagulation factors and activation of the fibrinolytic system. Microthrombi occur in the initial phase.

22.3 Hemorrhaging occurs because consumption of coagulation factors and activation of the fibrinolytic system result in lysis of microthrombi. Endotoxins are not associated with hemorrhage. Lysis of microemboli is the main reason. Lack of initiation of heparin and antifibrinolytics is not the main reason for developing hemorrhage.

23.1 Treating the underlying precipitating mechanism is the only way to stop the progression of DIC.

24.4 Blood transfusion is often needed during the hemorrhaging phase of DIC; because coagulation factors are consumed during the first phase of DIC, different factors are often needed to restore homeostasis. Limiting fluids is not a part of symptom treatment. Treatment of infection is not a symptom of DIC. Increasing activity is not a treatment because it can cause bleeding.

25.1 D-dimer is the most reliable and specific diagnostic test for DIC. Hemoglobin and hematocrit assess the oxygen-carrying component of RBCs and the percentage of RBCs. WBC count assesses infection. ABG assesses respiratory and metabolic status.

NCLEX® CHAPTER *11* ANSWERS

1.4 Heat or radiation sources are types of thermal burns. Chemical burns are the result of chemical substances. Electrical burns are caused by electricity. Ileal is not a type of burn.

2.2 The rule of 9s is used to determine the percentage or extent of a patient's burns. Depth is a determination of the length of healing. Pain is not a factor of extent because some burns are not painful. Being either a male or a female patient is not a factor of extent.

3.2 Full-thickness burns may be painless because nerves can be burnt. All the other types of burns listed are painful.

4.1 A co-morbid condition in burns is the age of the patient if the patient is over 55 years of age.

5.2 Dehydration, edema, and oliguria occur as plasma shifts into interstitial fluid. A generalized edema and no ileus can exist. Edema can cause weight gain with no tremendous output in urine.

6.3 Age, organ illnesses, and burns to the face and hands have the highest co-morbidity risk for burns. The 25-year-old patient is too young and has no co-morbidity factors. The 8 year old is also too young and has a small burned area. The 50 year old also has too small of a burned area.

7.4 To prevent a burned patient from being infected by the *Clostridium tetani* organism, tetanus toxoid may be given. This injection helps prevent tetanus from occurring. Vitamin K is for clotting problems. Vitamin B12 is given for the treatment of pernicious anemia. Mantoux injection tests for tuberculosis.

8.2 Contractures are a major complication of the musculoskeletal system in patients who have severe burns. Severe burns have burnt nerve endings; as a result, no pain is felt. Fractures are associated with the skeletal system and are not major complications. Severe burns are not complicated by muscle spasms.

9.4 The primary functions of the skin include protection, heat regulation, sensory perception, synthesis of vitamin D, and excretion of waste products. The skin does not absorb nutrients. This is the function of the small intestine. The skin acts as a protector from foreign invaders such as bacteria; it helps maintain homeostasis by being the container of the body and fluids and is responsible for sensory perception.

10.2 Adhesive tapes can cause dermal stripping of the skin if care is not taken to protect the skin with a barrier protectant before applying the tape or during its removal. Another option is the type of tape used during the securing of a dressing, which may include paper, hypoallergenic, or cloth tapes with microperforations that permit air flow and provide less adhesion. If irritation is eliminated, then breakdown is also eliminated. Applying a transparent dressing over reddened, bony prominences helps decrease friction. Heel or elbow protectors help protect the areas from trauma.

11.3 Partial-thickness loss of skin involving the epidermis or dermis (or both) is a stage II pressure ulcer. A stage I pressure ulcer appears as an alteration in the appearance of intact skin, usually nonblanchable. A stage III pressure ulcer involves damage of the subcutaneous tissue that may extend down to but not through the underlying fascia. A stage IV pressure ulcer is a full-thickness skin loss with extensive destruction of tissue that includes muscle, bone, or supporting structures.

12.2 A transparent dressing is best described as a clear, dressing sheet that is adhesive, waterproof, and allows for the transmission of oxygen and water vapor. A hydrocolloid is a dressing made of hydroactive and absorptive particles. A hydrogel is a starch- or glycerin-based compound that can insulate and provide a moist wound environment. An alginate is derived from the calcium salt of seaweed.

13.4 An antimicrobial dressing is a nonionic, silver-fused, transparent film that is effective against numerous fungi, yeast, and bacteria. A transparent dressing is a clear, film dressing, but it does not contain any antibacterial properties. A hydrogel is a wafer and is not classified as a film dressing. A composite dressing functions as a bacterial barrier and has excellent absorptive properties.

14.2 A specialty mattress replacement incorporates zoned air support that provides continuous air flow to maximize the potential for pressure relief over bony prominences. Foam mattresses were developed as an overlay and allow for pressure reduction. A static air mattress is an overlay but does not have a constant air flow through its chambers; additionally, it also provides only pressure reduction. Pressure reduction does not maximize the prevention of pressure; it only reduces the pressure.

15.1 Bariatric beds are specifically designed for patients weighing over 400 pounds and can facilitate body movement. Although possibly supporting the weight of a bariatric patient, water-fluid mediums do not usually accommodate the movement of a patient in and out of the bed. It is also difficult to move these beds from unit to unit. The potential for leaks is also a concern. A static-air bed does not support the weight or effectively decrease the pressure for capillary refill. Air-fluidized beds do not facilitate getting a patient in and out of bed.

16.4 The air-fluidized bed is best used for stage IV pressure ulcers that requiring flap surgery, which helps to maintain circulation and increase healing. Skin tears can be managed on hospital beds with frequent turning schedules. Stage II pressure ulcers can be managed on hospital beds with frequent turning schedules. Stage III pressure ulcers require a mattress that ensures pressure relief but not necessarily to the extent that an air-fluid bed provides.

17.1 Necrotizing fasciitis can affect any part of the body, including the abdominal wall, perianal groin area, face, neck, chest, and most commonly the extremities, particularly the legs. The extremities are the most common location.

18.1 The initial signs and symptoms of necrotizing fasciitis include the following: (a) the point of entry may be obvious, minor, or none; (b) the use of NSAIDs may delay the diagnosis by reducing inflammatory features; (c) fever; (d) exquisite pain that is local or referred; (e) disportionate pain to the appearing injury or condition; (f) ordinary flulike symptoms, nausea, weakness, malaise, diarrhea, and dizziness; (g) local erythema without sharp margins and hot, shiny, swollen skin; and (h) complaints of feeling very bad without the ability to explain why. Cough, headaches, and incontinence are not symptoms.

19.4 Immediate treatment of the more invasive necrotizing fasciitis is critical and requires prompt diagnosis and immediate action. Necrotizing fasciitis must be treated in the hospital with antibiotic IV therapy and aggressive débridement of the affected tissue beyond the involved gangrenous and undermined area(s) because of the rapidity with which the process can progress. Treatment needs to be implemented by medical personnel. Specific antibiotics are required for appropriate treatment. Rest does not delay progression.

20.2 Generally, those at higher risk for necrotizing fasciitis include patients with chronic illnesses (e.g., diabetes, cirrhosis, alcoholism, peripheral vascular disease, cancer); those who are abusing parenteral IV drugs, who are dependent on renal dialysis, who have impaired lymphatic drainage, and are chronically taking corticosteroids. Young children with varicella can be superinfected with group A streptococci and may place them at risk for necrotizing fasciitis. Immunization status geography and descent have no effect.

21.2 If necrotizing fasciitis is clearly suspected on clinical grounds with signs and symptoms such as deep patchy areas of surface hypoesthesia, crepitation, advancing erythema, bullae, and skin necrosis, direct operative intervention is indicated. This requires an immediate report to the physician and surgery.

22.1 The typical signs and symptoms of streptococcal toxic-shock syndrome (STSS) are chills, fever, a flat red rash over large areas of the body, confusion, vomiting, diarrhea, tachycardia, hypotension, renal impairment, decreasing level of consciousness with overwhelming infection, and multiorgan failure. Chest pain and shortness of breath are signs of pneumothorax. Pain is a sign of fracture. Incomplete lower spinal cord injury shows temperature changes and tactile changes.

23.3 Necrotizing fasciitis must be treated in the hospital with antibiotic IV therapy and aggressive débridement of the affected tissue beyond the involved gangrenous and undermined area(s) because of the rapidity with which the process can progress. As previously noted, surgical incisions must go beyond the area of involvement until the normal fascia is found, the necrotic fat and fascia is excised, the pus is drained, and the wound is left open. Reexploration of the wound is often necessary in 24 hours to ensure the initial débridement is adequate. Amputation may be necessary, and scarring may result. The fertility and auditory systems are not affected. No anaphylaxis occurs, except from the rare case of anesthesia.

24.1 Virulence factors of group A streptococci (GAS) organisms include: (1) special proteins for adherence and colonization, (2) the potential for an immunologic disguise along with the ability of antigenic variation and tolerance, (3) the ability to inhibit and kill phagocytes, (4) the ability to produce protein-splitting enzymes that allow for further spread of the bacteria, (5) the ability to release exotoxins, (6) and the ability to induce an exaggerated production of cytokines that contribute to the development of systemic toxicity. To add further injury to the host, an immune response and hemolysis can occur as a result of this bacteria. Circulating cross-reactive antibodies may be produced by the host during a streptococcal infection and may indirectly damage tissue. This autoimmune complication can continue even after the GAS organisms have been cleared. Finally, GAS usually are beta-hemolytic organisms and can cause complete lysis of RBCs surrounding the colony.

NCLEX® CHAPTER 12 ANSWERS

1.2 The patient may have an advanced directive that refuses resuscitation efforts. A patient's will has no bearings on what medical measures need or should be taken for resuscitation. Although laboratory results are important to assessing and treating the patient, you do not need to know the values if the patient warrants resuscitation. You must begin resuscitation efforts first. Disease state and prognosis may weigh into the length of time resuscitation continues, but it has no bearing on beginning resuscitation efforts.

2.3 In the secondary survey, one must search for and treat reversible causes. This is known as the D or the differential diagnosis. Defibrillation is the D for the primary survey. Drugs are a part of the C (circulation) for the secondary survey. Death is the termination of resuscitative efforts, which is to be avoided if not on the primary or secondary survey of the ECC algorithm.

3.4 VF is the most commonly seen arrest rhythm in adults. Asystole is often a terminal rhythm. PEA is not the first rhythm in most arrests. VT deteriorates into VF.

4.1 Defibrillation is the treatment of choice for VF and is included as the D in the primary survey. CPR may help, but defibrillation is the treatment of choice for VF. Drugs may help, but defibrillation is the treatment of choice for VF. Adequate ventilation may help resuscitative efforts, but defibrillation is the treatment of choice for VF.

5.3 The definition of PEA is normal electrical activity on the monitor and the patient is pulseless. VF is different from PEA. No electrical activity on the monitor describes asystole.

6.1 Epinephrine is the first drug to be administered in PEA, asystole, and pulseless VT or VF. Lidocaine is a second-line medication. Atropine is used in PEA and asystole. Aminodarone is a second-line medication.

7.4 It is critical to confirm asystole in a second lead. Although the code team is important, it is not one of the first things that must be checked when asystole is suspected. The status of the advanced directive on any patient should be known before a critical situation occurs. Although IV access is helpful, it is not the first thing that must be checked when asystole is suspected. The nurse must first know what rhythm he or she is treating.

8.2 Transcutaneous pacing attempts to create electrical activity in the heart. Asystole is the only rhythm that does not have electrical activity. The electricity that is used in VF is defibrillation. PEA is treated with medication; an attempt to determine the cause is made to ensure that the underlying mechanism is treated. Pulseless VT is treated like VF and uses defibrillation.

9.2 As health care treatments and procedures become increasingly effective, a greater number of patients are surviving traumatic insults. As a result, ICUs are treating more cases of MODS. Although cardiac monitoring is usually part of ICU nursing care, it is not the primary reason. The primary reason for the patient to be in the ICU is to receive aggressive support. ICUs are not the only nursing units with isolation capability. Patients with MODS may require isolation, depending on the organism. The patient is admitted to the ICU for aggressive support and does not require a laboratory report for this to be accomplished.

10.1 MODS is defined as the progressive dysfunction of more than one organ in patients that are critically ill or injured and most commonly results from a systemic infection. Usually MODS is the result of a bacterial infection, such as a gram-negative organism. Angioplasty and hypertensive crises have nothing directly to do with the cause of MODS.

11.4 Vascular occlusive events disrupt blood flow by enhancing the release of thromboxin, a potent vasoconstrictor, and by inhibiting synthesis of prostacycline, a vasodilating substance, thus resulting in an overall vasoconstrictive effect. The by-products cause effects in the vascular system. An increased intracellular oxygen demand occurs. The by-products cause effects in the vascular system.

12.3 Mortality of patients with MODS is high; however: it is not the expected outcome. To improve this prognosis, the diligent nurse minimizes risk for further complications.

13.3 Nutritional demands are significantly increased in this patient. Adequate nutrition must be provided throughout the duration of the illness. Caloric needs vary, depending on the patient's weight and metabolic demands. Nutritional support usually consists of IV or enteral feedings.

14.1 Emergently placed lines should be replaced in a controlled environment as soon as possible to reduce the risk of infection secondary to contaminated lines. Emergent placement of lines may result in possible contamination, which may lead to a nosocomial infection. Although the environment is important to consider when placing a line, the patient's need is the priority and lines placed emergently can be changed later.

15.3 Patients receiving tube feedings are at risk for aspiration of stomach contents. Aspiration pneumonia may lead to septic infection and potentially MODS. Tube feedings usually assist in preventing MODS because nutritional demands are being met. Tube feedings do provide adequate nutritional support. Although tube feedings may cause diarrhea and potentially dehydration, they do not directly contribute to the development of MODS.

16.1 The first line of defense is protection. Proper hand washing and aseptic techniques should always be used. Early recognition of symptoms by the vigilant nurse is the first step in the provision of appropriate treatment. Although the patient might be ventilated as a part of aggressive support, it is not the primary and most effective tool in combating MODS. Antibiotics are not administered unless appropriate, and dialysis is not ordered unless kidney function is compromised.

Index